Surgery and Salvation

STUDIES IN SOCIAL MEDICINE

Allan M. Brandt, Larry R. Churchill, and Jonathan Oberlander, *editors*

This series publishes books at the intersection of medicine, health, and society that further our understanding of how medicine and society shape one another historically, politically, and ethically. The series is grounded in the convictions that medicine is a social science, that medicine is humanistic and cultural as well as biological, and that it should be studied as a social, political, ethical, and economic force.

A complete list of books published in Studies in Social Medicine is available at https://uncpress.org/series/studies-social-medicine.

ELIZABETH O'BRIEN

Surgery and Salvation

The Roots of Reproductive Injustice in Mexico, 1770–1940

The University of North Carolina Press *Chapel Hill*

Set in Arno Pro by Westchester Publishing Services
Manufactured in the United States of America

Library of Congress Cataloging-in-Publication Data
Names: O'Brien, Elizabeth, 1987– author.
Title: Surgery and salvation : the roots of reproductive injustice in Mexico, 1770–1940 / Elizabeth O'Brien.
Other titles: Studies in social medicine.
Description: Chapel Hill : The University of North Carolina Press, [2023] | Series: Studies in social medicine | Includes bibliographical references and index.
Identifiers: LCCN 2023014318 | ISBN 9781469675862 (cloth ; alk. paper) | ISBN 9781469675879 (paperback ; alk. paper) | ISBN 9781469675886 (ebook)
Subjects: LCSH: Obstetrics—Surgery—Mexico—History. | Obstetrics—Surgery—Social aspects—Mexico. | Women's health services—Mexico—Religious aspects. | Racism in medicine—Mexico. | Human experimentation in medicine—Mexico—History. | Involuntary treatment—Mexico—History. | BISAC: SOCIAL SCIENCE / Ethnic Studies / Caribbean & Latin American Studies | SOCIAL SCIENCE / Gender Studies
Classification: LCC RG725 .O28 2023 | DDC 618.8—dc23/eng/20230503
LC record available at https://lccn.loc.gov/2023014318

Cover illustration: *Columbian Surgery: Caesarean Section*, Enrique Grau (1920–2004, Colombian), 1954. Acrylic painting on canvas. International Museum of Surgical Science, Chicago, Illinois. Collection number XX1995.814.3.

For Graciela

Contents

Tables

Acknowledgments

I owe a deep and ineffable debt to the historical actors whose stories play out across the following pages. The chapters evoke intimate moments of their lives and I hope to have done justice to their humanity. My gratitude is owed to those interlocutors who have helped me grapple with the ethical challenges of writing about people's experiences with reproductive health care. This book is also beholden to the mentors, scholars, archivists, activists, friends, editors, family members, and institutions who nurtured the ideas within while facilitating the research and writing. A heartfelt thanks to spectacular UNC editors, Andreína Fernández and Elaine Maisner, for their belief in this project. Thank you to Lindsay Starr, Dino Battista, Lucas Church, and the rest of UNC's design, production, and sales team, as well as to Allan Brandt, Larry Churchill, and Jonathan Oberlander for including the project in the Studies in Social Medicine Series. Many thanks to Anne Jones for her extraordinary copyediting, and to Jess Farr-Cox for providing tremendous indexing and proofing services. I am grateful to the International Museum of Surgical Science for allowing us to use Enrique Grau's 1844 painting as a cover image.

I will always be indebted to two peer reviewers who were supremely generous in their guidance and vision. I also wish to thank the following scholars for their wisdom and collegiality, with apologies to those I have missed: Nora Jaffary, Karin Rosemblatt, Laura Briggs, Jocelyn Olcott, Alexandra Minna Stern, Bianca Premo, Sonia Robles, Bonnie Lucero, Cassia Roth, Miriam Rich, Jacob Moses, Paola Bertucci, Ivano dal Prete, Farren Yero, Dillon Vrana, Deirdre Cooper Owens, Ana Barahona, Lina Rosa Berrio Palomo, David Carey Jr., Cara Delay, Erika Edwards, Julie Gibbings, Adam Warren, Laura Lopez Suárez y Guázo, Karen Graubart, Pamela Voekel, Bethany Moreton, Elizabeth Roberts, Ben Fallaw, Claudia Agostoni, Paola Siesa, Marcos Cueto, Martha Few, Raúl Necochea, Susan Deeds, Laura Shelton, Nicole Pacino, Hanni Jalil Paier, Jethro Hernández Berrones, Pablo Gómez, Alexandra Puerto, Ángelica Márquez-Osuna, Laura Isabel Serna, Rachel Nolan, Diana Montaño, Christina Ramos, Martha Liliana Espinosa, and Natalia Gasparowicz. I have enormous appreciation for Cristina Rivera Garza's brilliant corpus of work. My warm thanks to my friend and mentor Ana María Carrillo, who always shows me great kindness while sharing her incredible expertise.

Benjamin Smith, too, has offered decades of camaraderie. Ben introduced me to Gabriela Soto Laveaga when I was an undergraduate, and since then she has supported me as a person and as a researcher at every turn. My eternal thanks to them both.

Mentors at the University of Texas at Austin nourished this work for years. Special thanks are due to Matthew Butler, who was not only an exemplary dissertation supervisor, but who also modeled a rigorous and creative approach to interpreting the past. My profound gratitude is also owed to Seth Garfield, Ann Twinam, and Philippa Levine, who have sagely advised me through the book publication process and other milestones. To Julie Hardwick and Madeline Hsu: without your integrity and patience I would not have weathered the past year, much less finished this project. Additional support in Austin came from Virginia Garrard, John McKiernan Gónzalez, Susan Deans-Smith, Christen Smith, Frank Guridy, Bruce Hunt, and Martha Menchaca, as well as my cherished classmates Chloe Ireton, Eyal Weinberg, Christina Villarreal, Kristie Flannery, Altina Hoti, Adrian Masters, Sandy Chang, Renata Keller, Danielle Sánchez, Juandrea Bates, Claudia Rueda, Chris Heaney, Brian Stauffer, Eddie Shore, John Carranza, Jimena Perry, Sam Serrano, Tiana Wilson, Jess Osorio, and Nancy Preciado.

I am grateful for how this book transformed during the three years I spent in Baltimore as an assistant professor at Johns Hopkins University. I wish to recognize the wonderful community there, especially Alessandro Angelini, Ilil Benjamin, Nathaniel Comfort, Yulia Frumer, Mary Fissell, Jeremy Greene, Jessica Marie Johnson, Lan Li, Diane Horvath, Minkah Makalani, Graham Mooney, Nicole Labruto, Casey Lurtz, Silka Patel, Maria Portuondo, Randall Packard, Gianna Pomata, Ahmed and Soha Ragab, Erin Rowe, Christine Ruggere, Delida Sánchez, Bécquer Seguin, Carolyn Sufrin, Sasha Turner, Christy Thornton, and Sasha and Erica White. JHU's students have taught me more than they realize: thank you to S. J. Zanolini, Jessica Hester, Marlis Hinckley, Emily Xiao, Emily Rodríguez, Casey Reed, Emily Clark, Brooke Lansing, Darien Colson-Fearon, and many others, especially Juliana Márquez for her valuable research assistance. It humbles me to thank my new colleagues in the Department of History at the University of California Los Angeles, especially Soraya de Chadarevian, Benjamin Madley, Ted Porter, Bharat Venkhat, Kevin Terraciano, Robin Derby, Katherine Marino, and Fernando Pérez Montesinos.

Wonderful archivists, historians, and researchers in Mexico made this project possible. Thanks to Dr. Jesús Gabriel Sánchez Campa and Mstra. Elena Ramírez, whose Diplomado was a formative experience. Lic. Oscar Maya Corzo and Dra. María Xóchitl Martínez Barbosa expertly assisted in the Biblioteca

Nicolás León. Mtra. Patricia Guadalupe Alfaro Guerra, Patricia Olguín Alvarado, and Rogelio Vargas Olvera facilitated the investigation in the Archivo Historico de La Secretaría de Salubridad. In the LLILAS/Benson collection, I give special thanks to Adrian Johnson, Paloma Díaz, Adela Piñeda Franco, Linda Gill, and Jorge Salinas.

During research, the Rockefeller Foundation Archive Center and the Huntington Library generously allowed me access to their collections, and Steve Hindle was especially kind. Institutional support came from Fulbright-COMEXUS, the Tinker Foundation, the National Science Foundation, the American Council for Learned Societies, the Teresa Lozano Long Institute for Latin American Studies, the Department of History at UT Austin, Johns Hopkins University, the UNAM, and the National Endowment for the Humanities. Thank you to the FHHS, LASA-Siglo XIX, LASA-Mexico, the SHA, and Nursing Clio.

For years I've been afraid that I would omit a loved one from this list. With apologies for that inevitability, I extend love to my friends, especially Christine and Hugo, *querida* Alfonsina (who sacrificed a great deal in 2022 to give me writing time), Tatiana, Lynn, Adrienne, Sade, Paige and Sal, Amber and John, Kasey and Brian, Brad and Joy, Jairo, Sierra, Claudia, Eleuterio, Kellee, Patricia, Elaine, Chelz, Alysia, Tracy, Nina, Yolanda, Angelita, Rita, Enrique, Miguel, Chuck, Kai, Kara, Julie, Kelly, Olivia, Viviana, Melissa, Katie, Ester, Becky, Aubrey, and Zulma. My love and recognition go to my family: Freda, Mandy, Lynda, Erin, Fred, Alex, Daniel, Raegan, Chris, Jen, Katie, Louise, John, and Jim. Special thanks are due to my siblings, Sean and Grace, for their unconditional love. Thank you to those who enabled me to thrive when others did not believe in me.

I frequently insist that it was more challenging to finish a bachelor's degree than a PhD. I never would have been able to complete the former without Claribel's phenomenal friendship. I miss Claribel every day and will always admire her strength, determination, and grit. I dedicate this book to Claribel and also to my beloved daughter Graciela, my *corazón,* the sweetest and most generous person I know. Thank you for being so brave and patient and for always shining your light. I also dedicate this book to Claudia Meza for inspiring me to be OMS and not let anyone stand in my way. This book was written with love and admiration for my friend Raquel Padilla Ramos: may she rest in power and tranquility and may her legacy of fearless resistance help end gendered violence. Finally, I dedicate *Surgery and Salvation* to all the people, past and present, who have struggled to attain dignity and justice in all matters relating to sexual and reproductive health and well-being.

Surgery and Salvation

INTRODUCTION

The Young Woman of Devil's Alley

In the early morning hours of March 12, 1884, a pregnant eighteen-year-old walked on a derelict pathway in Mexico City. Known colloquially as Devil's Alley, the street has been featured in generations of ghost stories and urban legends. It was also infamous as a site of sexual commerce. Historians do not know what brought the girl to the backstreet, but we do know that her labor pains had not yet begun, nor was she in the midst of a medical complication. In the shadowy lane she encountered two women; they reportedly pitied the youth and persuaded her to accompany them to Mexico City's maternity clinic, la Casa de Maternidad.

Since 1806, la Casa de Maternidad had been a clinic for secret births: a place of refuge for so-called fallen women who wished to hide their pregnancies from friends, family, or the public.[1] By the 1880s, la Casa served women of all classes. Some paid for the comfort of a private room during their stay. Most, unable to pay, received free maternity care. Some patients were brought to the Casa by volunteers from societies like las Damas de la Caridad. The Damas organized philanthropic activities and collaborated with authorities to deliver food and medicine to the homes of people who were ill or destitute. In collaboration with the Sanitary Police, the religious women also roamed the city and detained women for imprisonment in hospitals.[2] By the 1910s, more than half the women patients in the General Hospital were carted into the establishment by the Sanitary Police; in the 1930s, nurses and social workers performed the same kind of door-to-door medico-moralization that compelled thousands of women to assent to state care.

When the young woman walked through the doors of the clinic in 1884, she was greeted by the lead physician on duty, José Torres Anzorena. He escorted her to an ample room with a bed, a fluffy cotton pillow, and clean white sheets. As he would later write, he sought to make her comfortable. The expectant mother may have been surprised by her reception in the clinic. She likely had little institutional familiarity with hospitals, as women rarely sought hospital obstetric care in the 1880s. The vast majority birthed at home or in sweat lodges called *temazcales*, with the assistance of midwives who provided herbal tinctures and teas to increase the strength of their contractions. Midwives also guided women in the use of birthing stools and saw to postpartum hygiene practices. The late nineteenth-century medicalization of childbirth brought with it the criminalization of popular and unlicensed midwifery; with fewer available midwives, more women sought health care in medical clinics. Midwives resisted with every means they had: by signing petitions, holding protests, and flouting licensing regulations.[3]

Other factors pushed people into the Mexico City's clinics by the last decades of the nineteenth century. Rapid industrialization prompted massive waves of migration to the city. By 1900, migrants from other states made up over one-half of the federal district's 500,000 inhabitants.[4] Hospitals provided recent arrivals with health care, shelter, and food. Obstetric patients came from all over the nation but especially from the states of Morelos, Guerrero, Oaxaca, and Veracruz. Others hailed from communities near and far, especially Toluca, Guadalajara, Querétaro, Jalisco, and the state of Mexico.

Public clinics were staffed by medical students and physicians of the Escuela Nacional Preparatoria (ENP), established in 1868. Medical education required a large number of patients on whom students and professors could practice examinations, diagnoses, surgeries, and autopsies. In fact, until 1936 students were required to design and perform medical research in Mexico City's clinics. Earning a medical degree required them to publish and defend their studies.

The medical school enjoyed massive funding from the cabinet of president Porfirio Díaz, who held office between 1876 and 1911. Díaz yearned to establish one of the biggest and most prestigious centers for scientific training in Latin America, one to rival the medical training of universities in Rio de Janeiro, Lima, and Bogotá, as well as Paris, Philadelphia, Boston, and Edinburgh. Outbreaks of diseases like cholera, bubonic plague, smallpox, measles, and typhus prompted public health officials to collaborate closely with physicians to address public health problems, including sex work. On the one hand, elites frequented upscale brothels, implying their tacit approval of sex work. On the other hand, rebellious "public women" degraded Mexico City's image, and officials increasingly sought to bring them under state control. Some of these women, pregnant and not, became obstetric and gynecologic patients for Mexico City's physicians in training.

It is impossible to know whether the eighteen-year-old of Devil's Alley was accused of sex work, but she clearly became an unwitting surgical patient. In the Casa de Maternidad she met the nation's most influential obstetrician, Dr. Juan María Rodríguez, who had been the clinic director and chief professor of obstetrics for fifteen years. She did not respond when Rodríguez and Anzorena addressed her. Perhaps she spoke an Indigenous language and could not understand their Spanish. Perhaps she refused to recognize their authority, and her silence signaled resistance. Or perhaps she suffered a disability and could not hear them or could not speak. Whatever the case, she almost certainly became perplexed by what happened next.

Drs. Rodríguez and Anzorena exited the room, and then returned in the company of another, younger man, who covered her face with a mask and held it there. Inhalation brought a pleasant odor and a burning, sweet taste. Chloroform incapacitated the patient, and then she was transported to the operating room where she underwent the first caesarean operation performed in a Mexican hospital for a medical purpose. She never awoke.

The national importance of this case prompted Dr. Rodríguez to write a short book about it and present his research findings widely. He partly built his professional reputation on making knowledge from the pregnant body of the girl from Devil's Alley. It is a sad irony that historians will never know the name of the woman whose experience marked such a turning point in surgery. Her family is unlikely to know to where she disappeared, or how her death contributed to modern surgical knowledge.

It is unsurprising that the operation took place in the 1880s, the so-called golden era of experimental surgery. Interventions remained dangerous in this decade due to the risk of hemorrhage, infection, and shock. Yet the Listerian use of antiseptic chemicals and the germ theory of specific disease had reduced postoperative infection rates while increasing patients' chances of survival.[5] Additionally, since the 1840s surgeons had employed gasses, especially chloroform and ether, to numb the nervous system while keeping patients tranquil and lessening their pain during operations. Such developments emboldened the performance of more interventions than before. Operations like neurosurgery, intestinal surgery, and cesarean section provided revolutionary insights into physiology as well as the pathological effects of disease on organs. Anatomists scrutinized the inner workings of the body and spent long hours mapping nervous systems, skeletal structures, and brain matter.

Historians working in the tradition of Georges Canguilhelm and his student Michel Foucault long ago pointed out that autopsies and advanced microscopes led nineteenth-century doctors to anatomize their patients, viewing their organs, tissues, and cells in increasingly greater detail. The perception of people as sets of organs, tissues, and cells contributed to the objectification of patients, the quantification of their ailments, and the silencing of their voices.[6] Previously, clinicians had needed to listen to a sufferer's narration of their symptoms and embodied experiences. By the nineteenth century, however, diseased tissue and vital measures like temperature and pulse did the talking. This was not a deliberate or nefarious silencing, but rather, the result of technological advancements and empiricism in medicine.

Meanwhile, anatomists' need for bodies gave way to the famous tradition of grave robbing in locations near medical schools throughout the United States and Western Europe. Graves in Mexico seemed to be much more carefully guarded than in places like Philadelphia, New York, and London. Tight security in Mexico City's cemeteries protected the dignity of the dead, but it also meant that anatomists there turned to live subjects instead of deceased ones.[7]

Although many nineteenth-century surgeons sought to explore or correct diseased or malfunctioning organs, the obstetricians who operated on the young woman from Devil's Alley had a different aim, which is explored in more detail below. Drawing on the early eugenics movement, they sought to prove that their subject was maternally deficient and racially unfit. While most surgeries aimed to uncover difficult-to-see organs, obstetric surgery unveiled different varieties of truths, especially those having to do with the creation of fetal life and the adjudication of maternal worth. After all, before the ultrasound technology of the mid-twentieth century, surgery remained the only means of gazing within a pregnant woman's womb, the only path to observing a fetus still attached to its mother.

Reproductive surgery was, and still is, philosophically, medically, and socially distinct from other kinds of surgery, partially because it invokes so many unknowns about the mother–infant dyad. The meanings of obstetric operations are profoundly intertwined with religious, racial, and gendered concerns, and have been for centuries. As a result, the notion of progress in reproductive surgery is contested in ways that are distinct from other surgical specialties. Yet, precisely how do surgeries acquire social and cultural meanings? And how do these shift or persist? This book addresses these questions through a long history of obstetric interventions, all of which sought to prove metaphysical claims, meaning those that are otherworldly, intangible, or ineffable. Because surgery manifests and reimagines the metaphysical, its history is imperative for understanding why racial and religious principles remain central to political conflicts about fetal life and maternal decision-making. This study explores the roots of these problems while historicizing contemporary debates about abortion, maternal mortality, the medicalization of birth, and present-day popular protest against obstetric violence.

The Tangled Ethics of Surgical Salvation

Surgery and Salvation illuminates the historical interplay between surgical politics and reproductive governance, a term that refers to the ways in which different actors and institutions use "legislative controls, economic inducements, moral injunctions, direct coercion, and ethical incitements to produce, monitor, and control reproductive behaviours and population practices."[8] The chapters interlace three main strands: how religious and theological ideas influenced obstetric surgery over time; how race and class became organizing logics for discourses about surgical advancement in Mexico; and how women experienced, and sometimes contested, the ways in which patriarchal medical authorities influenced their reproductive choices.

In all, the book argues that modern claims about fetal personhood are rooted in the use of surgical force against marginalized and racialized women, and that this history is key to understanding obstetric violence and obstetric racism today, in Mexico and elsewhere. Covering the mid-eighteenth century through the 1930s, the chapters examine an array of operations attendant to pregnant women and illnesses of the reproductive organs, including hysteria and sexually transmitted infections. Such operations include cesarean operation, ovariotomy (the extirpation of the ovaries), therapeutic abortion, hysterectomy, and eugenic sterilization via tubal ligation and vaginal bifurcation.

The title invokes authorities' paternalistic belief that they were redeeming women, children, the colony, and the nation by performing distinct kinds of surgery. Chapters refer to such episodes of meaning-making as "salvation through surgery," "surgical salvation," and "salvational surgery." For instance, while eighteenth-century priests performed cesarean surgery to save children's unborn souls through baptism, by the mid-nineteenth century, doctors endeavored to salvage some unmarried women's social reputations by practicing therapeutic abortions. In 1884, Rodríguez believed he was protecting the young woman of Devil's Alley from an obstetric emergency due to her deficient anatomy. He likely thought that he had saved her neighbors from the undesirable social consequences of her childbearing. (If Rodríguez held superstitious views, it is even possible that he told himself he was saving her from the devil, who ostensibly appeared nightly in the alleyway.) By the twentieth century, eugenic-minded physicians who performed sterilizations believed they were shielding the nation from supporting the children whose births they were preventing. In each era, surgeons' writings focused, intentionally or not, on the groups of women who obstaculized different governmental regimes: unchristianized Indigenous women in eighteenth century missions; elite women with hysteria during national debates about liberal rights; nuns exercising medical authority during state secularization; sex workers in the late nineteenth century urbanizing landscape; and women who asked doctors to help control their fertility at the height of eugenics. Obstetric knowledge was profoundly influenced by social currents.

The ideological or politicized use of bodies is a familiar theme for historians of medicine. Medical experimentation, far from being unique to particular regimes or antithetical to healing, is "embedded in the modern medical tradition."[9] For decades, scholars have demonstrated that the experimental use of bodies is a constitutive and integral aspect of clinical training and practice. Likewise, the trialing of new procedures and medicines was, and still is, part and parcel of scientific medicine itself. Although this book does not take bioethics as a central focus, it does identify some surgeries—such as the girl of Devil's Alley's cesarean operation—as exploratory and not therapeutically indicated. I use the word experimental to reference various procedural categories, including those of questionable curative utility, those that invoked dehumanizing logics, and those that prioritized the creation of politicized knowledge over improving a person's corporeal health. Sometimes doctors themselves referred to surgeries as experimental, especially when discussing novel forms of sterilizing operations in the twentieth century. I believe that many colonial cesarean surgeries were exploratory (if not precisely experimental) because they served a particular ideology (religious, in this case) and because officials expressly employed them in the prioritization of this knowledge over the survival of pregnant women.

I recognize that these designations are not straightforward, and I look forward to the conversations they provoke. I additionally wish to clarify that this book does not treat obstetric surgery as categorically harmful. Nor does it aim to make moral judgements about the actions of individual surgeons. In fact, it draws on examples in which women demanded hospitalization during childbirth, underscoring that not all patients saw medical spaces as fearsome and to be avoided. Moreover, women's demands for medicalized forms of fertility control underscore that patients were invested in changing the structure of clinical practice to respond to their own needs.

While attentive to the variability of individual's experiences, I avoid an anachronistic focus on liberal notions of women's individual consent. After all, hospital systems did not widely implement informed consent laws until after 1940.[10] Even leaving aside this legalistic definition, the agency of the patients in this book was severely curtailed, not only because they lived in an unfree world, but also because many experienced medical emergencies and unwanted pregnancies. Few things make people feel more powerless than a painful and unexpected life-threatening emergency, and such powerlessness often leads people to reflect on the other vulnerabilities they face. Instead of focusing on consent, this book probes the conditions that women encountered when they sought or received medical care despite the possibility of dire outcomes. What emerges are examples of how class prejudice, racialization, and social exclusion shaped their interactions with physicians and medical institutions, and how surgical politics became the tangible, embodied expressions of paternalistic, racist, and often coercive medical science. While recognizing patient agency wherever possible, this book underscores the constraints on women's options by illuminating how surgical politics exerted cultural and biopolitical influence over people during times of social change, under religious missions as well as during various waves of secularization and state formation.

Beyond individual circumstances, obstetrics was, and still is, overlaid by larger systems of patriarchal oppression, scaling from the local to the transnational.[11] This means that structural violence cannot be mitigated by well-intended practitioners, because institutions and economies make people's bodies crucial to the production of medical knowledge. The harshness of surgery in the pre-antibiotic era intensified due to power discrepancies between patients and physicians. Doctors were, by and large, buoyed by state power, and sometimes also empowered themselves to act outside the bounds of state prerogatives. Medical practice thus sometimes became medical violence, partially due to the social systems in which it took place. Structural violence exacerbates pre-existing vulnerabilities, including those related to racialization, class status, access to resources, disabilities or debilities, and the precarities of pregnancy itself. Discourses around both routine and emergency surgeries repeatedly drew on, reified, or exacerbated other forms of oppression.

This approach departs from several traditions in the history of surgery. Perhaps most importantly, historians rarely consider colonized and formerly colonized regions as important sites of surgical practice. This book centers Mexico and highlights the vast corpus of clinical knowledge produced by Mexican women, their bodies, and their health care providers. Far from being receptacles of European scientific practice and ideology, a range of Mexican actors conducted their own investigations and crafted their own theories. These theories were inherently transnational in that they arose from border-crossing networks and affected clinical practice elsewhere. Whenever possible, the book attends to the broader dimensions of obstetric knowledge while still focusing on its particular effects on Mexican women.

Obstetric research became particularly important in Latin America, where it metamorphosed into a source of post-colonial pride by the late nineteenth century. Nationalist surgeons decried the "backwards" colonial tradition of religious cesarean surgery and vowed to modernize the procedure. Many physicians believed that their countrywomen were anatomically deficient, and sought, for that reason, to become global leaders in correcting alleged hereditary reproductive deficiencies. Mexico City grew into an ideal setting for this research due to its population density, its well-organized public health system, and its abundance of hospitals, clinics, medical students, and patients. Social inequality, rapid urbanization, and high rates of hospitalization, institutionalization, and detention by the Sanitary Police created the conditions for clinical research to thrive by the late nineteenth century. In all, a view from colonial and postcolonial territories is key to understanding how medical ideologies come to reify, or contest, multiple forms of marginalization and exclusion.

There is also somewhat of a gendered gap in the literature on the medical use of bodies. Reproductive surgeries are sometimes separated from broader histories of exploratory and experimental treatments, although certainly there are many exceptions to this trend.[12] Questions about the moralization and exploitation of women's bodies have largely been taken up in a different historiography stemming from internationalist and women of color–led movements of the mid-to-late twentieth century. These struggles produced the reproductive justice framework, which is a rights-based concept that asserts the importance of women's and childbearing people's self-determination, including their right to bear children, to terminate unwanted pregnancies, and to raise families in safe and dignified environments.[13]

Reproductive justice–centered interventions have rightly anchored many historians' approaches to surgical history. Reproductive justice provides a structure through which to understand broad-based gendered harms to individuals and populations, enacted through interventions and prohibitions on childbearing, childbirth, and child-rearing. Chronology is one methodological challenge in this historiography. Because obstetric operations are largely modernist endeavors, the literature overwhelmingly focuses on the late nineteenth through twenty-first centuries. Medical experimentation writ large has long been associated with the twentieth century, and in particular with the ethical violations committed by researchers like those in Tuskegee or Nazi Germany. For these reasons, historians almost always study interventionist ideologies and ethics through secular sources produced by nation-states. This methodological bias tends to reproduce modernist paradigms, sometimes by privileging liberal debates about state-based rights and individual consent.

By looking back to the religious origins of the cesarean operation in Latin America, and by connecting this history to subsequent developments, *Surgery and Salvation* argues for a chronological broadening of how we understand meaning-making in obstetric surgery. Examining the theological origins of ideas about modern reproductive health care adds to a rich historiographic tradition that explores how authorities under distinct governments conceived of social interventions as pathways to moral salvation as well as biological regeneration. Because religion continued (and continues) to be a salient determinant in obstetric research, Mexico's archives provide a unique opportunity to bridge the metaphysical themes of the premodern era with the modern problem of population management. A simultaneous focus on religion and modern governance is more common in histories of Latin American reproduction, but less frequent in the historiography on surgery.[14] In all, the history of surgery in Latin America helps elucidate why religion remains so closely tied to maternal and fetal health care today.

Defining Obstetric Violence

A history of reproductive surgery in Mexico helps us understand the theological, patriarchal, and epistemological roots of a phenomenon that feminist activists call obstetric violence. This term refers to harm inflicted during or in relation to pregnancy, childbearing, and the postpartum period. Generally used in public health, medical ethics, and reproductive justice literatures, the phrase is less frequently invoked in *historical* analyses of reproduction.[15]

Childbearing-based violence can be both interpersonal and structural, arising from the actions of health care providers as well as from broader political and economic arrangements that disproportionately harm marginalized populations. It manifests in many forms, including physical abuse, injury resulting from unnecessary or excessive intervention or medical neglect, nonconsented care, nonconfidential care, nondignified care, discrimination, abandonment, and detention in facilities. Though an imprecise semantic category, obstetric violence nonetheless has immense value as a conceptual framework. As anthropologist Paola Sesia underscores, framing diverse violations under this umbrella shifts the discourse away from that of individualized, accidental, or random medical malpractice, to a critique of structural conditions that infringe on the well-being of childbearing people as a whole.[16] A historical approach illuminates how medical practices can simultaneously reflect and amplify social oppression.

The phrase "obstetric violence" was first invoked by physician James Blundell in an 1827 article in *The Lancet*.[17] Patients, reformers, and physicians have referred to the concept since then, though it did not gain prominence until its popularization by Latin American human rights activists in the 1990s. Although I do not impose this term onto past situations, it is a key concept inasmuch as the book features the voices of people who spoke out against harm done to women's bodies during both emergency and exploratory medical procedures. Many also insisted that to deny access to needed health care is itself a form of violence.

I wish to underscore that obstetric violence is not somehow inherently worse in the Global South than the Global North.[18] Preventable maternal mortality and reproductive inequality are worldwide phenomena that disproportionately affect racialized, impoverished, and marginalized groups, even—and sometimes especially—in the Global North. These problems relate to the structural inequalities wrought by colonialism, slavery, and settler-colonialism, and they contextualize why oppressed groups suffer health disparities even when treated within the same medical systems as privileged people. Reproductive injustice stems from power disparities; it is not caused by, nor is it a symptom of, deficient scientific progress. Mexico is not predisposed to medical violence, and the history of obstetrics should never be pathologized, exotified, or weaponized to reify xenophobic, racist, or Eurocentric narratives about surgical "backwardness," "Western progress," or gendered medical "machismo."

Relatedly, I have opted to refrain from dichotomizing medical practice as "Western" versus "non-Western." Not only is Mexico in the Western hemisphere, but the nation's surgeons have, whenever possible, used the most advanced biomedical technologies. (This was true even in the eighteenth century, before Mexico was a nation, and when priests were the most likely to perform cesarean surgery). In Mexico as elsewhere, only historical analysis can explain how reproductive governance became embedded in systems of racism, classism, and patriarchy, and why these entanglements are harmful for women's health outcomes.

Latin American organizing against gender violence is part of a regional legacy to hold states and regimes accountable for abuses of human rights and dignity. Writing in the twenty-first century, the Mexican activist group GIRE (Grupo de Información en Reproducción Elegida, or Reproductive Choice

Educational Collective) refers to a broad range of harms as a "continuum of violence facing women." These include adolescent pregnancy; a broad-based lack of access to fertility control and abortion, especially for Indigenous women; sexual violence; obstetric violence; maternal mortality; and deficient social support for mothers and families with young children. GIRE asserts a strong and radical narrative, insisting that the state is responsible for eradicating these forms of gendered structural violence and that the state has the duty to ensure women's dignified and safe access to all forms of reproductive health care.[19] Inspiring this focus on redress are civil demands for reconciliation and accountability, which arose in the aftermath of late Cold War era authoritarianism and genocide. But just because the movements were born in a rights-based context does not mean that they will stay there. As the Colombian legal scholar Ana Cristina Vélez González says, it is now time to look to the postcolonial world for lessons about the future of reproductive health care.[20]

And yet, questions of accountability are always complicated. GIRE, for their part, does not believe that individual practitioners should be held responsible for deficiencies in public health funding and access to resources; in fact, criminalizing individual practitioners could absolve the state of its rightful burden to address health inequities. While these debates are not unique to any one region, Latin Americans' vision, analysis, and critique are important because they come from a particular history and because they push global debates about reproductive injustice into new territory. This book historicizes these debates in one of the most surgically significant countries in the Global South.

Obstetric Racism in Historical Perspective

The topic of obstetric violence brings us back to the young woman of Devil's Alley. Racism, colorism, classism, and sexism all influenced medical interpretations of the girl's body and mind, making her particularly vulnerable to experimental forms of surgical intervention. Her surgeon, Rodríguez, made clear that the girl became an instructional subject and that she had no choice in the matter. As soon as his colleague Dr. Anzorena saw her, he "happily announced that he had found the ideal patient for that day's medical lesson." Enthused, Rodríguez entered the room and "greeted her warmly, to win her favor." When she only responded with nods, he "resolved to proceed without directing another word at her."[21]

Rodríguez's and Anzorena's descriptions of the patient evinced a tripart aglomeration of modern racism: their words were anti-Indigenous, anti-Black, and orientalist. Their words were violent, and this violence is painful to witness. Rodríguez wrote that the girl of Devil's Alley was dark-skinned and that she had "a vague, stupid, inexpressive gaze." Her spine was "somewhat hunchbacked," and she apparently had the "angular face of an Indian," as well as "small and unfriendly eyes, which slanted like those of the Japanese." He weaponized racist language to disparage her other physical characteristics as well, noting that she had "a wide and short nose, big dark lips that stuck out, and an awkward head plopped on a thick trunk." Insisting that the woman had been a "victim of the savage man who sexually devoured her," his narrative seemed to symbolically deny her child's paternity while insisting that only the state could fill that biopolitical gap.[22]

The girl from Devil's Alley was marked by the erasure that so often accompanies racism.[23] Her reproductive acts made her a key focus of the medical landscape and implicated her intimately in the national project of scientific development. At the same time, the medical elite believed that she did not display the requisite biological fitness for reproducing the nation's citizens. Physicians pathologized and denigrated the characteristics that marked her as a woman, taking part in late nineteenth-century discourses that demarcated femininity within the boundaries of whiteness. In contrast, elites invoked specters of monstrosity, pathology, masculinity, and infantilism when referencing Black and Brown women's bodies. Furthermore, the girl of Devil's Alley was silenced in Rodríguez's celebrated book and through the act of surgery itself. While this silence is an important part of the history of obstetric racism and obstetric violence, resistance echoes in the archives and its historical legacies.[24]

Following his examination, Rodríguez officially diagnosed the young woman with "infantilism," a racially charged term that denoted incomplete or unsatisfactory physical and intellectual development resulting from evolutionary degeneration. Her narrow pelvis formed a key component of his diagnosis, as he believed it would make vaginal birth impossible. In Rodríguez's words, "we decided that if we did not perform a caesarean operation, she and her child would become cadavers right before our eyes." Ironically, they did become cadavers right before their eyes because mother and child died while a group of medical students stood around the operating table in observation. The young woman and her child were erased by the same origin story they made. In a further irony, Rodríguez's autopsy report noted that the woman's pelvis did not meet the scientific criteria for infantilism after all.[25]

But she met other criteria. The opening and deconstruction of this patient's body represented much more than the pursuit of information about her pelvic size: this became a quest for an intimate scientific truth about Mexico. Inspired by positivism, physicians sought to discover rules about the nation's biological roots and about the organic composition of those who were allegedly stymying national progress.[26] They argued that racialized women's bodies were irrationally organized and therefore in need of scientific correction.

Historians of medicine have long been concerned with pain, that ineffable, immeasurable, and nontransferable category of human experience. The episode with the young woman of Devil's Alley is painful in more than one way. It was violent to her body and dignity and destructive to her life and that of her child. It surely wrought grief onto her family and community, who likely wondered why their loved one had disappeared. It harmed the medical students, who learned that this was proper therapeutic care for public patients and an appropriate way to extract medical knowledge from others. These words are painful for readers of this history, who know that this young woman's life contained much more than what this scene entails. She had loved ones, joys, sadnesses, relations, and a life beyond her pregnancy. Medical archives can only give us limited glimpses of patients' lives, and this alienates and desensitizes us from the injustices they faced.

The development of obstetric science, the "science of woman," is inseparable from the politics of race, class, color, and the de facto exclusion of many, even in the context of liberal citizenship and inclusion laws.[27] The history of surgery sheds light on the place of Mexican women's bodies in the creation of obstetric knowledge while also calling attention to the paradoxes of state projects that exacerbated anti-Indigenous prejudices even while romanticizing *indigenísmo*. If Mexico is a nation of "enemies within," reproduction figures as a key realm within which to track bias.[28] And as Laura Briggs tells us that "all politics are reproductive politics," this study shows that reproductive politics and their concomitant metaphysical debates inflected on political conflicts throughout modern Mexican history.[29]

Key here is Dána-Ain Davis's analysis of obstetric racism, a form of gendered and racialized discrimination exacerbated by medical, legal, and social vulnerability during the childbearing experience.[30] Because race functions as a distinct signifier in different times and places, histories of obstetric racism vary in important ways. For example, US physicians viewed African Americans as simultaneously biologically pathological and as medical superbodies, desensitized to the pain experienced by White bodies. Mexican obstetricians eagerly consumed the studies written by foreign practitioners and sent their own back on trains and boats to the United States and elsewhere throughout the world.[31]

At the same time, Mexican obstetricians created unique medical epistemologies about impoverished Mexicans' frailty, deformity, disorganization, and lack of sensitivity to pain. Because the idea of race—an ideology of power, a biologized category of difference, and everything in between—is so slippery, phenotype, language, place of origin, and the amorphous notion of "culture" often became markers of racial difference. Mexican obstetric racism was flexible, pernicious, and parasitic. It drew, as we have seen, on an amalgam of tropes about class, culture, education, biology, hygiene, and worth. Racism made race, not vice versa.[32]

Though Rodríguez's words comprised a pastiche of racist tropes, he spoke to Mexico's complex racial history, which is all too briefly summarized here. A majority of Mexicans are of predominantly Indigenous descent, although it is, of course, a colonially rooted overgeneralization to lump together the nation's many ethnically and linguistically diverse Indigenous groups. Approximately one quarter of a million Spaniards migrated to Mexico during 300 years of colonization (1521–1821), during which time the government imposed a racialized hierarchical caste system. The classificatory schema was rooted in sixteenth-century Spanish claims to "purity of blood" (*limpieza de sangre*), invoked by Christians to differentiate themselves from Muslims, the Moors who had conquered the Iberian peninsula, Jewish people, converts, and so-called "pagans."[33]

Of course, Spaniards were not the only newcomers to Latin America. Significantly, more than a quarter million enslaved Africans worked on haciendas and in urban slavery in New Spain. Many escaped or purchased their freedom, and a sizable number formed maroon communities with Indigenous people. Mexico has been the recipient of substantial Asian migration, though it is underresearched and seldom recognized. Filipinos came to New Spain during the colonial period, and by the late nineteenth century Chinese migration had increased substantially as well, leading to a large twentieth-century boom that provoked violent episodes of Sinophobia. Mexico strongly encouraged European migration in the late nineteenth century, during which time the nation invited migration from many religious and separatist communities. The nineteenth century additionally saw an influx of African Americans who in Mexico escaped slavery and Jim Crow laws. By the twentieth century, the nation received large groups of migrants and refugees; in the 1930s, for example, 25,000 Spaniards fled Franco's fascist regime and resettled in Mexico City. In sum, Mexico's self-designation as a "mestizo nation" elides the cultural and genetic diversity of its people.

When one doctor estimated Mexico's national population in 1891, then standing at around 11.68 million people, he guessed that 18 percent of the nation's population descended from Europeans and were "white." Thirty-three percent were "of the pure Indigenous race," 47 percent were "mixed," and only 2 percent were "of the purely Black race or of African origin." The author did not hide his racial prejudice, stating that those of "the white race [were] intellectually and socially superior," while "the rest" were allegedly "indolent and apathetic" due to "traditional social factors" as well as "climate and geography."[34] Although many cited in this book held similar prejudices, they often held back on commenting forthrightly about the ethnicity and identity of their patients. As Karin Rosemblatt has demonstrated in her transnational study of racial politics, scientists in the United States also struggled to concretize notions around race and racial groups, and racial classifications were contested in both countries; they were not inherently firmer or more entrenched in the United States than in Mexico.[35]

Doctors' ambiguous terminology reflected this messiness. Physicians frequently employed coded racialized language, like the term "outsider" for newcomers from other states or countries. Surgeons routinely referred to impoverished women with moralizing and denigrating words, including "dirty," "shameless," "disgraceful," and "unfortunate." They did not use those phrases when writing about upper-class, elite, or otherwise privileged women, for whom they used respectful language like the word *señora* instead of *muger*.

Others spoke of culture to refer to ethnic and class designations, even embedding these into formal mechanisms such as patient charts. Jesús Andrade took note of women's "culture" in his 1927 thesis on labor pain. Conflating notions of class and culture, he made a chart with notes on nineteen birthing patients. Two had given birth at home, and the other seventeen birthed at the Hospital Juárez. Fourteen were domestic servants who worked in Mexico City homes and hailed from the states of Toluca, Texcoco, Hidalgo, Chiapas, and Oaxaca—places with multiple and distinct understandings of culture and class. Andrade designated his patients in reductionist terms, referring to the "Indigenous class," "humble class," "medium class," and "high class." Not only did this erase African-descendent and Black Mexicans, but it also placed Indigenous Mexicans, quite literally, in a class of their own. Andrade categorized women according to four scales of "culture": none, rudimentary, medium, or elevated.[36] He deemed Indigenous women to have rudimentary culture, at best.

Such obscurities do not diminish the importance of racialized concepts as signifiers. As anthropologist Deborah Poole notes, "we might argue that this ambiguity distinguishes the concept of race and lends it its singular power to mobilize older social prejudices and modes of understanding difference, reworking them to fit the exigencies of changing social and political landscapes—always present but never quite the same."[37] Others have called this "racecraft."[38] The history of surgery is important because of the ways in which reproductive health care interfaced with the politics of racism, class, and belonging in Mexico. Although women of all racialized groups and social classes are featured in the chapters, throughout we see that surgery often became a fault line demarcating inclusion, exclusion, and embodied prejudice.

Women, Gender, and Medicine in Mexico

There is a rich literature on women and gender in Mexico's colonial and postcolonial periods. Yet relatively few historians have turned to "operation-based histories," which examine surgery as fundamental "in the medicalisation of women, through which cultural notions of femininity were embedded into surgical practice."[39] Although historians have foregrounded important issues like sex work, eugenics, education, nursing, disease, religion, and activism, we know relatively little about how Mexican women experienced different clinical treatments across time.

Surgery and Salvation draws inspiration from and is indebted to Nora Jaffary's *Reproduction and Its Discontents in Mexico,* which explores the private reproductive worlds of many eighteenth- and nineteenth-century women by analyzing their experiences with contraception, abortion, midwifery, and infanticide. Whereas *Reproduction and Its Discontents* offers compelling and intimate portraits of how childbirth transformed from an "unremarkable and private matter at the end of the colonial period to an event of intense public concern by the close of the nineteenth century," *Surgery and Salvation* focuses on moments in which authorities reconceptualized surgical technologies to stake claim over women and unborn subjects.[40]

Many histories of reproductive politics draw on records written by twentieth-century eugenicists, who were determined to affect the course of human heredity by influencing reproduction. Eugenics offered powerful scientific and policy-based tools in the service of national projects, including those that increased fertility, reduced women's autonomous use of fertility control, and mitigated high rates of infant mortality. Scholars of eugenics have explored the crossroads of scientific racism and women's reproduction through many realms, including public health campaigns and institutions such as foundling asylums and poorhouses.

Inspired by Nancy Stepan's classic work on eugenics, historians have explored how policy, legislation, and medical practice shifted in response to scientific and medical writings about racial regeneration as well as social and biological improvement. In Mexico, these debates were strongly influenced by the Mexican Eugenics Society.[41] Later chapters of this book engage with this important historiography. In contrast to other works, I focus primarily on the religious valences of obstetric practice in the midst of pitched cultural battles about authority and secularization. This adds to recent conversations about Catholic eugenics as well as the confluence of secular paternalism and Catholicism in the modernization of patriarchy.[42]

Scholars of slavery have shown that the monetization and commodification of enslaved women's reproduction lies at the core of the modern Atlantic world as well as white supremacist capitalism. It is no coincidence that that the majority of cesarean sections in nineteenth-century America were performed on enslaved women, or that slave-holding doctors like J. Marion Sims first trialed vaginal fistula-repair surgeries on women in bondage. It is also no coincidence that he did so without using available pain control methods.[43] Like the girl of Devil's Alley, enslaved women's corporeal service to the state extended to the medical use of their bodies. Furthermore, and as we saw previously, anti-Black medical racism in the United States reinforced and exacerbated medical racism elsewhere, including in Mexico. In other words, nineteenth century anti-Indigenous racism was influenced by global anti-Blackness. This book adds to literature on the medicalized commodification of women's bodies by showing that obstetric violence also lies at the heart of claims about fetal souls, maternal worth, and the inclusion of marginalized groups into national projects in Mexico and beyond.[44] The origins of religious, political, and cultural claims on mothers and their unborn are surgical as well as metaphysical because authorities invoked surgery while making assertions about life, death, and the soul. Their contentions, in turn, bolstered patriarchal forms of governance.

Such analysis is inspired by the feminist scholarly tradition of writing history through the body. It also contributes to larger debates about how the unborn came to be understood as rights-bearing citizens who stand in spiritual, legal, biological, and ontological opposition to their mothers.[45] Reproductive injustice in Mexico is dually rooted in religious paternalism and racial prejudice, and that politicized claims about reproduction were co-produced by church and state authorities, even when those authorities were in conflict. Examining historical efforts to imbue surgeries with spiritualized, racialized, and politicized meaning provides additional insight into how these ideologies affected people's lives.

Source Selection, Methodology, and Terminology

Surgery and Salvation draws on a range of religious, medical, and state-based sources, including theological tomes, ecclesiastical records, mission records, and writings by medical students, clinicians, and public health officials. The later chapters feature complaints by women themselves. The book first addresses the religious use of the cesarean operation. Complementing prior studies of the cesarean surgery in Peru, Guatemala, Puerto Rico, and Sicily, I pay special attention to the operation's history in colonial Mexico.[46]

Spatially, the book starts in Indigenous missions and becomes increasingly focused on Mexico City. By the mid-nineteenth century it centers on central Mexico. Finally, by the 1930s, most sources derive from Mexico City's Hospital General, which was where the vast majority of reproductive surgeries took place, and which also was a key site of conflict about reproduction. Because surgical practices became increasingly centralized and nationalized over the course of the period under study, this latitudinal narrowing simply results from the source base.

The 1880s witnessed a quantitative explosion of Mexico's medical literature, especially in the form of student theses. Students' writings are particularly useful for how they espoused political alliances, religious beliefs, and social prejudices and for how they commented on patients' economic status, phenotype, and class. Between 1861 and 1936, 4,146 Mexican medical students published theses. They varied in length, ranging between around fifty and 350 pages. In 1936 the medical school dropped its requirement for students to perform research in Mexico City hospitals before graduation.

Although they are problematic in many ways, student writings were closer to the ground than those by their professors. Students were often more genuine, more critical, and less attuned to the careful and diplomatic omissions their professors chose. They frequently said the "quiet part out loud," exposing prejudices and conflicts that their textbooks silenced. I deliberately treat medical students as actors with clinical importance because they interfaced with large numbers of surgical patients during their time working in hospitals. They held clear influence in the clinic, where they performed surgery and wrote about their endeavors. Because my main concern is how that affected ideas women's health care options, I do not dwell excessively on the biographies of medical students or doctors.

Research led me to read the majority of student theses on reproductive surgery produced between 1880 and 1940. Nonetheless, there were many deserving topics that I could not address at length, such as puerperal fever, spinal anesthesia, Indigenous herbs and chemical drugs, and the use of X-rays for fetal and pelvic imaging. There is also much more to say about sex work, contraception, midwifery, and miscarriage. Whereas others have examined the nuances of these themes, I wanted to focus primarily on surgery, where ideology melded and clashed with clinical practice in dramatic ways and where metaphysics became manifest. Two intertwined themes guided my reading of primary sources: metaphysical and salvational discourses on the one hand, and racial pathologization and its connections to eugenic practice on the other.

Some questions on terminology and language deserve mention. Referring to unborn children is complicated; indeed, ideas about the unborn have not only changed over time but have been complex in each historical era. Whenever possible, I refer to the unborn with the actor's categories used by people in the past. Yet even those terms—product of conception, product, fetus, embryo, baby, infant, and child—are ambiguous in their own ways, then as they are now. The boundary between an embryo and a fetus is unclear, and it was even more so throughout history. I often write "product of conception," not only because it was the most common way to refer to the unborn but also because it is accurate at any stage of pregnancy. On questions of language, I should include the customary note that all translations in the book are my own; that is, none of the primary sources I consulted have been published in English.

Lexicological complexities regarding gender and sex are always relevant to the history of reproductive medicine. I use the term "women" critically, recognizing that the modern category of woman was itself shaped by gendered medical violence as well as sociocultural ideologies promulgated by state, scientific, and religious institutions. While reproductive governance is a gendered form of social hegemony that marginalizes non-men in particular ways, I am wary of reifying the gender binary or suggesting that only women-identified people became pregnant in the period under study.

Gender norms affected the medical profession as well as the patient population. Male medical students authored the vast majority of medical theses focusing on reproductive surgery in Mexico. Although 116 women graduated from the national medical school between 1887 and 1947, only one authored a thesis cited in this book.[47] It may initially seem curious or ironic, but this gender imbalance underscores the masculinization of the surgical specialty.

Surgeons were prized for masculine characteristics, such as bold, brash, and decisive action, especially in the preanesthetic era when brute force was needed to amputate limbs as quickly as possible, and often in less than ten seconds. The field certainly needs more research about masculinity, emotion, affect, performance, and surgery in Mexico and Latin America.

As mentioned earlier, decades of medical historians have faced the problem of accessing and understanding the patient's voice. Indeed, modern medical practice and record-keeping technologies and practices quite literally erased patients' voices from the medical record.[48] Following traditions in feminist theory, especially as developed by historians of slavery, when possible I have endeavored to read sources against the grain by imagining aspects of medical history from the patient's narrative perspective. While imperfect, this method sought to develop more empathy for their positionality and to underscore that their experiences should figure centrally in the history of reproductive surgery.[49]

Chapter Descriptions

Nine chapters, organized in five chronological sections, address surgery under the rubric of different forms of salvation: religious (1745–1840), postcolonial (1840–76), positivist (1876–1911), and revolutionary (1911–40). The last section includes the epilogue and focuses on resistance. Each section contains two chapters that together historicize reproductive surgery—first in theory, then in policy, and finally, in clinical practice.

Part I, "Surgery and Religious Salvation," begins in the eighteenth century when the Spanish empire required that priests perform caesarean operations on dead and dying women so that they could extract unborn fetuses, baptize them, and make them subjects of the Crown. Chapter 1 underscores that cesarean surgery was essential to the then-radical and contentious claim that life begins shortly after fecundation. Demonstrating that the operation was more common than historians have believed, chapter 2 examines the cesarean in the context of colonialism. As a whole, this section argues that Bourbon authorities envisaged a surgical technique that would spiritually incorporate the Indigenous groups that they wished to assimilate into the state. Colonial hegemony became central to cesarean surgery, especially in the violent and highly contested borderlands between colonial New Spain and settler-colonial US territory.

Part II, "Surgery and Postcolonial Salvation," turns to reproductive medicine in the context of nineteenth-century republican state formation, analyzing women as both reproductive subjects and as medical professionals with expertise in reproductive science. This was the era of Mexico's liberal reform laws (*la reforma*), a time that witnessed a series of military and cultural battles between liberals and conservatives who held competing visions of the nation. Chapter 3 examines the medicalization of the hysteria diagnosis within the secularization of Mexico City's clinics. Chapter 4 looks at issues of class, honor, and hysteria in debates about therapeutic abortion and artificially induced premature labor. Both consider questions of gender as well as liberal notions about useful citizens in Mexico's postcolonial national project.

By the late nineteenth century, the bacteriological revolution and advancements in germ theory contributed to developments in surgical procedures. Part III, "Racial Science and Surgical Salvation," examines the intensification of racial prejudice in obstetric ideology and practice. In Chapter 5, Porfirian obstetricians began to claim that Indigenous women were biologically inferior due to their small pelvises. Chapter 6 explores how racial science provided a widespread rationale for experimental surgeries. The availability of patients was facilitated by the newly revived Sanitary Police, which by the end of the century brought thousands of women per year into Mexico City's clinics. Midcentury medical concerns about morality, affect, and biological regeneration became racialized in new ways.

Part IV, "Surgery and Revolutionary Salvation," analyzes eugenic sterilization and fertility control after Mexico's social revolution of 1917. This section challenges a long-standing assumption that Mexican eugenics was not surgically interventionist or that Mexican eugenicists did not sterilize large numbers of women. Chapter 7 shows that many twentieth-century physicians reified racialized prejudices in medicine to legitimize the surgical prevention of birth. Chapter 8 examines vaginal bifurcation, a form of temporary sterilization that reconciled eugenics and fertility control with 1930s papal politics. These chapters underscore that eugenic physicians espoused salvational politics, even when they were decidedly anticlerical.

Part V, "Resistance," focuses on this elusive but all-too-important theme, in part by highlighting patients' complaints and other ground-level voices, as in chapter 9. A scandal of leadership in the General Hospital attracted the attention of the prominent feminist activist Elvia Carrillo Puerto, who showed sympathy with the complainants; presumably her activism for fertility control and women's rights influenced—and was influenced by—her visits.[50] By the 1930s, popular feminist struggles spoke to the relationship between health care and patient dignity.

The conclusion/epilogue discusses contemporary feminist activism around reproductive injustice. Among its sources are recent reports from GIRE, which has relentlessly advocated for reproductive rights since the 1990s. In 2016, Mexico's national survey on the dynamics of household relationships included questions on women's recent childbearing experiences. The results were concerning: of the 8.7 million women who delivered at least once between 2011 and 2016 in Mexico, 33.4 percent reported having suffered abuse by health providers. Such stark nationwide data allowed for a broad evaluation of the scope and variables associated with obstetric violence and prompted some states to address the problem legislatively.[51]

Though grueling, advocacy and activist efforts have been enormously successful in Latin America. Feminists in recent years have succeeded in legalizing access to pregnancy termination in Mexico, Colombia, and Argentina. At the same time, access to reproductive health is under dire attack in the United States, where the question of premodern Catholic views of fetal personhood were central to the Supreme Court's 2022 ruling in *Dobbs v. Jackson Women's Health Organization*. Justice Samuel Alito cited an eighteenth-century case to argue that the right to abortion was not deeply rooted in the national traditions, helping to fuel a nationwide conversation about the uses and misuses of history. The first section of *Surgery and Salvation* turns to the eighteenth century to examine surgery and the roots of the modern fetal personhood debate colonial New Spain.

Part I
Surgery and Religious Salvation

CHAPTER ONE

As Small as a Grain of Barley

The Catholic Enlightenment and the Cesarean Operation, 1745–1835

Beginning in 1749, Catholic authorities throughout the Spanish empire implemented legislation requiring priests to perform cesarean operations on dead and dying women. The surgery enabled clerics to baptize infants who would otherwise have perished in utero without receiving the sacrament. Before the eighteenth century, the cesarean operation served a different purpose: for centuries, medical and religious authorities had performed surgery to save the corporal lives of women and infants.[1] Although priests, surgeons, and midwives had baptized the infants they extracted whenever possible, spiritual salvation was not their only—or even their primary—aim.

During the eighteenth century, however, Catholic authorities repurposed the surgery and insisted on the removal of small products of conception. Extracting and baptizing miniscule fetuses was completely novel: never before had authorities required priests to perform surgery to save the spiritual life of an embryonic being. This chapter argues that Catholic theologians transformed the cesarean operation into a salvation-based surgery, and that they did so to advance the then-radical and contentious claim that life begins shortly after fecundation. Such claims gave way to new definitions of personhood, new rituals with which to reform the baptismal sacrament, and new ideas about pregnant women's obligation to undergo surgery. The cesarean operation facilitated Catholic claims that the unborn were ensouled and endowed with spiritual personhood, and that their baptism was of utmost importance even if it entailed the death of their mother. Some theologians emphasized that a reproductive person's duty was to bear, protect, and birth the unborn, even at the cost of her own life.

Theologians additionally advanced scientific claims about embryology, the study of fetal development. A closely related concept was ensoulment, a term referring to the time at which the unborn are considered to be in possession of their own (human and rational) soul. In Spanish-language writings, ensoulment was referred to as *animación,* or "animation." Ensoulment and animation were distinct from quickening, which refers to the time during which women first felt fetal movements in utero. Quickening is a key concept in the history of reproduction due to the fact that pre-modern women frequently practiced menstrual regulation (the restoration of menstruation) and abortion in the months before quickening.[2] Eighteenth-century Catholic authorities shifted their focus from quickening to ensoulment, thereby politicizing matters of maternal and fetal life and death in new ways.

What follows is an intellectual history that focuses on physicians, theologians, and colonial officials who wrote about the cesarean operation in the Catholic world and the Spanish empire. It illuminates how religious authorities drew on Enlightenment discourses to argue that surgery, a scientific technology, could perfect the baptismal sacrament. Many of their ideas stemmed from Enlightenment Catholicism, a movement that sought to reform religion by reconciling metaphysics with modernity, progress, and reason.[3] Debates about humanity's capacity for the use of reason were particularly relevant to Enlightenment colonial projects. Indeed, Iberian deliberations about rationality dated to the conquest in the fifteenth century, when colonizers like Bartolomé de las Casas questioned whether paganism prevented the possession of natural reason, and accordingly, whether Indigenous people or Africans possessed a rational personhood that exempted them from slavery. By the eighteenth century, surgery offered priests an applied science with which to address centuries-old colonial questions about rationality and the soul.

This chapter first analyzes an early cesarean surgery performed in Spain in 1750, which was motivated by concern for the mother's life and not the child's soul. In doing so, it establishes a baseline from which to compare later operations. The second and third sections examine theologies regarding baptism and ensoulment, with a particular focus on the metaphysics of diagnosing maternal and infant death. A main argument is that theological claims about embryonic ensoulment radicalized in the Latin American context, and over the course of the eighteenth century. Finally, the last section examines the gendered ideas concomitant with the cesarean operation in Latin America, where the ideology underpinning surgery as salvation intensified over time.

From Mythologized Surgery to Medicalized Operation

Like all forms of technology, the cesarean operation has acquired and disinherited many distinct meanings throughout time. From antiquity through the medieval period, authorities viewed it as an unsettling surgery, associated with the unnatural, the supernatural, and the cult of the virgin saint Rocamadour.[4] Mythological iconography in the Middle Ages depicted both saints and devils extracting the unborn through abdominal incision.[5]

The first legal effort to promote postmortem caesarean surgery came in 715 B.C., when King Numa Pompilius made it unlawful to bury a pregnant woman without attempting to cut out the child to save its life. The Roman emperor Caesar Augustus later renamed this legislation *lex caesarea*.[6] Centuries later, the Parisian archbishop Odon de Sully (1196–1208) apparently became the first church official to recommend the procedure; yet he emphasized that surgery could only occur when the child might survive the mother's death. He wrote: "Those who have died in childbirth should be cut open when the child is believed to still be alive; however, it has to be well-established that they [the mothers] are dead."[7] At this time, canon law forbade clergy from performing procedures that involved the shedding of blood, so cesarean surgery was left to midwives and lay surgeons.[8] "Cesarean operation" did not become a medical term until 1581, when French physician François Rousset invoked religious imagery to claim that he "baptized" the surgery by naming it *opération césarienne*.[9] Despite substantial debate regarding their usefulness, medical cesareans became increasingly common by the sixteenth and seventeenth centuries. Sadly, in these centuries the only alternative for ending an otherwise hopeless labor (in which mother and child were both likely to die) was embryotomy. During this procedure, a practitioner would puncture the infant's skull and remove the dismembered child with the hope of saving the childbearing person's life. Since very few births were attended by doctors before the twentieth century, this gruesome task was associated with midwives. The cesarean operation offered hope for delivering a live child despite an arduous labor; however, a dearth of pain control made this daunting indeed for live women.[10]

When Spanish physician Jaime Alcalá y Martínez performed a cesarean section in 1750, his rationale seemed to have been more corporeal than religious.[11] A midwife by the name of Vicenta Iñego summoned him to assist María Ivañez, a forty-year-old woman who had become fatigued during childbirth. Iñego had requested the doctor's assistance because the child, a boy, appeared unable to move in the womb. Labor seemed obstructed because only the child's hand, not his head, was visible in the cervix. Alcalá y Martínez attempted to retrieve the fetus with a speculum, a curved piece of metal that increased intravaginal visibility. When he had no success with this method, the physician called for a conference with another practitioner and Iñego. He apparently respected the midwife's clinical skills, judging by his consultation of her opinion on the case. Iñego, the midwife, believed that mother and child would die without surgical intervention, and she begged Alcalá y Martínez to perform a cesarean. Perhaps she felt that her professional reputation was at stake. By this time, both María and her child seemed close to death due to a steady hemorrhaging of blood from María's uterus.

In 1750 cesarean surgery was contentious enough that a doctor's opinions alone were insufficient to justify surgery. In order to operate, Alcalá y Martínez was obligated to consult with a representative from the Protomedicato, a board of physicians who oversaw and administered medical practice in Spain and throughout the Spanish empire. Since 1628, the board had been responsible for coordinating public health initiatives, granting and renewing medical degrees, and supervising hospital administration and medical practice.[12] After considering the circumstances, Protomedicato authority Dr. Valencia Gómez asserted, "The proposal [to operate] was just and rational. It was also pious, and loyal to reason, law, and justice. Our conscience obligates us to perform the surgery."[13] Alcalá y Martínez and Valencia Gómez both emphasized that the operation was "rationally conceived," based on observation, experimentation, and science. The physician clearly hoped to appeal to Enlightenment-minded intellectuals; by contrasting Enlightenment science with barbarity, he implied that superstition and medieval medical practice could be reformed by modern surgical techniques.[14]

Both the midwife Iñego and the doctor Alcalá y Martínez believed that María should undergo a cesarean while still alive. Some of the censors who wrote introductions to Alcalá y Martínez's text disagreed with this stance, insisting that a woman must already be deceased before a surgery could occur. Alcalá y Martínez dissented from the censors' opinions in his tract, quoting Hippocrates at length and explaining that, whenever possible, "[he] expect[s] to save both [mother and child]."[15] His motives were both medical and religious: in this case, he saw surgery as the "only pious path" and as "the only hope of restoring [María's] natural ability to give life."[16]

In his explanation Alcalá y Martínez characterized the womb as a "natural cavity," likely in response to prohibitions against surgery by canon law. By arguing that the uterus was already a natural penetration—a cavity—he portrayed the penetrant knife as no more invasive than the hollow that already shaped women's bodies. Because the uterus represented a naturalized kind of incision, cutting into it arguably did not violate canon law prohibiting surgical mutilation. Furthermore, he insisted that the incision was a "simple" one because it was allegedly close to the surface. The doctor's discussion mirrored the then very-recent 1749 Sicilian law requiring surgeons to bypass the canonical prohibition on the opening of cadavers in their efforts to save a fetus. The law, too, rested on the argument that the cesarean was not a surgery per se because it only required one incision and because the uterus already constituted a penetration of the body. Thus, the 1749 Sicilian legislation required surgeons to make "a single cut" when they deemed it possible to save both mother and child during a difficult childbirth.[17]

Midwife Iñego and physician Alcalá y Martínez's 1750 performance of a medicalized cesarean is important precisely because fetal baptism was not their dominant priority: though baptism became a fortunate side effect, it was never their fundamental goal. In fact, Alcalá y Martínez did not send the child to the church for baptism until the day after the surgery, which was the day of María's death.[18] Despite Alcalá y Martínez's emphasis on progress, reason, and the Enlightenment, religion did not motivate him to perform cesarean surgery. This would change substantially with the dissemination of colonial and Catholic theology and legislation.

Spiritualizing the Caesarean Operation: Generation and Regeneration in Catholic Theology

If Iñego and Alcalá y Martínez performed surgery to save the corporal lives of María Ivañez and her son, other eighteenth-century surgeons acted on explicitly religious motivations. One of the most important theologians to write about religious cesarean surgery was the Italian priest Francesco Emanuele Cangiamila (1702–63), whose book, *Sacred Embryology*, was first published in 1745. Over the next century, Cangiamila's 120,000-word work was translated into eight languages and distributed throughout the world, sometimes in abridged form.[19] Many historians who have examined cesarean surgery have emphasized the importance of Cangiamila's work, which is widely recognized as one of the most important Enlightenment-era texts on fetal personhood. *Sacred Embryology* directly influenced the Catholic Church's position on fetal ensoulment, which by 1869 declared unequivocally that the church considered life to begin at conception.[20] This chapter contributes to the literature by elucidating *Sacred Embryology*'s theological rationale, which rested on a metaphysical redefinition of human generation and on a reconceptualization of childbirth as a precursor to spiritual regeneration.

Cangiamila's enthusiasm for the caesarean operation commenced in 1736, when he surgically extracted a living infant from a parishioner who died during childbirth in his parish in Palermo, Sicily. His success surprised the birth attendants, a midwife and a surgeon, who insisted the child had already died.[21] Encouraged by this, the priest took part in over two dozen operations over the next decade while he penned *Sacred Embryology*. Though initially contentious and hotly debated, Cangiamila's book soon gained the support of Charles III and Pope Benedict XIV, who demanded that priests perform the operation and declared that a failure to do so would result in charges of homicide.[22] As historian Adam Warren has noted, Cangiamila's ideas were so influential that after writing *Sacred Embryology* the priest gained political prominence and became the head inquisitor for the kingdom of Sicily.[23]

Sacred Embryology emphasized that baptism provided recipients with regeneration (spiritual rebirth) as well as spiritual parentage, thereby constructing a supernatural God as a paternal figure for the newly baptized. The necessity for this stemmed from original sin, which Cangiamila described with scientific language, likening it to contagion, disease, and infection.[24] Similarly, his work sustained that only surgery offered a path to spiritual regeneration for the unborn trapped in their mother's wombs. The baptismal sacrament provided another kind of deliverance, as well: that which saved souls from the devil and death. This was salvation through surgery indeed.

A key point in Cangiamila's text was that baptized people experienced not two births (birth and regeneration) but three: ensoulment, birth, and regeneration. The first, ensoulment, was a metaphysical occurrence in the womb; this was the "real" birth because it represented the child's spiritual creation: "In this moment," Cangiamila insisted, "God creates a body that is rational, meaning that is it well-organized enough to receive a soul."[25] Less important was the physical act of birth, which simply took place when the fetus emerged into the light. This meant that women did not give birth; rather, birth was given by God and facilitated either by nature (natural birth) or science (cesarean operation). Women were passive participants, while "men, so vigorous and healthy, climb out of the prison of their mother's wombs without any assistance."[26]

This theorization of baptism necessitated a rejection of Saint Augustine's insistence that unbaptized children go to limbo. Saint Augustine argued that fetuses did not need to receive the sacrament because they gained spiritual rebirth through their mother's baptism and the umbilical cord that connected them.[27] Cangiamila disagreed, explaining that "the child is not truly *part* of the mother. That is, he does not form a physical part of her; indeed, he is distinguishable as separate because he is a man, himself, and must be baptized separately."[28] The point of debate was whether an unborn fetus could be considered individuated from its mother.

Older practices of baptism thus became unacceptable. Previously, when doctors, midwives, and priests sought to baptize the unborn, they injected a syringe filled with holy water through the cervix and into the womb. In 1733, theologians at the Sorbonne in Paris called this method "in-womb baptism," and obstetricians in many nations and colonies adopted the practice enthusiastically.[29] Cangiamila disputed the assumptions underlying in-womb baptism, arguing that fetuses could not receive the sacrament in the womb and that they needed to be birthed by surgery instead.

Because the cesarean operation rarely produced a living child, Cangiamila proposed the use of conditional baptism, under which a priest would proclaim "if you are human and capable of receiving the sacrament, I baptize you."[30] Conditional baptism allowed for new flexibility in definitions of life, death, and their interstices. The "apparently nonliving"—fetuses qualifying for conditional baptism—included those who had lived but died, those who were never alive, and monstrous fetuses, which did not appear human at all but arguably still merited baptism.

Modifying a sacrament was no small matter. Cangiamila justified it at length, devoting many pages to prescribing the correct kind of baptism for different situations. If, for example, the head of the fetus was showing and the fetus was in danger of death, the head was to be baptized.[31] Here the head symbolizes the presence of a soul; in fact the author referred to the head as the "seat of the soul," aligning his thought with a dominant trend in Enlightenment science that focused on the brain as the foremost symbol of rationality.[32] Even a miniscule embryo "must be baptized," Cangiamila asserted, "even if it is no larger than a grain of barley" and "no matter how little time has elapsed since the moment of conception, although it may not show any signs of movement to indicate life." If found within the amniotic sac, priests were to open the sac and perform yet another baptism. When inseparable from the sac, the products were to be baptized via immersion in a glass of water.[33]

As I will emphasize, *Sacred Embryology* originated and inspired new metaphysical claims to reconceptualize the status of the unborn. Even unborn and apparently dead fetuses could achieve eternal grace thanks to conditional baptism, a shift in sacramental procedure. This meant that theological innovations and surgery allowed Catholic authorities to alter definitions of both temporal and spiritual life, thereby bolstering these authorities' quest for authority and influence in scientific, legal, and religious deliberations about unborn personhood.

Making Embryology Sacred

Defining personhood thus became a predominant focus for theologians writing about the cesarean operation. Because a true subject was required in order for the baptismal ritual to be valid, Cangiamila and others strove to prove that the unborn should be considered an ensouled human subject, no matter how small. The ancient philosopher Aristotle penned one of the earliest known writings on ensoulment, *De Anima,* in 350 B.C., though the work was not published until the thirteenth century. Even as Aristotle developed theories on ensoulment, he recognized that attaining "any assured knowledge about the soul is one of the most difficult things in the world."[34] Is the soul potential or actual? Is it divisible? Aristotle could not answer these questions, and arguably no one can. But he did insist, for his part, that the soul requires a body to be acted upon as an essential condition of its existence, meaning that a soul could not exist prior to the formation of a body to receive it.

Aristotle believed that fetuses came to possess three souls over the course of their generation. Small products of conception first possessed "vegetative" souls, which simply absorbed nutrition and did not move on their own accord. The second was an "animal" soul, which moved but did not possess human sentience or rationality. Aristotle believed that male fetuses held such a soul after forty days of gestation; females did not gain the animal soul until ninety days, allegedly because the embryonic female's body was "hotter" and so its internal matter would take longer to solidify. Around an unidentified time close to birth, Aristotle postulated, fetuses developed rational souls that employed the use of imagination.[35] For him, the soul was the formal cause of life and was something generated internally, not inhaled or absorbed. Aristotle's theories influenced Church fathers like Augustine of Hippo (354 B.C.–430 B.C.), who did not differentiate between the animal and rational souls. Late Roman law also drew directly from Aristotle, regarding the fetus as neither *Homo* (human), nor even *Infans* (speechless, or infantile), but only as *Spes animantis,* or "potentially ensouled."[36]

Another immensely influential theologian, Thomas Aquinas (1227–74), proposed that a fetus's vegetative and sentient souls perished in turn before the endowment of a rational soul. Unborn life thus metamorphosed through multiple deaths as well as multiple rebirths. Apart from these reiterations of Aristotelian thought, historian Joseph Needham insists that "embryology has very little history" until the sixteenth century.[37] In part, this was because anatomists generally lacked access to embryos and fetuses to study. Though surgeons and others performed a handful of dissections, eviscerations, and caesarean operations between the thirteenth and sixteenth centuries, physicians rarely acquired these anatomical specimens or others, such as products of miscarriage.[38]

Leonardo da Vinci (1452–1519), one of the most prominent Renaissance anatomists, took a standard approach to the question of ensoulment. Da

Vinci insisted that small products of conception had no heartbeat and that they only had a derivative maternal soul instead of an individuated one. He wrote, "Nature places in the bodies of animals the soul, the composer of the body, i.e. the soul of the mother, which first composes, in the womb, the shape of man, and in due time awakens the soul which shall be the inhabitant thereof, which first remains asleep and under the tutelage of the soul of the mother, which through the umbilical vein nourishes and vivifies it."[39] For da Vinci, the child's soul was a creation of "nature," which existed under the "tutelage" of the mother's soul and was not fully "awake" until the child was outside of the womb and functioned as an individual. As late as the eighteenth century, Dr. Juan Marcos, the leading university physician in Prague and an acquaintance of Cangiamila, believed that "the rational soul does not exist before birth," but rather that "the child is infused with a soul only when he is born, and when he begins to breathe."[40]

DaVinci insisted that because the unborn cannot respire, they depend upon their mother to receive the air that sustains life. Cangiamila concurred: "For those who understand 'soul' to mean '*soplo*,' the air that is necessary for respiration, this is an undeniable truth." Indeed, Marcos cited his intellectual debt to Plato, the Greek physician Asclepiades of Bithynia, and the pre-Socratic Greek philosopher Protagoras. For these thinkers, the child was part of the mother's body until it could breathe independently, and the concept "soul" was best translated as "*soplo*," or air.

As this brief overview has shown, before the mid-eighteenth century there existed no scholarly or theological consensus regarding embryology, the fetal soul, or a supernatural role in these metaphysical matters. Embryology did not become an official branch of scientific inquiry until the eighteenth century, when the Enlightenment provided the ideal intellectual climate in which to endow personhood with new meaning, and, in doing so, to shift the Church's stance on the matter of unborn life. Although Cangiamila yearned to argue that ensoulment occurred early in a pregnancy, he was prohibited from taking this stance because the Catholic Church had not yet solidified its position on the matter. Cangiamila thus conceded, "It is impossible to prove anything regarding such an obscure subject." He admitted that "canon law has not yet decided whether the fetus is fully formed before it can be endowed with a soul."[41]

Historian Ulrich Lehner has related Cangiamila's claims to Pope Clement XI's 1708 decision to add the feast of the Immaculate Conception to the liturgical calendar, and his insistence that the feast must occur nine months before the birthday of Mary. Clement XI's logic held that because God had endowed Mary with grace and preserved her from original sin, she must have been a full human person from the first moment of her being. Clement implored theologians to explore the notion that if "Mary was a human person with a soul from conception on, then it was likely that all human life began at conception."[42] Though Cangiamila responded to Clement XI's request more forcefully than any other theologian at the time, he could not make unequivocal statements on ensoulment.

In the absence of ideological coherence, it became important for priests to feign certainty on the topic. Cangiamila stated that priests should aim to convince their flocks that there was, in fact, theological consensus on ensoulment, and that a priest should "tell his flock that it is probable that the embryo is alive from the first few days after conception, and maybe even from the moment of conception."[43] Even so, in 1745 Cangiamila wrote that it would be "impossible" to obligate surgeons in hospitals to perform the cesarean operation before the fortieth day of pregnancy, but that it was "reasonable" to promote the operation as "highly advisable" after the twentieth day of gestation.[44]

Cangiamila insisted on refuting da Vinci's notion that the child's soul was under the tutelage of its mother's soul and that fetuses had neither a heartbeat nor respiratory capacity while in utero. Emphasizing corporeal individuation, he claimed that a "child does not subsist on the life of its mother, but rather his life absolutely belongs to him."[45] For evidence of this, Cangiamila scrutinized fetal arterial and circulatory systems, hoping to disprove da Vinci's belief that the mother's body executed these tasks on the behalf of the fetus. In a fifteen-page discussion Cangiamila argued that fetuses not only had a heartbeat but also received a kind of "breath" in the womb via the circulatory system. Cangiamila evinced a nuanced understanding of fetal development, likely due to the embryonic material that he had acquired from one dozen recent caesarean operations. *Sacred Embryology* included portraits of nineteen stages of embryonic growth and discussed the products' shape, size, color, texture, and malleability.

Catholics authorities' overarching motivation, according to Cangiamila and others, was to save the souls of unfortunate infants and convert them into angels in heaven. Yet, the scientific discussions in *Sacred Embryology* implied that proponents of salvation through surgery wanted priests to produce scientific research that would bolster Catholic-inspired embryological authority. Indeed, Cangiamila's "theological embryology" took part in defining embryology as a scientific field: the priest was evidently the first to combine the Latin *embrio* with the suffix *logía,* though etymologists have wrongly dated the word to 1825.[46] Spanish physician Antonio Joseph Rodríguez also contributed to Catholic embryology in his 1760 dissertation about respiration, which proposed that priests in the Americas should aid in the "noble, Christian, and scientific project to identify physiological differences between Indian and European fetal stages of development."[47] At this time, priests additionally commanded midwives to practice cesarean operations on animals, to ensure both that they possessed the proper tools for surgical operations and that they were brave and confident enough to complete the task on human subjects.[48]

Sacred Embryology was in dialogue with dozens of medico-theological works—on reproduction, caesarean surgery, and the unborn—that circulated widely throughout the Spanish empire. I will discuss the writings of four public intellectuals within this genre: Antonio Medina of Spain (1750), Francisco González Laguna of the viceroyalty of Peru (1781), José Alzate Ramírez of New Spain (1800) and Vicente Francisco Sarría of Alta California in New Spain (1830). The discussion will proceed thematically, first focusing on fetal ensoulment, and then on maternal death. The 1800 letter from José Alzate Ramírez is a key source for the discussion of diagnosing maternal death, inasmuch as it makes clear that some clerics resisted their duty to perform the operation based on the matter's uncertainty. I will pay particular attention to how these physicians' and theologians' ideas diverged from those in *Sacred Embryology*, arguing that Cangiamila's ideas became radicalized in the American context and over time.

Like Cangiamila, the physician Antonio Medina considered the question of fetal ensoulment, although his approach was oriented toward medical thought and not theology.[49] Medina, a leading eighteenth-century obstetrician in Spain, wrote abundantly about gestation, pregnancy, and midwifery. Because the Protomedicato approved his material for the instruction of midwives in New Spain, his work offers a unique perspective on how theological doctrine dialogued—and sometimes conflicted—with concurrent medical ideologies and how these translated into policy and practice. Similarly to Alcalá y Martínez (who operated on María Ivañez), Medina wrote in 1750, prior to the popularization of Cangiamila's ideas. Therefore his work, too, serves as a precedent from which to compare later ideas about unborn life.

Medina rejected the claim that ensoulment occurred at conception because he believed that all products of conception began life as small lumps of flesh, not in human form. The physician insisted that fetuses "begin as a small mass of meat with indistinct parts, and require nine months of proper nutrition to develop a perfect and rational body." This means that the physician rejected preformationism, echoing instead Aristotle's insistence that matter preceded form, and that form needed an outside infusion of energy to host animated life. Catholic theologians such as González Laguna and Vicente Sarría believed that the unborn received their souls by means of divine intervention. The difference, they believed, was that the product of conception was perfectly formed, perhaps even inside the spermatozoa, and so that form preceded the growth of matter. Medina likewise chose not to use the term "embryo" and opted instead for the pre-Cangiamilan designation "fetus." He was not convinced that the embryo deserved its own categorical representation.

In fact, Medina presented a clear-eyed opinion on fetal ensoulment. He titled a key chapter of his work "How Long Does a Fetus Take to Develop a Rational Soul?" "The official response," he explained, "would be that this [fetal animation] occurs in a matter of days, and the laws follow this dictate." By "laws" Medina presumably referred to caesarean section mandates. Yet he was not convinced that products of conception were immediately ensouled. He wrote, "In such a murky matter, it is better to affirm that a fetus has a soul only when it has developed all of its parts and only when they are well organized." Medina similarly asserted that a fetus was only ensouled when "capable of exercising its vital functions." This was a clear rejection of the idea that small embryos were animated or possessed rationality. He further explained, "This [ensoulment] is what makes the creature a man, and it could occur earlier in some fetuses than in others, depending on the natural processes of reproduction."[50] Nature was too miraculous for a fixed or dogmatic understanding of the matter.

Further evidence of Medina's treatment of fetal animation appears in his discussion of "molar pregnancies" (*molas*), nonviable masses or tumors. In the eighteenth century it was impossible to know whether a pregnancy was molar before the expulsion of the product, so questions about the baptism of these masses were contentious. Without knowing whether a pregnancy was molar, Cangiamila insisted on baptism or conditional baptism. Medina took a different approach, underscoring that *molas* were not alive, but "aborted masses of meat." This echoed contemporary definitions of molar pregnancies.[51]

Writing several decades after Cangiamila, in 1781, the priest González Laguna advocated a much more doctrinaire understanding of fetal animation than both Medina and Cangiamila. As noted, Cangiamila had suggested that early fetal ensoulment was possible, and that priests should err on the side of caution by assuming that ensoulment at conception was "very probable."[52] González Laguna, on the other hand, insisted that "both [male and female embryos] are animated since the moment of conception."[53] As historians

Ulrich Lehner and Marina Caffiero have demonstrated, it was in the 1780s when theologians began to make this argument; the priest from Lima was thus at the forefront of this trend.[54]

González Laguna also questioned the logic that the products of molar pregnancies were not ensouled, insisting that caesarean operations had brought to light *molas* containing fully formed fetuses. The *limeño* priest explained, "If, instead of a fetus you find a *mola,* as has happened to us several times, you must not abandon your task. Open it, and perhaps inside you will find what you seek."[55] When humans were hidden within masses of meat, scientific inquiry could unveil the supernaturally made creatures within. Medina, on the other hand, argued that molar pregnancies were not rational, human, or meant to survive. While some moved, and while some had human body parts, he assured readers that most did not. Likewise, he contended that while most *molas* were expelled after three or four months of pregnancy, a few remained in the uterus for up to two years. This, Medina insisted, was proof that they were not human: because God and nature had given all mammals fixed gestational cycles, any mass that deviated from this norm could not be ensouled.[56]

Relatedly, Medina believed that doctors and priests should not manipulate the human gestational period, which led him to oppose the use of preterm caesarean operations. The physician insisted that it would be "against nature" for "fetuses [to] stay in the womb for less than nine months." Although Medina recognized that the crown had begun to insist on caesarean surgery—and although he agreed that midwives should be trained to operate on an emergency basis—he considered the removal of preterm and nonviable fetuses as unnecessary and against nature.[57]

In Mexico, Vicente Francisco Sarría (1767–1835) resolutely advocated for the performance of the caesarean. Sarría—who was a *peninsular,* born in Vizcaya in 1767—performed caesarean surgery in the California mission of San Carlos Borromeo on September 25, 1822, where native groups including the Sargantroc, Guachirron and Kalendaruc lived. Sarría's experience executing surgery prompted him to write, in 1830, a treatise entitled "The Caesarean Operation and California Missionaries."[58] In general terms, Sarría's mission was to render Cangiamila's tome into accessible terms for parish priests while convincing missionaries to make the caesarean a "regular procedure" that would open "the gates of eternal salvation to aborted children."[59] Sarría's work was printed alongside Father Antonio José Rodríguez's treatise on the method of performing the operation, which was endorsed by other mission priests and church authorities, including Ramón Abella, Felipe Arroyo de la Cuesta, Juan

Moreno, José Viader, Narciso Durán, Tómas Esténaga, Juan Amorós, and Buenaventura Fortuni. Sarría, for his part, emphasized that small products of conception were alive, even if he did not declare them to have been ensouled. For example, he insisted that the operation "ought to be performed even in the case of women of doubtful pregnancy, for one should and can baptize the live fetus, even if it is no more than an embryo."[60] Sarría's writing underscores that the Catholic Church's official position on ensoulment shifted gradually and interwove a diversity of voices from colonial territories.

Physicians and theologians debated another metaphysical issue as well, that is, diagnosing the moment of death in both mother and child. This was pressing because policy dictated that a caesarean should only be performed on a woman who was already dead and should aim to save fetuses that were still alive. However, some priests operated before the childbearing person had deceased. In 1804, the Bourbon era Spanish King Charles IV recognized the following: "It is true that some women, apparently dead but still alive, have been victim of the ignorance of those who have executed the operation." Likewise, in the second edition of his tome, Cangiamila noted, "I have seen many priests who were erroneously persuaded that the first incision of a caesarean operation must be made before the woman draws her last breath."[61] Such actions owed, as mentioned above, to medieval thought on respiration, still prominent in the eighteenth century, which claimed that because the mother was the source of the child's oxygen supply, the fetus would suffocate soon after the woman's last breath.[62]

Cangiamila and González Laguna were hesitant to disregard this long-standing respiratory theory. While González Laguna advised priests to open the dead woman's mouth to provide the fetus with fresh air, Cangiamila recommended inserting hollowed sugar canes into the woman's throat and vagina to facilitate the transmission of oxygen to the fetus. Although he recognized that physicians increasingly contested the claims behind the practice, Cangiamila reasoned that it was "always prudent to take precautions." Even if it did not provide oxygen to the fetus, the sugar cane might "facilitate the exit of putrid particles that would endanger the life of the child if left inside."[63] According to Cangiamila, this practice was first mandated in 1528 and 1550. The first objections to the practice were published in the eighteenth century by physicians Ambrosio Paréo and Lorenzana Heister, who emphasized that because the child was enclosed in the embryonic membranes, it did not have a connective pathway to the mother's trachea.

Cangiamila, for his part, proposed that a key moment for diagnosing death occurred when blood ceased to circulate. At this point, he asserted, "the patient ceases to exist." Yet ceasing to exist was not the same as death. The true and verifiable arrival of death was "difficult to diagnose." In fact, as the priest asserted, "putrefaction is the only sure sign of death."[64] Cangiamila recommended shaking, yelling, and striking a person to ascertain her status; irritating their nose and trying to make them sneeze might serve the same purpose. At the same time, he generally evidenced a more conservative approach by counseling caution before surgery: "If the light in her eyes has not extinguished, and if her limbs are still flexible, the operation should be suspended, even if she has appeared to be dead for days."[65]

Just as González Laguna exhibited a more radical approach toward the topic of ensoulment than Cangiamila, so did the two theologians diverge on the issue of maternal death. Because González Laguna advocated strongly for the caesarean's immediate performance on the arrival of death, he embarked on a lengthy discussion of the "unmistakable signs with which to declare the death of the pregnant woman."[66] In accordance with Charles IV, González Laguna noted that "the inability to discern the moment in which a pregnant woman is truly dead is what provokes qualms for priests."[67] While admitting that the matter was complicated, and while echoing Cangiamila's comment about putrefaction, González Laguna endeavored to define how the signs of death related to the caesarean operation. Although there were five such signs, he asserted, only three of them were "valid for [all] pregnant women." The first of these was discoloration, such as greyness, yellowness, or paleness of the face.[68] The second sign included a "slack jaw," as well as "stiffness in the limbs and difficulty in flexing those, even before the body has lost its heat." The third was "glazed and slack eyes [which had] lost their light and had become completely dark."[69]

The other signs of death were more ambiguous, such as stillness and stiffness of the body, cold sweat, and severe hand tremor. González Laguna encouraged priests to attend births regularly so that they might become familiar with the process and so that they would learn to recognize death. The last diagnostic criterion proposed by González Laguna was explicitly racialized: "Indians produce a shrill, continual moan, whereas Black women exhibit great coldness in the limbs, as well as a loss of *pullo*."[70]

Of course, it is counterintuitive that death could be diagnosed in the presence of any noise made by the woman or in the presence of any movement, such as a hand tremor. Here, González Laguna departed from Cangiamila's treatment in several respects. Not only was he quicker to ascertain the absence of life, but he also adapted the theme to the Latin American context by mentioning Indigenous and African-descendent women. Whereas Cangiamila's conceptualization of "others" invoked religious categories like infidel, Muslim, Jewish, and pagan, González Laguna echoed racial theories of the kind popularized by the French Enlightenment naturalist George-Louis Buffon.[71] These differences surely owed to their distinct locations: Cangiamila's Europe, on the one hand, and González Laguna's predominantly Indigenous Andes, on the other.

González Laguna insisted that if death was certain, a priest must not let pass "more than a few moments" before commencing the operation, for fear that the child may perish. The dead woman was to be held by two people, "who should preferably be women." If no women were present to sustain the body, the ailing person was to be lifted onto a table. The priest, for his part, needed to "maintain a steady hand in his execution of the incision." While many apparently thought it fitting that "the incision itself to be in the form of a cross," González Laguna offered an opposing suggestion: "It should be a long incision. Not just because this is easier, but also because if the signs of death have not been properly interpreted, and if the woman resists because she is not dead, a [long wound] will heal more easily."[72] This is suggestive evidence that not only was the surgery implemented on live women, but that some of those women resisted the procedure while on the brink of death.[73]

González Laguna's perspective clearly took hold, at least in the Latin American context. Twenty-three years after the Peruvian publication, Charles IV's 1804 pragmatic sanction endorsed the idea that the absence of overt signs of life could prove death. Charles recommended an application of "an alkaline gas" on a cloth near the mouth, nose, and eyes. Furthermore, he suggested that a needle be inserted between the fingernail and "the meat" of the finger. If these did not provoke a reaction, the woman was to be immediately subjected to the operation.[74]

Theologians were not alone in expressing support for the caesarean operation and emphasizing the urgency of its performance on dying and recently dead women. One notable proponent of the operation was Manuel Antonio Valdés (1742–1814), whose public letter about maternal death and the cesarean operation provides one of the most provocative sources on the topic. In order to understand the significance of Valdés's letter, it is first necessary to underscore the weight of his intellectual influence in the Spanish Crown.

Between 1784 and 1809, Valdés was the editor and principal author of Mexico City's *La Gazeta de México*. Although *la Gazeta* was a nonstate organ, it generally served as the voice of the Bourbon state. By publishing civil and ecclesiastical proclamations, decrees, and reports, *la Gazeta* streamlined the communicative efforts of governors and local officials such as mayors. Valdés additionally wrote to influence his readers in favor of the Bourbon administration's efforts to modernize, improve, and reform the colonies.[75] By providing access to the latest scientific and social information, and by doing so in an often-entertaining manner, Valdés's voice loomed large in the formation of public opinion.

Valdés worked with Father José Antonio de Alzate Ramírez (1737–1799), whose role as the science editor of *la Gazeta de México* almost certainly gave him authority over the publication of articles and reports regarding the caesarean surgery.[76] Alzate Ramírez possessed profound scientific knowledge, as evidenced by his publications on topics including botany, cartography, and astronomy; he offered an influential enlightenment perspective on the use of science to improve society and religion. Apart from his prolific scientific writing, he was also a secular priest in the archdiocese of Mexico.[77]

In 1769, Archbishop Francisco Antonio de Lorenzana—an archbishop who epitomized Enlightenment politics—ordered Alzate Ramírez to produce the policy recommendations for Bourbon efforts to restructure the regular parish (*doctrina*) system, affording him a crucial role in the reconceptualization of priests' responsibilities.[78] This gave him a platform to advocate for clerics' participation in scientifically minded tasks such as surgery.

In one article in *la Gazeta*, Valdés and Alzate Ramírez spoke out against baptism via the injection of holy water into the womb by means of a syringe. Dr. Joseph García Jove, a member of the Mexico City Protomedicato, had strongly advocated for this nonsurgical method. Yet Valdés and Alzate Ramírez claimed in *la Gazeta* that baptism via injection only "frustrated" the baptismal effort. In their words, it would mean that "only the womb receives the baptism, and its intended subject remains unsaved." "Only the caesarean operation," they claimed, could bring "eternal happiness" to unborn children, and such a task would be impossible without new heights of priestly zeal.[79]

Priests must have voiced ethical, legal, and logistical concerns about these demands, although echoes of their resistance surface rarely in the archive. Valdés and Alzate Ramírez spoke to such clerical refusal in a letter published in *la Gazeta de México* on September 22, 1800. Their commentary challenged the protestations of one ecclesiastic who refused to perform the surgery, although their admonition did not reveal the priest's identity.[80] The piece, entitled "Letter Written to a Priest from This City Regarding His Obligation to Perform the Caesarean Operation," amply illustrates the Crown's attitude toward disobedient clerics.

Valdés and Alzate Ramírez addressed the anonymous dissenting priest in a familiar tone. They referred to a "mutual friend" who informed them that a nonconforming priest had received "informational documents that promoted the duty of pastors and priests to perform the caesarean operation on deceased women." Perhaps he had received the short document authored by Josef Manuel Rodríguez in 1772. Apparently, the anonymous priest was not convinced by the literature, and he "spurned the entire endeavor for the sole reason that it may be difficult to ascertain the true point of [a woman's] physical death." The recalcitrant priest emphasized that he was not willing to perform surgery on women while they were still alive. Valdés and Alzate Ramírez admonished his resistance as "scandalous," and lamented that this cleric's relatively high status in the Church lent credence to his dissent.

Valdés and Alzate Ramírez reminded the uncooperative priest that he could use "inquiries and observations with which to ascertain the moment of death." Although they did not specify which inquiries and observations were meant to provide proof of death, they mentioned that a surgical subject would cry out in pain if cut open while alive. In Valdés and Alzate Ramírez's words: "in the process of making the first careful incisions, one would see signs of life if they were present." Underscoring that the priest's words presented "grave harm" to the crown, Valdés and Alzate Ramírez asked the hypothetical question: "If you are not willing to open the womb of a woman to avoid the possibility of killing her, in what conscience, and by what rationale, are you willing to bury her?" They even insisted that Jesus Christ would support the caesarean operation—that he would say, "in the last throes of His agony . . . 'From the moment you decided to bury her, you must resolve to open her.'" Valdés and Alzate Ramírez ventriloquized Jesus Christ to publicly shame a priest for worrying that surgery would kill a woman who may have lived otherwise.

Alzate Ramírez and Valdés advanced a spiritualized definition of the "true" death of a body. They asserted, "In opening the womb, there is only a slight fear regarding the death of a body. Yet, by not opening her, you will facilitate the moral death of the child's soul and its body." They alleged that in the first scenario—the death of a woman's body—the priest was "clinging to the fear of an imagined truth." The irony, of course, is that the body is real and not at all imagined. However, the editors explained that they "called it an 'imagined truth' because Bishops in Italy have threatened ecclesiastics with excommunication for refusing to perform the operation . . . as prudent and wise as they are, prelates would not obligate us to perform an operation that would require us to commit a sin." They continued, jesting about the priest's protestations over performing premortem surgery: "where is the barbarity, the cruelty, and the inhumanity in he who performs a caesarean section with his heart full of piety, love, and compassion?"

Alzate Ramírez and Valdés continued, explaining that in the second scenario—"the moral death of the child's soul and its body"—the priest would be guilty of "both a homicide and a true occurrence." Alzate Ramírez and Valdés advanced a spiritualized definition of the "true" death of a body. The editors' approach de-emphasized positive definitions of the body as a physical unit comprising flesh and organs; instead, their "alternative truth" prioritized a theologized understanding of life in which corporal death was "imagined"—inconsequential, unproven, or unnecessary—and in which only the soul was "true" because it had an eternal life and because it could be saved, and thus perfected, by a familiar, dependable, and enforceable ritual. They insisted that priests were better off risking the sin of homicide than abandoning an infant's potential life, writing, "I declare, and I will repeat, that without hesitation and without fail, we must perform this service [the caesarean operation] because we are charged with responsibility for the corporal and spiritual life of these poor creatures [the unborn]. . . . Sir, you must obey: It is better to risk the sin of homicide than to abandon a [fetal] soul."

As regarding the unborn, the logic went thus: first, infants were no longer eligible for limbo; second, a priestly failure to baptize the infant would be homicide, and as such it would be a severe moral crime. This is, perhaps, the most drastic way in which the Bourbon religious reforms intensified priestly responsibilities in life and death matters. Meanwhile, the corporal death of a pregnant woman was merely an "imagined truth," because the priest might kill her body, but he could not kill her soul. The body's death was of no importance if the soul lived. This meant that, for Valdés and Alzate Ramírez, dissenting priests engaged in "impertinent scruples, and childish tantrums." It also meant that Crown's new logic regarding infants' souls was intertwined with the use of coercion, and sometimes violence, onto women's bodies.

The uncooperative priest evidently referred to the premortem caesarean as barbarous, cruel, and inhumane. Cangiamila and González Laguna, too, addressed this perception among some priests. Perhaps the most eloquent reference is from González Laguna, who lamented: "How many times we have had to convert razors into hands to overcome the resistance of our fingers, the censorship of strangers, the critique of priests, and above all else, the rude distractions of lazy university physicians?"[81] For González Laguna, only Enlightened priests could truly understand the theological and temporal significance of the surgery, while dissenters were cowardly, lazy, and ignorant—especially "university physicians," perhaps including Antonio Medina.

Another theme was prominent—albeit, suggestively—in the editorial admonition of the cleric's dissent. This was a repeated reference to the presbyter's "regularity," and alternately, to his "irregularity." This language appears throughout the letter, as when the editors mentioned the presbyter's "more than regular" career and when they offered the following admonishment: "You claim that to be 'irregular' would be less offensive than death itself: but you should, instead, dare to become irregular before you should abandon a soul." Valdés and Alzate Ramírez made eight references to "irregularity" in just three paragraphs.

The dissenting priest may have referred to the ecclesiastical *irregularidades,* or violations of canon law, occasioned by the practice of the caesarean. This was a real concern because, as mentioned, the surgery violated Catholic prohibitions on the mutilation of the womb as well as those that disallowed priests from practicing surgery. Canon law referred to these prohibitions as *irregularidades.*[82] However, the sarcastic tone of the editor's public response, and the accusation that the dissenter was childish, scandalous, and belligerent, evidences a derisive and mocking play on the terms "regular" and "irregular." The editors seemed to jest that the dissenting cleric was a priest of the *ir*regulars, and hence that he resisted the surgery because he was loyal to the church's regular orders and not the Crown. As will be discussed more in chapter 2, this is fitting because the Bourbon state's insistence on priestly performance of surgery partially owed to their efforts to exert heightened control over the regular orders.

Whereas Indigenous conceptualizations of death placed great emphasis on the adult, proponents of the theological caesarean did not; because the mother was presumably already baptized (or, at least, absolved), the fetus gained priority. Cangiamila's and González Laguna's deliberations on diagnosing the death of an infant followed this trend, as evidenced by their extensive investigation into, and confirmation of, the death of an infant. When a child was extracted lacking signs of life, both recommended that it may have drowned in the mother's amniotic sac. As such, priests were instructed to hang a "drowned" child by the feet. They might blow through a hollowed sugar cane into the mouth of the child while plugging its nose so that the air could travel to its lungs. Cangiamila additionally suggested that sucking on the left nipple of the child could stimulate the nerves and provoke movement; likewise, rubbing the bottom of an infant's feet, or tickling them with a feather, might produce a reaction and revive the child from death.

Cangiamila instructed priests to immerse a newborn in water after placing rosemary cooked in wine around its neck. If this was ineffective, they were to burn the placenta next to the baby (while he or she was still connected via the umbilical cord) and bathe him in its smoke. Another option was to blow smoke from a pipe through the rectum and into the intestines with a hollowed-out sugar cane. Midwives in Sicily apparently sometimes placed the beak of a chicken inside the infant's rectum, which reportedly caused the subject to awake "quickly" even after three or four hours of lifelessness. Of course, one might wonder whether this more violent accusation was leveled at midwives due to their lesser social status as compared to physicians. Another recourse was to warm the baby's body extensively and to slowly drain it of blood via the umbilical cord.[83]

Debates about conception, life, death, and the soul—its arrival and its departure—were contentious and invoked medico-religious teachings developed by Catholic theologians during the Enlightenment. Just as the physician Antonio Medina disagreed with theological assertions about fetal ensoulment, he also advocated for the use of firm medical criteria in diagnosing pregnancy. For him, the mere absence of a menstrual cycle was not enough: a true diagnosis would invoke medicalized signs of pregnancy, such as aversions to foods, headache, pain in the umbilical area or hips, a round and firm stomach, raised and enlarged breasts, and changes in the cervix.

These diagnostic criteria showed more moderation and credibility than Friar González Laguna's and missionary Vicente Sarría's take on the matter, given their assertion, discussed below, that the existence of a pregnancy could be assumed based on gossip. As we have seen, theological debates influenced the trajectory of scientific and medical inquiry. No doubt they reverberated on a grassroots level, in that priests invoked these ideas when they provided public and private justifications for the surgery, and when they attempted to secure premature surgical consent from women who were potentially pregnant.

Fertility Control, Honor, and Maternal Subjectivity

A final theme is that physicians and theologians writing about the cesarean surgery emphasized women's societal value vis-à-vis their relationship to the potential production of life. An Enlightenment era focus on mothers was accompanied by the expectation that women should bear children for the colony or the nation, which, as Lehner points out, imagined them, in political terms at least, as "breeders."[84] During this time, European and colonial authorities began to express moral outrage about what they perceived as declining birth rates due to contraception and abortion. Lehner further suggests that "early modern Catholic parents sometimes deliberately caused the death of their children by neglect, usually from the fifth child onward." Some used passive terms to describe such behavior, likening death via neglect as a "bringing into heaven"; an abortionist, likewise, was often "called an 'angel maker.'"[85] Meanwhile, women's frequent use of herbs for fertility control and menstrual regulation provoked anxiety for priests as well as colonial authorities. This influenced scientific and surgical politics because authorities broadly prioritized the spiritual subjectivity of the fetus over the corporal life of its mother.

Cangiamila, for his part, took a milder view on abortion than some of his successors would. He explained, "We have not proposed to impose harsher penalties on abortion, we merely seek the eternal salvation of these fetuses by means of the baptismal sacrament." At the same time, he insisted that physicians, pharmacists, bloodletters, and midwives "all sin gravely if they help a woman to abort."[86] Nonetheless, Cangiamila recognized that abortion was widespread, especially among unmarried women, and that women often helped each other terminate unwanted pregnancies. He seemed resigned to this, and although his focus on the fetal soul permitted a criminalizing view of abortion, it did not seem to be his major impetus.

Cangiamila believed it was important that women take physical precautions to shield their offspring during pregnancy. This put pregnant women's behavior under scrutiny because neglect allegedly resulted in miscarriage, or spontaneous abortion. Women were to protect themselves from harmful emotions, foods, and activities, under threat of excommunication. Although Cangiamila contested some humoral medical theories, here he reiterated premodern claims that if a woman had improper nutrition, exercise, or rest, the resulting humoral imbalance could cause suffocation and malnutrition for the fetus. Here it is important to define abortion, because eighteenth century understandings of the term distinguished "accidental abortion" (which we would now deem miscarriage) from intentional or "criminal" abortion. Even "accidental abortion" could be interpreted as the childbearing person's fault if it resulted from her excessive work, uncontrolled emotions, or unbalanced humors. González Laguna claimed that "abortion is, unfortunately, extremely common amongst wealthy people, due to their unorganized lifestyle, and due to the frequency with which they gift the womb and Venus amongst themselves."[87] Presumably, Venus refers to the genitalia, and the "gift" is an insinuation of promiscuity. It was, therefore, the job of priests to promote marriage and to provoke patriarchs' consternation about the "fall" of their daughters.

Equally crucial to Cangiamila, González Laguna, and Sarría was a person's willingness to die during a cesarean operation to save the spiritual life of her unborn child. Refusing to do so, Cangiamila insisted, would constitute "spiritual homicide," which was "just as bad as corporal homicide," and indeed was often inseparable from it. Underscoring this point, he declared, "Important authors have defended the idea that a woman is obligated to suffer through the cesarean operation, even when it presents a risk to her life." The risk of surgery was "acceptable as long as it is not sure to kill her, and as long as the risk might mitigate the possibility that her fruit will die unbaptized."[88]

Sometimes, then, priests sought to execute the caesarean prior to a woman's death. And more disturbingly, some proposed that authorities should allow women to perish without medical assistance so that their children could receive baptism. Some contemporaries were horrified by this notion, as Cangiamila acknowledged in his Book 1: "Many will voice the objection, perhaps, that it is cruel that a pregnant woman should die while deprived of the assistance that a doctor could well provide. I confess that this is cruel, yes." He conceded that it was "violent, and [therefore] impractical" to obligate surgeons to "tie a woman to a table to practice the operation against her will."[89] Yet the author believed it was God's will for some women to perish without medical assistance; that the "eternal salvation of a child is of such superior importance to the life of a mother, that we must prioritize the former over the latter"; and that women should model themselves after the sacrifices of Virgin Mary and uphold their public honor by living for their children and not themselves. The rationalization of the embryonic soul prompted a brand of necropolitics in which the church claimed the right to alter women's corporeal and spiritual subjectivities by taking their lives. Surgery ultimately facilitated a new era in the relationship between the Spanish empire, religious corporations, and their subjects.

Priests became responsible for impressing this new social dynamic upon the women in their communities. They instructed pregnant women to confess regularly to avoid dying in a state of sin, to participate enthusiastically in pious rituals, and to "to make a daily offering to God, by means of the Holy Virgin, that they should offer him the fruit they carry in their wombs."[90] Mandates such as these did not just seek to alter women's religious practices, they sought to change how women approached childbirth: they were to seek out a priest and receive Eucharist. This was to provide strength in the face of a physical challenge; yet Cangiamila added that it ensured that a priest was nearby in case a caesarean operation became necessary.

Theologians also seemed to believe that the idea of undergoing cesarean surgery could curb promiscuity, especially in unmarried women.[91] González Laguna focused on this point on this point more extensively than Cangiamila, meaning that the Latin American priest furthered the spiritualization of caesarean doctrine in terms of its sociopolitical application as well as its medico-theological view of fetal ensoulment. González Laguna strongly encouraged priests to investigate local women's sexual activity, with the stated goal of coercing their agreement for a hypothetical caesarean.

Confession was the first recourse for procuring this agreement. Accordingly, González Laguna insisted that confession "must be practiced, even more so when there is reason for suspicion—or, reason to fear—that the woman is hiding a pregnancy." On the other hand, there was always reason to suspect pregnancy when "an unmarried woman is accused of carnal sin." In cases in which a parishioner "confesses to be pregnant," a priest "must command her to confess this outside of confession." After procuring a confession, "if the woman dies, the eternal loss of the offspring might be recuperated; [salvation of the unborn] will take precedence over any ill-reputation or lack of respect there may be [regarding the woman's honor]." Finally, González Laguna stated that if the woman refused to confess to sexual activity and potential pregnancy, "she may not be absolved."[92]

In cases in which priests failed to acquire such information during confession, gossip became a highly effective strategy of inquiry. "Just asking one question, in passing, has proven to be useful, because women discuss everything between themselves, and because they know everything about each other," González Laguna explained.[93] In this way, priests were implicitly trying to break the seal of the confessional to do the crown's bidding and subject women to the operation. They broke one sacrament (penance) to prioritize another (baptism).

Due to the importance of honor in the pre-modern world, the spreading of rumors that questioned a woman's sexual activity must have fostered resentment among community members. González Laguna underscored this point, commenting, "if there is a hidden pregnancy, or reason to believe that there is one, someone is sure to arrive shortly with the news or the suspicion." He continued, "If this suspicion or news is founded, that person must be told to guard the secret, and because of the secret, the incision must be used, but with utmost care to make witnesses stay at a distance, by providing some kind of excuse, before the woman is dead."[94] It is disturbing that the priest would make an excuse or a lie to send the family members away before "making the incision," and that he chillingly prescribed that the witnesses be sent off "before the woman is dead." In this way, González Laguna suggested that priests must employ the operation to convey to women that they must beware becoming pregnant outside of marriage—for fear that they could be submitted to this practice. This was likely to harm interpersonal relations: a woman's family might blame the performance of a surgery on the unscrupulous person who revealed to the priest that she was pregnant.

Surgery implied that the women and children of the community pertained to colonial authorities—priests, as proxies of the state—instead of belonging to the family and group unit. Indeed, if the spiritualized caesarean was a topic of discussion between priests and parishioners, the prospect that surgery would result from pregnancy must have entered the purview of everyday conversation as well. It is even possible that the topic affected people's reproductive decisions. Importantly, it signaled that the unborn were animated and autonomous subjects from conception and hence subject to the Christian state.

The writings examined above, by Cangiamila, González Laguna, Alzate y Ramírez, Sarría, and Medina, suggest that Bourbon ecclesiastics intensified their oversight of parishioners' sexual activity and reproductive decisions when the Crown mandated cesarean operations in the late eighteenth and early nineteenth centuries. In the confessional, especially, priests sought information about the sexual activity of the confessee to deduce whether she was a potential candidate for salvation through surgery. Such a conversation, of course, awkwardly presumed the woman's death even when it was not foretold. When priests learned, or inferred, that a woman may be pregnant and therefore that the surgery would be warranted under certain circumstances, they asked for the woman's preemptive permission to operate; women who refused to consent to a hypothetical procedure could be denied absolution. In practice, this meant that all women of childbearing age were under the continual suspicion of pregnancy, and ecclesiastics in rebellious Indigenous communities may have wielded the threat of surgery as a kind of social discipline.

Surgery promised to stake a claim over the future generation, no matter how noncompliant with Catholic values their parents may have been, such as in the case of Indigenous "pagans." Priests encouraged women from all classes to preserve their honor and abstain from premarital sex because an illegitimate pregnancy could be revealed through a postmortem caesarean section. The threat to an unmarried woman's honor now extended beyond her temporal life—if she were pregnant, or even suspected of that status, her body could be opened to reveal a product of conception within. This might shame a woman's family by offering undeniable proof of her dishonorable behavior during life. Caesarean surgery thus highlights how Bourbon reformers and priests sought to enact patriarchal controls over women through corporal dominance and punishment, and how these measures were underpinned by Catholic claims about the individuated fetal soul.

As this chapter has explored, the theology of salvation through cesarean surgery sought to revise the definition of birth itself, as well as to propose systematic changes to the baptismal sacrament. The new definition of birth insisted that prebirth humans had in fact already been born—by virtue of their ensoulment by God; they then awaited rebirth, which was regeneration, actuated by baptism, performed by a priest, and authored by God, Jesus, and the Holy Spirit. The actual, physical birth that took place between these two "spiritual" births—the human journey from womb to exterior—was a mere "manifestation" and was, therefore, the least important of the three births.

By this new definition, so-called natural birth no longer constituted a major ontological shift during which the unborn became a human manifest in the world. Surgery shifted to salvation with the argument that physical birth was of little consequence for a child's arrival—in fact, it became the only birth (of the three) that science could replace. By rationalizing the theologies behind human generation and childbirth, theologians opened a new rhetorical and epistemological space in which the caesarean operation became necessary as early as conception.

The salvational caesarean meant to conceptualize and uphold a new social category: the unborn man. In the process, it offered Catholics a new technology with which to extend the baptismal sacrament to the unborn. It contributed to the creation of a sacramental variation—the conditional baptism—and expanded the definition of personhood to include not only the unborn but monstrous and molar pregnancies, as well. These points connected to another goal of Enlightened Catholics, which was to develop a sustained focus on the individual human as a rational being, a divinely created entity, and a renewed subject of scientific and theological inquiry.

By popularizing new insights regarding generation and gestation, and by scientizing the long-standing metaphysical mystery of the soul, the use of surgery also helped to promote an emphasis on modern rationality. Finally, authorities emphasized the individual's ability to improve his or her social and spiritual status. The "lost souls" recovered via surgery could enjoy spiritual salvation when exposed to exceptionally pious zeal. Because many adults were capable of performing surgery (provided that they owned a shaving razor or other sharp instrument), the potential for this improvement was implicitly within popular reach.

Francesco Cangiamila and other theologians sought to verify that a reformed Church could force the caesarean out of its historical association with evil, mutilation, and the devil, and recuperate its place as a miraculous surgery performed by saints and angels who blessed children with and good fortune. In doing so, they deviated from historical precedent, which had always emphasized the caesarean's utility for saving the lives of pregnant people, and insisted instead that the spiritual life of the fetus was the primary concern of religion and the colonial state.

CHAPTER TWO

Ramón Neonato

Colonialism and the Cesarean Section in New Spain

In the century following the publication of Francesco Cangiamila's *Sacred Embryology*, a surprising number of priests in New Spain heeded his call to "save the lost souls trapped in their mother's wombs." When Father Ramón López commanded a local midwife and a retired military sergeant to perform the surgery (in Sonora, in 1798), he explained that he acted "according to Cangiamila's instructions."[1] The priest dictated surgical directives from his copy of *Sacred Embryology* while he stood beside the body of María Antonia Zapatito, who had presumably just perished. Also present was María's husband, Cristóbal Bravo, who was an Indigenous Pima like his wife. It is unclear whether María or Cristóbal had been baptized, or whether they had previously interacted with the priest, Ramón López. After sergeant Francisco López de Xeres opened María's body with a shaving razor, the midwife extracted a girl who survived for eight minutes. Although the sergeant and the midwife were the surgeons in this scenario, it fell to Ramón López to baptize the child before she died. The priest later noted enthusiastically that the three had become "agents of the operation," in accordance with Cangiamila's exhortations. Indeed, the surgery afforded the Catholic church a unique opportunity in the context of late Bourbon colonialism. In the Americas, priests increasingly became scientific agents of the state, empowered to extract and examine the unborn. Many believed that Spain's flailing colonies could be saved by Enlightenment science, and only priests could be trusted to wield a surgicalized show of force in the name of religion and the state.

As other historians have shown, clerics practiced religiously mandated surgery throughout the Spanish empire, including in Puerto Rico and the Caribbean, the Philippines, Sicily, and Central and South America.[2] Turning from the subject of chapter 1—the philosophical underpinnings of the religious cesarean—this chapter examines its implementation on the ground in New Spain: first in legislation and policy, and then in practice. One of the chapter's findings is that priests in New Spain appear to have performed more cesarean operations than historians previously realized. In fact, eighteen of twenty-eight missionaries in Alta California practiced the surgery, and six of those did so more than once.[3]

As Spain's largest viceroyalty, New Spain covered a vast expanse of land, from the current border of Guatemala in the south through all of Mexico, Arizona, New Mexico, and Texas; the territory stretched far north, to northern California and into Colorado. There were hundreds of Indigenous groups on this land. Whereas most Indigenous people in central Mexico had been incorporated into Spanish missions for centuries, this was not so in the contested northern borders. There, many were relatively autonomous into the eighteenth century: some were not yet colonized, made to live on missions, or Christianized. Indigenous people were also under attack by multiple empires, including the French, the British, and the United States. Colonization forced Indigenous people into a pattern of warfare, in which some made frequent raids on mission posts and suffered deadly retribution. Often, first contact with settlers and missionaries provoked outbreaks of deadly epidemic disease, including smallpox, measles, mumps, influenzas, and coronaviruses.[4] Cesarean surgery acquired heightened importance in the midst of warfare, settler-colonialism, and epidemiological decimation. As this chapter demonstrates, the operation sometimes became a technology of colonial warfare that allowed missionaries to coercively Christianize Indigenous people and claim them as colonial subjects. Throughout Bourbon New Spain, some priests employed religious surgery as a means of forcible salvation.

Meanwhile, colonial authorities hailed the surgery's utility for individualizing the spiritual relationship between the Crown and the souls of its subjects. This sheds new light on Pamela Voekel's contention that Bourbon authorities envisioned modern subjects with an individualized relationship with God. Voekel suggests that an Enlightened modernity was to be achieved via disciplined worship and unmediated, individuated spirituality.[5] Here I emphasize that, Bourbon authorities pursued another kind of individual relationship: that between God and the unborn. When priests performed surgical salvation, even embryonic subjects could become vassals of the Crown and children of the king. This reinforced other Bourbon policies, including the 1794 decree that made all orphans children of the king.[6] In all, Catholic authorities and Bourbon reformers envisaged a surgical technique that would help them spiritually reform the Indigenous groups that they aimed to incorporate into New Spain.

Cesarean Surgery Policy in Colonial New Spain

The caesarean operation dialogued with Bourbon monarchs' efforts to subordinate the regular clergy and convert priests into a professional class of scientifically minded, spiritual specialists.[7] In this way, the state's insistence that priests perform surgery focused a new lens onto an important eighteenth-century question: Who could become a surgeon? In Spain's American colonies, priests became important practitioners in a field that has long been seen as divided between barber-surgeons and learned physicians. These efforts corresponded to the goals of the Enlightenment. Clerical reform and parish administration took root under King Charles III, who believed that the decline of Spanish "morality and economic strength" was due to intellectual darkness and superstition, making a reform of Catholicism necessary.[8] Yet the goals of Enlightenment Catholicism did not map neatly onto the Bourbon reform effort, in large part because the absolutist state sowed tension by subjugating the church, and because absolutism compromised the philosophical bases of the Catholic Enlightenment.[9]

One main goal of Bourbon religious reforms was to force clerical administration under the Crown's authority. This was largely accomplished by secularization—that is, limiting and altering the judicial and administrative roles filled by the regular clergy. Because the regular clergy had acquired independent funding, and with it, relative autonomy and privilege, the Bourbons saw the regular orders as excessively powerful, wealthy, and disobedient. As such, the Crown sought to dismantle the regular clergy's Indigenous parishes (*doctrinas*) and to replace Franciscans, Dominicans, and Augustinians with secular priests. They claimed that the regulars were not only disloyal to the Crown, but that they were lenient in terms of religious practice. According to the Bourbons, Indigenous vassals would never reach an Enlightened state under such deficient spiritual authority.[10]

In the state's eyes, obligating clergy to perform surgery was an extreme test of priests' loyalties. Clerics, for their part, had mixed reactions to the state's efforts to transform them into obstetric surgeons. Some were eager to prove their usefulness, so they performed the operation as often as possible, carefully recording their compliance. While the priestly zeal for caesarean operations was particularly immense in Diocese of Sonora and in California, priests in all regions, both religious and secular, practiced the surgery.

Most priests appear to have accepted the religious rationale underpinning the procedure, best demonstrated by the production of numerous pamphlet-sized renditions of theological treatises that intended to popularize the surgery and its metaphysical logic.[11] Additional evidence of their compliance derives from royal decrees, ecclesiastical commentary by prelates, and articles from New Spain's most prominent publication, *La Gazeta de México*. In addition to pastoral circulars and theological writings, this chapter also draws on baptismal records, which provide the most satisfactory, if still imperfect, way of mapping the incidence of caesarean operations onto Latin American history.

THE FIRST CROWN AUTHORITY to show avid support for the caesarean section was King Charles III, the ruler who initiated the Bourbon reforms in the Americas.[12] As historian Adam Warren has demonstrated, Charles read Cangiamila's work in 1761 and subsequently issued a pragmatic sanction obligating priests to employ cesarean surgery "to ensure the spiritual and temporal salvation of children, both born and unborn."[13] Such mandates resulted in 225 operations in just two years on the islands of Sicily, and fifty-two caesarean surgeries in Spain between 1777 and 1806.[14] At the same time, Charles III instructed Sicilian bishops to distribute the information contained in Cangiamila's *Sacred Embryology* while urging priests to model the surgery for others.[15]

In 1772, Viceroy Bucareli of New Spain (former governor and captain general of Cuba), was the first to require parish priests to perform the operation in Spain's colonial territories.[16] His mandate came shortly after his arrival in New Spain. In support of Bucareli's initiative, Friar Josef Manuel Rodríguez translated parts of Cangiamila's tome into Spanish and offered an introduction tailored to the Latin American context, which essentially extracted and summarized the main ideas from Cangiamila's original. Whereas Viceroy Bucareli's decree had refrained from proposing punishment for priests in New Spain who refused to perform the operation, Rodríguez disagreed. He wrote, "I would like to insist that this jurisdiction requires the operation's performance, and that it be practiced as soon as possible [during an obstetric emergency], under penalty of 500 pesos."[17]

The Church agreed with this proposal. Archbishop Alonso Núñez de Haro y Peralta supported Rodríguez's position, declaring that any person who prevented the performance of surgery should be charged with homicide, and that the individual must also "be treated as a criminal." Such interference generally came from family members of the deceased. This lead Haro y Peralta to insist that priests take measures to "lessen the horror associated with this surgery." Finally, he offered an indulgence of eighty days to clerics who complied with the order to perform surgery.[18]

A key furtherance occurred in 1804, when Charles IV wrote a strongly worded *cédula* (executive order) in support of the archbishop's 1779 decree. As previously mentioned, now Charles IV ordered that priests must not allow the burial of a woman unless he first ascertained whether she was pregnant, no matter how long she had been deceased. Even if the woman was merely rumored to have been pregnant, the priest was obligated to open her womb. The *cédula* clarified that priests were to view an unborn child of any size as ensouled, even if it were as small as one "grain of barley." The use of the word barley parroted text from Cangiamila's tract, which asserted that, under the penalty of mortal crime, one must "baptize any mass that can reasonably be considered an embryo, even if it is no larger than a grain of barley."[19]

Unsurprisingly perhaps, Charles IV's 1804 *cédula* expanded considerably on previous mandates. He ordered that if a priest had allowed the burial of a woman, and then subsequently learned that she may have been pregnant at the time of her burial, then he was to exhume her corpse from its burial place and open her womb before allowing her to be reinterred. Charles IV additionally ordered that caesarean surgery be executed on all women: not just in missions, but in rural areas and hospitals as well. Accordingly, he approved Viceroy Bucareli's requests to amplify hospitals and construct cemeteries.[20] These measures demonstrated that King Charles IV took the most extreme religious view conceivable. The details also explain why priests would resent the obligation to perform such an onerous duty.

Additional social and institutional context for these reforms can be found in the fourth Mexican Provincial Council in January 1771, which was overseen by the ultra-regalist Archbishop Lorenzana. Called by Charles III, the council was attended by all the prelates of New Spain to consider some twenty points proposed by the King.[21] His basic motive for convoking the council was his search for ways of improving the religious establishment, with a particular concern for greater efficiency and stricter observance of regulations.[22] The result was a list of structural, bureaucratic, and spiritual mandates that sought to increase oversight over the regular clergy while fostering the development of a disciplined and rational Church presence in the New World. Article 17, for example, affirmed the Crown's intent to "ensure the subordination of the regular orders, as much in their public conduct" as in the "administration of the sacraments or control of the missions in their charge."[23]

Beyond the caesarean operation, the Crown invoked the baptismal sacrament in other aspects of parish reform. First, priests were to exert increased oversight over midwives, a measure that aimed not only to curb the autonomy of midwives but also to empower priests in their place.[24] Specifically, curates examined midwives to ascertain their knowledge of emergency baptismal procedures. They were required to ascertain that midwives were familiar with Christian doctrine and to confirm that they were "good Catholics" who possessed a Christian preoccupation for mother and child. Priests assumed the task of forcing midwives to respect restrictions on abortions and making sure that they did not assist any woman in terminating a pregnancy, even if that pregnancy threatened a woman's life. Priests also attempted to prevent midwives from facilitating the informal adoption of illegitimate children to protect the honor of an unmarried woman.

Finally, the council prohibited midwives from disposing of the malformed and miscarried unborn products sometimes referred to as monsters. Instead, they were required to preserve the product until the priest could examine the body and baptize it if any signs of rational organization or life were present. In addition, the fourth provincial council stressed that priests should prevent midwives from baptizing infants unless an emergency baptism was warranted. Reformers echoed this recommendation in 1803, when they officially prohibited midwives from baptizing any infant that was not in immediate danger of death. Although the Crown needed midwives' familiarity with reproductive bodies, because they were powerful women it was key that they be prevented from attaining too much spiritual authority.

Distributed to parish priests in New Spain, the prohibition read as follows: "Under threat of penalty from the Bishop, midwives are prohibited from engaging in their profession without examination by an ecclesiastical judge . . . and they must have a written license from the judge to perform baptisms. . . . To midwives who are approved, we warn them: They commit a grave sin by baptizing an infant that is not in danger of death. If they do perform a baptism, they should attempt to ensure the presence of two women who will testify that they heard the correct words pronounced when a parish priest examines them to discern whether the child is baptized." In this way, the spiritualization of the caesarean and the Bourbon religious reforms sought to obligate midwives to conform to Catholic theological dictates, which they had to reconcile with the requests of community members who often asked them to perform nonorthodox tasks.[25]

The fourth provincial council stated that the regular clergy was obligated to root out and punish popular rituals and illicit baptismal practices. For the Crown, such rituals epitomized Indigenous superstition, idolatry, and false beliefs. For example, some laypeople believed that children could receive "two baptisms," and that perhaps, as a result, they could have "two Christianities." At least twelve Inquisition "re-baptism" cases were tried between 1719 and 1807; the majority of these occurred in the last quarter of the eighteenth century.[26]

One was the 1775 case of María Guadalupe, a midwife accused of rebaptizing her child. When inquisitors examined her husband, he proclaimed that he did not understand why the rebaptism of a healthy child posed a problem; furthermore, he was acquainted with many people who secretly took their children for a rebaptism due to *bautismos malos*—apparently, this was a popular recourse when the first baptism was spiritually unsatisfactory. María admitted to procuring the double baptism but claimed that she was unaware of prohibitions against the practice. She even postulated that double baptism "could not possibly be a bad thing, because it was a godly act," and it would beneficially provide "two christianities" to the recipient. These inquisition cases underscore that baptism was a source of increasing metaphysical struggle between popular actors and Bourbon officials.

Bourbon reformers worried that regular priests actively participated in the depreciation of Catholic orthodoxy when they allowed impurities of the faith. Such was the case when the Inquisition investigated two clergymen accused of participating in doll baptisms. This case echoed others featuring dolls that were baptized in elaborate ceremonies and that were made to represent priests, parents, and infants.[27] Reportedly, the celebrant performing the ceremony would say, "In the name of the rooster and the hen, I give you the name *clabellina*."

Surprisingly, the use of this phrase was not a one-time occurrence, nor was it limited to one group or region: rather, inquisition records show a broad geographic distribution of the term, from the Chichimecs of Sonora to the Totonac of Veracruz and the Zapotecs of Oaxaca. This baptismal practice could be interpreted as a classic example of so-called syncretism, the strategic and ritualistic combination of Indigenous and Catholic religious ideas and practices. Alternatively, it may be interpreted as what William Taylor calls "pagan resistance," in that Indigenous people seemingly mocked the importance of the baptismal ritual. The baptisms took place en masse at elaborate parties, during which midwives and other community authorities would ceremonially distribute the dolls to young expectant women. In three related cases, inquisitorial authorities interrogated midwives for having furnished the dolls, sewn their clothes, or performed the baptismal services.[28] Crown authorities believed that midwives needed increased surveillance and reform because they catered to popular reproductive desires, rituals, and practices.

In March 1771, just months after the Fourth Provincial Council ordered greater oversight and subordination of the clergy, a deputy appointed by the office of the Inquisition in Guadalajara responded to these prompts by producing a report on unorthodox and bastardized baptisms.[29] The deputy wrote to the head inquisitor of New Spain to advise him that unlawful baptismal practices occurred regularly on haciendas, and that, in these, midwives and curanderos baptized Indigenous people in erroneous ways.

Emphasizing that he was willing to do whatever was necessary to suppress illicit baptisms, the deputy requested inquisitorial support in this mission. He referred to those who performed illicit baptisms as "bad Christians" and accused them of practicing a range of spells. Indigenous people, he said, "are inclined to moral depravity due to their ancient pagan customs. When midwives and popular healers provide them with such a bad example, their spiritual ruin continues, even though we wish for them to experience a complete and total conversion." The deputy grumbled that Indigenous people on haciendas baptized each other in erroneous ways, such as by saying, "I baptize you in the name of the cock and the hen," instead of in the name of the Father, Son, and the Holy Spirit. He concluded, "It is extremely onerous for us to sort out this mess to prevent the spiritual ruin of Indigenous on haciendas."

Bourbon reformers were primarily concerned with the "spiritual ruin" of Indigenous Mexicans, and as such, the Crown was desperate for a way to root out such decay and Christianize children before they were subjected to ungodly and ruinous rituals. Indeed, in their view there was no shortage of ways in which children became corrupted by demonic influences shortly after childbirth. In Sonora, for example, a Jesuit missionary lamented that newborn infants underwent ritual tattooing of the eyelids and face soon after birth. For Indigenous peoples, tattooing blessed future warriors; for reformers, it exemplified how paganism placed visible claims on the bodies and the souls of the newly born.[30]

The Crown's most effective and scientific way to forestall such spiritual ruin was the salvational cesarean operation. Not only did the operation ensure a completely novel form of evangelization via the Christianization of the unborn, but it reached children in the root of society's supposed spiritual ruin: the wombs of Indigenous women, who were incubators of culture and tradition, and who could not be trusted to alter their allegiances. Indigenous women's influence over their children's spiritual fate could be interrupted, but only if priests' reach penetrated sufficiently.

Surgical Salvation in Practice

The use of reason and science to enforce social control was precisely what Bourbons envisioned when they ordered the subjugation of the regular orders and a purification of the faith. As expressed in the Fourth Provincial Council, priests were to exert influence over Mexicans by any means necessary.

Although "the preferable option was to lead by example and constant instruction," the provincial council also "granted priests the right to use harsh treatment of non-Christian Indians."[31] The council stressed that priests should bureaucratize maternity by maintaining more accurate and complete records of parishioner's marital and reproductive statuses. This section builds on those themes by documenting the prevalence of cesarean sections in Mexico, underscoring that Bourbon officials valued the operation's utility for asserting hegemony over Indigenous people through surgical force. It does so by analyzing forty-three caesarean operations performed in late eighteenth-century and early nineteenth-century New Spain, which are listed in table 2.1.

A note about the documentary sourcebase for understanding the colonial surgery: most of the cases discussed below are from the Franciscan missions of Alta California, Baja California, and Sonora. Our knowledge of these cases is owed to the efforts of the Huntington Library in California and University of Arizona's mission databases to preserve and organize colonial mission records. As a result, this skewed regional distribution of operations is document generated and thus may be somewhat of an optical illusion for understanding how the caesarean surgery was implemented in New Spain as a whole. Priests clearly performed surgery in New Spain more frequently than historians have assumed, but their reporting methods were so inconsistent that a more accurate number will likely never be known.

Even a painstaking review of the death records of colonial parishes presents methodological challenges and opaque evidence of the procedure, strongly indicating that priests in New Spain performed caesarean surgeries without recording them. When priests noted a surgical operation, they often did so by scrawling "opn" or "o.pn." This signified *operación*, but it was not always accompanied by the word *cesarea*. Due to the poor legibility of many death registers, it is likely that those who compile mission databases have missed this designation and therefore did not include it in the notes of a database entry. Likewise, researchers who review death records on microfilm are likely to miss the barely legible note "opn" scrawled in the margins.

There is suggestive evidence that priests who performed surgeries did not leave any record of having done so, even with the cursory "opn." Declining to note "operación," priests instead appear to have recorded the performance of a caesarean by assigning some variation of the name Ramón Neonato (Newborn Ramón) to the products that they extracted. Variations on the theme included such names as Ramón/Ramón(a) Neonato(a), Ramón(a) Nonacido(a), and Ramón(a) Nonat(a).

TABLE 2.1 Products of conception removed via cesarean operation in colonial and postcolonial Mexico

No.	Date	Location	Surgeon	Name
1	1766, January 9	Arizpe Arizona	Manuel Fernandez Carrera (Jesuit)	Criatura
2	1779, May 29	Santa Clara Mission, CA	Two missionaries	Unstated
3	1795, January 21	Panotlan, Zacualtipan Hidalgo	Parish priest	Criatura
4	1795, January 21	Panotlan, Zacualtipan Hidalgo	Parish priest	Criatura
5	1795, January 21	Panotlan, Zacualtipan Hidalgo	Ecclesiastical judge	Criatura
6	1795, January 21	Panotlan, Zacualtipan Hidalgo	Barber surgeon	Criatura
7	1795, June 20	Chiautla de Sal, Puebla	Parish priest	Unstated
8	1798, September	San Antonio de Oquita, Sonora	Three participants: Priest Ramón López; a midwife; and a sergeant, Francisco López de Xeres	Unstated
9	Unknown	Unknown	Francisco Moyano	Unstated
10	1799, January 26	Santa Clara Mission, CA	José Viader	Unstated
11	1801, October 25	San Carlos Borromeo Mission, CA	José Viñals	Buenabentura
12	1801, December 26	Caborca Arizona	Fray Andres Sánchez	Unstated
13	1802, February 19	San Antonio de Padua Mission, CA	Florencio Ybañez	Ramon Nonato
14	1802, March 17	San Antonio de Padua Mission, CA	Florencio Ybañez	Ramona Cavallero
15	1802, April 23	San José Mission, CA	Jose Antonio de Uria	Unstated
16	1802, November 4	San Carlos Borromeo Mission, CA	Baltasar Carnicer	Buenaventura
17	1805, August 27	San José Mission, CA	Jose Antonio de Uria	Unstated
18	1805, November 12	San Francisco de Asis Mission and Presidio, CA	Ramon Abella	Ramona

(*continued*)

TABLE 2.1 *(continued)*

No.	*Date*	*Location*	*Surgeon*	*Name*
19	1806, March 16	San Miguel Arcangel Mission, CA	Pedro Muñoz	Ramon Nonat
20	1807, June	Unstated	Miguel Priego and a physician	Teresa de Jesus
21	Unstated	Unstated	Miguel Priego and a physician	Unstated
22	1807, January	Cristoval Carrillo, Oaxaca	Dr. Briones	Unstated
23	1808, January 8	Santa Ynes Mission, CA	Luis Gil de Taboada	Baltasara
24	1808, January 8	Santa Ynes Mission, CA	Luis Gil de Taboada	Buenaventura
25	1808, March 23	San José Mission, CA	Narciso Duran	Infant *de razón*
26	1809, May	San Miguel Coyuca, Guerrero	Francisco Patiño	Unstated
27	1809, December	Unstated	Priest Francisco Patiño	Unstated
28	1811, August 6	Santa Barbara Mission California	Luis Gil de Taboada	Unstated
29	1819, July 23	San Antonio de Padua Mission, CA	Juan Bautista Sancho	Ramona Nonacida
30	1821, May 18	Santa Barbara Mission, CA	Antonio Ripoll	Unstated
31	1821, July 28	San Antonio de Padua Mission, CA	Pedro Cabot	Beatriz Fages
32	1822, September 25	San Carlos Borromeo Mission, CA	Vicente Francisco de Sarria	Getrudis
33	1825, January 15	San Diego Mission, CA	Vicente Oliva	Ramona
34	1825, December 21	San José Mission, CA	Priest Narciso Duran and two barber surgeons, Nazale and Silvestre	Unstated
35	1826, November 15	Santa Cruz Mission, CA	Luis de Taboada	Joseph
36	1826, November 15	Santa Cruz Mission, CA	Luis de Taboada	Maria

No.	*Date*	*Location*	*Surgeon*	*Name*
37	1829, March 28	San José Mission, CA	Narciso Duran (priest), Silvestre (surgeon)	Unstated
38	1832, January 29	San José Mission, CA	Narciso Duran	Unstated
39	1832, April 27	San Carlos Borromeo Mission, CA	Ramon Abella	Unstated
40	1836	Mexico City	Unnamed doctor	Unstated
41	1836	Mexico City	Unnamed doctor	Unstated
42	1841, December 28	Santa Clara Mission, CA	Jesus Maria Vasquez del Mercado	Maria Juana
43	1845, December 11	San José Mission, CA	Suares del Real and Jose Maria del Refugio	Unstated

Source: The Early California Population Project of the Huntington Library; La Gaceta de México; León, *La obstetricia en México* (1910), and the University of Arizona Mission Databases Information project. Following Kuepper-Valle (1974), the enumeration reflects the number of infants extracted, not the number of women who underwent surgery. Therefore, twins are listed as separate products.

Taking one data set as an example, the Early California Population Project database registers the death of 17,646 newborns in the colonial missions of Baja California and Alta California between December 29, 1782, and December 2, 1848. Of these, 153 bore a variation of the name Ramón Neonato, such as Ramón Nonat, Ramona, Ramona No Nacida, and Nonacida. Ramón Neonato translates as Newborn Ramón, but the other second-name variants—Nonat, No Nacida, and Nonacida—all translate literally to "unborn." Ramón and Ramona are references to the caesarean operation as a "Roman Ritual," due to its association with Roman liturgy.[32]

It is quite suggestive that 58 percent (153 of 201) of those infants named with some variation of Ramón were born to dead mothers *and* died shortly after birth. Such mortality would be expected if they were born by caesarean operation because, as far as historians know, no infants extracted via surgery in the California missions survived. Other names provide potential points of comparison. For example, of 2,941 infants born between 1782 and 1848 who were named Juan or Juana, only four of these were born to deceased mothers *and* died during or shortly after birth. The rate here is 0.01 percent, which is hardly comparable to the 58 percent incidence of Ramón-named infants who were born to deceased mothers and themselves died. Thus, it seems highly likely that priests delivered these infants surgically. This evidence suggests that priests performed around 200 caesarean operations in Alta and Baja California between 1790 and 1848. Furthermore, those were just the ones that found their way into the records, so they may only represent a small percentage of religious surgeries.

Table 2.1 shows that priests assigned names to sixteen of the thirty-eight infants extracted via caesarean operation in New Spain. Nineteen of the infants have no recorded name. The death registers for sixteen simply read "unstated"; one reads *criatura* (meaning "infant") and the other states *criatura de razón*. The literal translation of "de razón" is "to have reason" or "to be rational," which stems from the Catholic notion that unbaptized Indigenous people were so-called pagan and so lacked rationality before undergoing baptism and Christianization. Of 17,646 deceased infants in the California missions (1782–1848), 137 were given no name. Of those sixteen, six bore a version of the name Ramón Nonato; the other ten were named Buenaventura (three times), María (two times), Teresa de Jesús, Beatriz, Gertrudis, Baltasara, and Joseph. Approximately half of the named infants born by cesarean who were *not* named Ramón were given names with a Christian reference, such as Teresa de Jesús, Joseph, or María.

The name *No Nacido* (literally unborn, not born, or not birthed) was less common than Ramón Neonato, and carried a stronger connotation of having been priest-born. Only three deceased infants were buried under the name No Nacido in the California missions. Of these, two were the product of caesarean operations and appear in table 2.1. The third was the child of a mother who "died during childbirth, and for this reason her body was not buried for three days."[33] Because there is no mention of a caesarean operation on the woman's death register, it is impossible to know whether she underwent the surgery. However, it seems likely that a caesarean operation occurred because the priest denoted an individualized death record for the child. This is more suggestive evidence that priests regularly performed surgery without recording it as such. Even the alternate scenario—that the infant was buried while inside of the womb—would support the thesis that Bourbon reformers sought to individuate the fetal soul, and that priests responded favorably to this directive.

"Buenaventura" is another name that was sometimes attributed to the products of caesarean sections, and there is some cause to believe that it signified that an operation had occurred. Of 48,746 deceased individuals in the

Early California Population Project database, 205 of these were named Buenaventura. Yet much like those named "Ramón Neonato," more than half (110) of those named Buenaventura died as newborns, meaning that some may have been born via caesarean as well. Then there was the newborn who died at birth, for whom the following notes were recorded in the database: "The priest wrote, 'I named her Cesarea,' and in the margin of her baptismal and burial records she is also referred to as 'Cesarea.'"[34]

Only the death record for one infant was consistent with this description (died before or immediately after birth and named some variation of "unborn") but definitely did not refer to a caesarean surgery. The child in question, a girl named Ramóna Nonata, was born to an Indigenous couple, Silvano María and Antonia María, both of whom were unbaptized and unchristianized. The infant was allegedly strangled in strips of clothing and fed to the pigs near her house; as such, the parish priest documented her death as an abortion, though arguably infanticide would have been a more accurate term, unless Silvano and Antonia had a miscarriage and pigs consumed the aborted product.[35] Perhaps the missionary priest decided to designate the infant as a timeless "newborn" because she had died before receiving the baptismal sacrament. Apart from this lone case, the use of the name Ramón Neonato and its variations appears to have been a strong indicator that a child was removed via caesarean, even if the recording priest did not note the operation as such.

Documented caesarean cases became more common as the nineteenth century progressed. Of forty-three surgeries in table 2.1, thirty-three transpired after 1800. The uptick in operations is likely owed to three intertwined factors. First, it may have taken several decades for knowledge of the cesarean to circulate among all priests of New Spain and post-independence Mexico. Second, the colonial mandates apparently generated a cultural shift that gradually made the caesarean operation more acceptable—and perhaps even appealing—for priests and parishioners. Third, some priests choose to perform and document more surgeries than others. Indeed, six priests in table 2.1 performed multiple operations, meaning that their enthusiasm tips the overall chronological balance.

As the nineteenth century progressed, a greater number of operations occurred earlier in the pregnancy; by midcentury, most occurred around six and seven months of pregnancy. One possibility is that priests' records became more accurate and consistent as the nineteenth century progressed. An examination of some holes in the record might support this theory. For example, the California mission records show 48,746 deaths total between 1782 and 1848. Of these, as already noted, 17,646 (36 percent) represent the deaths of a *párvulo*, or infant. It is strange, then, that only sixty-seven women were listed as having died during childbirth during this time. Surely the number must have been higher.

Typically, the women listed as having died in childbirth had more complete death records. These read "deceased during birth," "deceased due to difficulty during birth," or "deceased due to excessively long childbirth." The vast majority of such documents were generated after 1830; in other words, before 1830, late eighteenth-century and early nineteenth-century death registers almost never listed detailed accounts when women died during birth.

It is conceivable that priests only recorded cesarean surgeries when they viewed their efforts as successful. González Laguna's words certainly support this notion. He wrote, "It is better to perform the operation on one hundred women, without results, than to let a single fetus suffocate miserably as it perishes in the maternal womb."[36] González Laguna echoed Charles IV's insistence that priests disinter corpses to search for products of conception in their wombs. If a priest's surgery yielded "no results," he would probably leave no paper trail because the stakes of operating were so high. Priests knew that failing to undertake a cesarean operation or interfering in its performance could incur charges of homicide. Thus, it was likely more sensible to feign the absence of an operation than to admit that one had failed to produce a child. These circumstances likely encouraged clerics to record only successful attempts at surgery.

The Northern Borderlands of Colonial New Spain

Religious zeal for converting Indigenous subjects made the Spanish borderlands an ideal location for the implementation of a risky surgical technique. For example, San Antonio Oquitoa—where María Antonia Zapatito underwent surgery by Father Ramón López—was one of the mission towns founded in the late seventeenth century by Jesuit priests, during what historians have called "the second conquest" of the Spanish empire in the Americas. At the time, missionary towns in Sonora were home to a diverse array of Indigenous groups, including the Apache, Pima, Comanche, Guaymas, Yuma, Yavapai, Opata, Papaga, and Seri. Jesuit missionaries may have felt cursed in their efforts to convert individuals from these groups into subjects of the Spanish Crown. Rebellions and attacks on missions were common, especially from the Seri, Apache, and Pima, who resisted the deepening encroachment of Spanish colonialism.

Disease and illness were also prevalent and devastating. Between 1723 and 1750, nine measles and smallpox epidemics devastated the missions of the northern borderlands and their surrounding communities. This made Catholic authorities focus on saving as many souls as possible. The final blow to Jesuits came in 1767, when they were expelled by the Spanish Crown and replaced by Franciscan priests. Despite this turmoil, colonial missions were not dusty intellectual backwaters. The caesarean operation converted missions into an important site of early surgical practice in the Americas.

One such site was the Diocese of Sonora, an ecclesiastic division of the vast Archdiocese of Mexico that encompassed the present-day states of Sinaloa, Sonora, Baja California, and Alta California. As a group, the Sonoran priest-surgeons shared many traits with Vicente Francisco Sarría, whose views on fetal souls were examined in chapter 1. The Sonoran priests were largely Spanish-born and occupied influential positions in the frontier missions. They were well connected to central Mexico because they traveled frequently to Mexico City and spent time in colleges there.

There are some possible explanations for the prevalence of the surgery in Mexico's northernmost diocese. The Spanish empire was preoccupied with these territories due to encroachments from US and French imperial powers in the borderlands. Protecting the border was challenging because northern New Spain was home to many Indigenous groups and nations that were autonomous and invested in protecting their own territories. Other Indigenous groups were being forcibly relocated by the US settler-colonial state. Because rebellious Indigenous people threatened the stability of the Spanish empire during the precarious pre-independence period, evangelization was an important step in the assimilation and subordination of Indigenous nations. The Crown placed particular emphasis on the evangelization of Indigenous people in missions that were far-removed from the seat of New Spain. The caesarean operation was a way for the colonial government and clergy to assert corporal dominance over rebellious and unincorporated Indigenous groups, thereby advancing a religious and colonial civilizing mission. Some missionaries believed that Indigenous peoples would only be subdued by the application of rationalized and modernized tactics of colonial rule.

The first of New Spain's caesarean surgeries occurred in 1766 in the mission of Arizpe, Sonora, in present-day Arizona. As seen previously, the mandates ordering the operation had not yet been issued for the Spanish colonies. Against that background, the very early occurrence of this surgery lends credence to González Laguna's assertions that the operation was already in use in the Spanish colonies before its popularization by Bourbon officials.

In any case, the 1766 operation was due to a magistrate named Manuel Fernández de la Carrera, whose job was to perform legal services for the area missions. Fernández de la Carrera had learned of the surgery from the prominent Jesuit missionary Juan Nentvig, who supervised five Sonoran *presidios*.[37]

Nentvig was born in Schlessen, Germany (now Poland), in 1713, and entered the Society of Jesus around 1734. He arrived in New Spain around 1750 and acted as the superior in Guásabas (Huásabas) from 1759 until 1767, where he became a prominent missionary. Nentvig died on September 11, 1768, en route to Guadalajara after having been informed of the banishment of the Jesuit order from New Spain. As a surgeon and judge, Fernández de la Carrera enjoyed a close relationship with Nentvig, gaining such authority in the region that he became the friars' attorney in by the 1780s, even after the Jesuit's expulsion.[38]

De la Carrera's surgical subject was a woman named Agueda, who confessed before her death and was anointed with oil preceding her burial in the church. Agueda's child lived for a short time after he or she was extracted. The word "operation" did not appear in Agueda's death register. Instead, De la Carrera referred to the surgery in a rather casual manner, noting, "After her death she was cut open and her unborn infant was removed."[39] While de la Carrera left little commentary regarding his efforts, his close ally Nentvig extensively documented the social and political context of the province of Sonora.[40] Nentvig's 145-page report offered an important panorama of the Sonoran region, illuminating the social aspects of the missions where priests sometimes became surgeons.[41] The Sonoran missions stretched from present-day west Texas through Arizona and Baja California, and were home to several large Indigenous nations, including the Pimas Altos and Bajos, Opatas, Eudebes, Jovas, Seris and their confederates, the Apaches and Tarahumara.

Nentvig believed that the subjugation and Christianization of the local inhabitants would only be achieved through scientific means. He also thought that military might would be an important factor in the Spanish war against rebellious nations, and especially against Apaches. He explained, "I am of the opinion that in addition [to Christianization] we should employ the means which prudence, experience, and military art dictate. . . . We should not be content with the first course only [prayer] and expect the scourge to be lifted through miracles." Only by putting their faith in technology—and not miracles—would the Spanish prevail over the autonomous nations. Evangelization would only be possible, in his view, through military domination: "Then, Sonora being somewhat recovered, some thought could be given to converting the Apaches to Christianity or subjugating them by force."

At times, Nentvig's ample commentary on Sonoran Indigenous nations assumed a hopeful tone regarding their capacity for reason and potential to assimilate into Christianity. This was especially evident in his praise of the Opatas' and Eudebes' craftwork, agriculture, architecture, and trade networks. As historian Laura Shelton notes, Nentvig believed that Indigenous people could "escape barbarity," but only in segregated parishes, isolated from the Spanish and Mestizos.[42] Nentvig thus became a vocal opponent of parish secularization.

Much of Nentvig's commentary on Indigenous peoples dripped with disgust, and even hatred. His ire likely stemmed from witnessing a massive Indigenous rebellion in Sonora, which began on November 21, 1751. The last chapter of Nentvig's book, entitled "How to Punish the Enemy and Prevent the Ruin of Sonora," made a case for the immediate deportation of the Seris and the Pimas. The chapter concluded, "The only remedy is to remove the Seris from our midst so completely that not a single one remains in this section of the country. They are so blood-thirsty that so long as the seed remains, the evil cannot be rooted out." Of the Pimas, he wrote, "there is as little hope of converting them to the faith as there is of converting the Seris. . . . Because they are delinquents, apostates, incorrigible, and obstinately harmful to the Crown and the public, they should be deported or made to serve as oarsmen in the Royal galleys." The missionary insisted that the expense of such a deportation program would be offset by the potential economic benefit to colonial mining settlements, pearl fisheries, and haciendas, which had apparently been abandoned due to Indigenous resistance. Nentvig further insisted that Spain needed to *exterminate* the Apaches, who made regular raids on mission societies, taking hostages and easily defeating Spanish troops in war.

Nentvig's distinction between assimilable, unassimilable, and "savage" Indigenous groups was common among eighteenth century Enlightenment thinkers, who, following the French naturalist Georges-Louis Buffon, generally believed that groups possessed varying levels of reason, intelligence, and civilization. As Nentvig admits, "In general the nature of the Indigenous is so variable that it is hard to explain." Even so, the Jesuit opined that the "nature" of Indigenous peoples could be interpreted on the basis of "four traits, each more despicable than the one that follows: ignorance, ingratitude, inconstancy, and laziness. Their lives revolve around these peculiarities." As David Weber tells us, by 1804 such notions were so common that Miguel Lastarria devised a schema in which he divided Indigenous into fourteen stages of progress toward the "adult stage of civilization."[43]

For Nentvig, Indigenous views on the soul proved their ignorance and lack of reason. He reported that when an Indigenous Pima, Seri, or Apache person died, "the body is left undisturbed for three days while the relatives wait for the frightened soul, supposedly hovering about, to reenter the body." After three days, the deceased person's relatives would bury the cadaver along with *pinole* (roasted ground maize mixed with cacao), and wild greens. Nentvig referred to this religious ritual as evidence of "the drollery and the silliness of the Indigenous people." While priests and missionaries interpreted Indigenous metaphysics as "superstitious and literal-minded," a "blurred" line between life and death was reasonable indeed: at the time, scientific authorities lacked clear diagnostic criteria for death.[44]

In light of this philosophical tension, the caesarean operation functioned as a lesson in orthodoxy for groups who believed, for example, that life after death consisted of an underworld, and not hell or eternal damnation. Given that late colonial priests "repeatedly complained that they had difficulty instilling a fear of death and hell in their Indian communicants,"[45] priests' insistence that the operation was necessary to save unborn souls from eternal damnation likely found little resonance with some parishioners. Likewise, the idea that opposing the operation was "evil" likely rang false among Indigenous peoples. After all, Indigenous religions tended to locate both good and evil in singular deities or saints. Furthermore, given the widespread belief that the soul encircled the body for three days, and that the desecration of a recently deceased person was an affront to the deep importance of ancestor worship, Indigenous Mexicans were likely to interpret the sacralized use of surgery as a kind of spiritualized violence that violated their worldview.[46]

The Indigenous worldview was seemingly inconsequential to priests who were focused on saving unborn children's souls. Franciscan missionary Narcisco Durán (1776–1846) was the most enthusiastic surgeon in the northern missions, where he performed three operations and oversaw one more between 1808 and 1832. All four of Durán's surgeries took place in mission San José, where he spent the majority of his forty years in California. A vocal opponent of parish secularization, the Spanish-born Durán became the vicar forane and ecclesiastical judge for Alta California in 1832. He then became president of the missions from 1833 to 1838, and commissary prefect after 1838.[47]

Durán had only been in Mexico for two years when he first endeavored to remove an infant from its deceased mother's womb. Durán's report of this initial surgery was less boastful than the subsequent ones would be. He simply noted: "child was removed from mother's body following her death." He listed De Razón as the infant's name, as if to assert that the infant had been baptized and definitely had a soul. De Razón's father was unidentified, and his or her mother was Teodora Zalazár, an unmarried and unbaptized Indigenous woman.

Seventeen years passed before another caesarean operation took place in the mission of San José. Although Narcisco Durán was also the officiant in this case, the surgery bore little resemblance to the first. This time—December 1825—Durán decided that a woman who was only four or five months pregnant needed to undergo the surgery. However, he was reluctant to execute the task himself and thus ordered two unbaptized barbers—Nazale and Silvestre—to extract the infant instead. Because the unnamed child showed neither signs of life nor movement, Durán performed a conditional baptism. The deceased mother was also an Indigenous woman, onto whom Durán posthumously imposed the Christianized name Clara. Four years later, Narciso Durán once again ordered the Indigenous barber Silvestre to extract the unnamed product of an unbaptized woman who he called Cristina. Cristina was presumably deceased before Durán ordered Silvestre to operate; even so, this time Durán did not note whether this was the case. His commentary simply read: "The woman was pregnant; Silvestre, a neophyte, performed a caesarean operation. We removed the product, and I baptized it conditionally."

In January 1832, Durán oversaw his final surgery in San José. This time, he hurried to arrive at the woman's bedside, and he did not convey the nature of her obstetric emergency: "The woman was in labor," he wrote, "and so I went immediately. She received the sacraments and then died. We performed the caesarean operation and extracted the infant, which was baptized conditionally." "We" seems to reference Durán's tendency to order Indigenous people to operate on his behalf. This case stands out due to its seemingly rushed manner. Not only did Durán report hurrying to the woman's side, but he also listed the cause of death as both "childbirth," and "caesarean operation." It is unclear whether the surgical subject was, in fact, already deceased, and Durán's notes leave some ambiguity in the matter.

It was relatively common for missionaries to undertake multiple surgeries in short sequence. This is a fitting description of Franciscan priest Florencio Ibáñez, who arrived in California from Spain in 1801.[48] Although Ibáñez only resided in the San Antonio de Padua Mission for two years, he performed two caesareans during that time. The first woman to undergo his shaving razor's incision was Facunda Cifre, an Indigenous woman married to Magin Figuerola. Facunda's "ineffective" labor resulted in her death, and so she "was opened" (*fue abierta*) on February 19, 1802. The child was "removed via caesarean operation" and lived for one hour and a half. In the previous examples,

Narcisco Durán chose not to name the products of his surgical efforts; Father Ibáñez, on the other hand, preferred to do so. He chose Ramón Nonato as the name of the first child; less than one month later, on March 17, 1802, he named a second child Ramóna Cavallero after extracting her from the womb of her eight-months pregnant mother. Both children's death records expressed some ambiguity concerning whether they had been "born": not only was the boy named "unborn Ramón," but he noted in Ramóna's death record that she was both "not born" and was also thirty-seven hours old. On the whole, these cases demonstrate that Indigenous women and children were more likely to die during cesarean surgeries, and their perspectives, unlike those of elite women, were rarely if ever recorded.

Central Territory of Colonial New Spain

If the missionaries of Sonora documented their surgical exploits with increasing frequency, central Mexican priests did not do the same. Perhaps most emblematic of this is a January 1795 note in *la Gazeta de México* regarding four salvational surgeries in the small Indigenous town of Panotlán, which is located in the central Mexican state of Hidalgo. The note was casual and relatively devoid of detail: "Four infants were successfully baptized by means of the caesarean operation." The report continued, "Two operations were performed by the parish priest; the vicar (ecclesiastical judge) also completed a caesarean surgery, and finally, so did a surgeon."[49]

The bare report provokes many questions, including: How did three men perform four surgeries in the tiny village of Panotlán? Did the surgeries all occur on the same day? With such scant detail it is only possible to speculate about the four operations. Given its diminutive size, it seems unlikely that Panotlán would have been home to a priest, a vicar, *and* a surgeon, even if the latter was a popular surgeon and not a licensed one. It is unlikely that four women would have perished in such close succession. Perhaps the unnamed vicar, priest, and surgeon were traversing Indigenous communities in search of recently deceased women from which they could extract unborn products of conception. Such a strange grave-robbing pilgrimage certainly would have terrorized Indigenous peoples and conveyed to them that colonial authorities claimed them in life and death. It is suggestive that *la Gazeta de México* casually mentioned the spate of corpse-cutting, giving the impression that it could have been a regular occurrence in central Mexico.

Although *la Gazeta de México* almost never reported on caesareans in frontier missions or Indigenous communities, it triumphantly disseminated news of the surgery when realized on middle-class or elite women. One such case transpired in 1807, when the parish priest Miguel Priego and a local physician traveled to a woman's home where she had struggled to give birth.[50] A man informed the doctor and the priest that the woman had been dead for three and a half hours. Priego and the physician "began to run, and decided that if no one was daring enough to do so, [they] would attempt the caesarean operation." When they arrived, "everyone insisted that the child was dead," but Priego "refused to believe them." Encouraged by the physician's presence, Priego explained, "We performed the operation, but not without a great deal of horror: first we baptized the child conditionally, before extracting her from the uterus, because we doubted that she was alive." To their surprise, the girl was still breathing, and survived for fifteen minutes after baptism.

Priego likely succeeded due to the doctor's presence—indeed, he mentioned that his previous (solo) attempt at surgery ended disastrously. He wrote, "Even though this operation was so noble that it is worthy of imitation, I will not mention its antithesis: I was part of quite the opposite situation a few years ago, and it was so terrible and scandalous that it should never again be mentioned. In fact, it should remain buried in silence." It is easy—though unpleasant—to imagine the mishaps that could have befallen Priego's first surgical effort. Perhaps he opened the woman's body fruitlessly and could not locate the unborn, despite considerable gore. Or it is possible that he operated before the woman's death—such a decision would have done little to sway the public toward salvational surgery.

Bourbon officials and the press apparently respected Priego's attempt to bury the operation in silence, because it received no coverage. Yet, it may have been representative of the norm. Not only was it atypical for a priest to be aided by a physician, but it was rare that the child was alive upon extraction. It was additionally remarkable that locals from Priego's flock came to alert him of the incident, considering that his last surgery floundered. Finally, Valdés and Alzate Ramírez's decision to omit coverage of Priego's first operation emphasizes that *la Gazeta*—and priests themselves—often neglected to mention religious surgery, either due to its routinization or its failure.

La Gazeta reported several other surgeries practiced on the wives of politicians, elites, and soldiers. In May 1809, for example, in the small mountainous *pueblo* of San Miguel Coyuca (Guerrero), María Teodosia Ramírez died in the early stages of childbirth.[51] Parish priest Francisco Patiño noted in his account that he was hesitant to perform the operation due to his lack of medical and surgical experience. Patiño also affirmed that he first had to convince María's family that the surgery was urgent and necessary. Such persuasion may have invoked an element of coercion since resistance on their part risked incurring charges of homicide.

Although Patiño may have preferred to ask a local doctor, midwife, or barber to extract the child, none was available. However, the priest did have a very small pamphlet entitled "Theological-Moral Guide." Written by Father Félix Eguía, it contained excerpts from *Sacred Embryology*, and it had been distributed throughout Latin American to promote the surgery. Despite his apprehension, Patiño was so "inspired by a holy zeal to fulfill the duties of his ministry" that he extracted a living child, which he baptized, allegedly before its death. Several months later, when a woman named Narcisa del Carmen died during her seventh month of pregnancy, Patiño operated once more. This time, the priest "had the satisfaction of seeing the infant live for an hour after he extracted it." *La Gazeta de México* praised Patiño's actions and deemed him "so zealous and commendable that we can only hope others will imitate his dignified actions."[52]

In 1799, *la Gazeta de México* offered similar compliments to Father Francisco Moyano. He had operated on Ignacia Martínez, who was the wife of soldier Manuel Moreno and eight months pregnant at the time. The child, a girl, survived one half-hour after her baptism. "This brought great relief to the woman's family," *la Gazeta* noted, "who had expressed strong resistance to the idea that priests would execute this operation. Perhaps they were unaware of the procedure, or perhaps they believed that it should only be performed by physicians."[53] Whereas Bourbon authorities failed to note Indigenous resistance or other reactions to the caesarean operation, they did believe that central Mexican elite reactions were noteworthy. Their reports replicated a familiar narrative arc, in which clerics first had to convince the family to allow surgery. Cesarean operations on non-Indigenous women were much more likely to benefit from a physician's assistance, and mother and child were both more likely to survive. Middle class and elite families allegedly responded to surgical salvation with gratitude, relief, and an enlightened surge of piety. Meanwhile, official Crown publications silenced Indigenous perspectives on cesarean surgery while creating a racialized narrative about well-heeled families deserving of deliverance.

Cesarean Operations in Postcolonial Mexico

Although salvational surgery in the Americas grew from the politics of colonization, its effects would reverberate into Mexico's national era. By 1836, writings in the *Periódico de la Academia de Medicina en México* exhibited medics' shifting attitudes towards the surgery. Surgeons and physicians now seemed to uniformly accept the operation, but their discourse increasingly focused on science as well as salvation. In-womb fetal survival following maternal death garnered particular interest. For example, in 1836 one Mexico City doctor described an infant that continued to draw oxygen from the placenta, and through the umbilical cord, for five minutes after its birth. "I have cited this incident," the physician explained, "to demonstrate the point to which fetuses have independent circulation, and to prove that the caesarean operation should be practiced during a much longer period following maternal death than what is generally presumed." "Fortunately," he continued, "this operation is rare, but as it now has the support of our highest medical authorities, and as it is one of the oldest and most well-proven tactics, it is important to consider how long after maternal death the operation can be successful." He then provided examples of two operations: the first of which occurred an hour after maternal death, and the second, thirteen minutes after. In both cases, the infants allegedly survived but then perished soon after leaving the womb.[54]

It is particularly interesting that the doctor described the operation as "one of the oldest and most well-proven tactics." This represents a shift from the standpoint of some late eighteenth-century physicians who believed that the caesarean section was futile, especially when the viability of cesarean-born infants was near zero. By 1836, a Catholic medico-cultural approach to cesarean surgery had prevailed, and the nation's highest doctors drew on the latest scientific evidence to support its use.

Meanwhile, priests continued to perform caesarean operations, even if they now did so in the service of the Republican state, not the Spanish Crown. When Vicente Francisco Sarría wrote about the operation in 1836, he invoked the question of honor. Refusing to accept that the sight of naked flesh would dishonor anyone involved, Sarría argued that the uncovering and opening of a woman's body would, instead, provoke a divine epiphany for the surgeon. In his view, "the opposite of evil thoughts" would occur during surgery. The priest "will be uncovering such marvels of the omnipotence of our Creator, in the structure and organization of the human body, [and in] the enclosure and formation of the fetus, [and so] there cannot help but occur to him a thousand good thoughts concerning the wisdom and power of the Lord our God." For Sarría, such meditations would even challenge the "vanity and arrogance of men" and would encourage them, instead, to show greater appreciation for humility.

Sarría's rhetoric was uniform with a broader intellectual push of the 1820s and 1830s toward natural metaphysics.[55] Beyond that, his politicization of reproductive surgery could not have evinced a more Republican tone. Instead of insisting on the surgery as a means with which to offer vassals to the king, now Sarría used the operation itself as a way to insult royalty by writing that gazing within the interior of a womb would awaken the political conscience of priest-surgeons. He wrote: "For he will see and he will feel that the exalted state of pontiffs; the haughty grandeur and pride of emperors, and of kings and princes; the insolence of tyrants, and in sum, all those conceited ones who, it seems, forever strut about the world—all these had their origins in the filthiest place in nature, and lived there for a period of nine months."[56] In this attack on both monarchal politics, the pope, and the womb, Sarría insisted that the haughtiest and most arrogant of all men were those associated with the Church and Crown. For him, elites and royalty were no better than commoners because all had a common origin: inside the body cavity of another human. Even kings, Sarría insisted, had their origins in the "filthiest places in nature."

The mid-nineteenth century also saw a fascinating episode that evidenced the popular uptake of caesarean surgery. As Nora Jaffary has documented, this case took place in June 1844, when two women from Camargo (a small city in the eastern part of Chihuahua) used a sharp shaving razor to extract a child from its mother's womb. Because the mother of the child still lived, they first intoxicated her with a mixture of *aguardiente* (sugar cane liquor) and an undefined narcotic substance. The women chose to make a longitudinal incision on the left side, resembling the form that was recommended by proponents of religious surgery and theological embryology.[57]

National newspapers speculated about the potential motives of the "brutal operation." Some opined that the mother had wished to abort the child, but cesarean surgery would have been a highly unusual manner of aborting a pregnancy. Both mother and child perished approximately one month after the operation. One of the surgeon's was reportedly the subject's aunt; it was "apparently jealousy [that] moved her to commit this premeditated crime." When the local priest arrived to administer the woman's last rights, a "fetid smell" led him to discover that she had undergone the operation and that it had been hidden from community members. Although the priest was horrified to discover the "disgusting" incision, perhaps he should not have been. After approximately six decades of Crown efforts to convince the public that ceasarean surgery best substantiated one's dedication to the salvation of innocent children, it is unsurprising that women would attempt to employ the operation for their own reasons as well.[58]

It is fitting to end this chapter by highlighting that religious leaders' efforts to promote the religious surgery persisted through the mid nineteenth century. In 1853, Bishop Juan María Luciano Becerra y Jiménez issued a pastoral to the parish priests and clergy of his diocese, insisting that they continue to practice the surgery. On November 11 of that year, the "Carta Pastoral" occupied half the front page of the widely read newspaper *El Siglo Diez y Nueve*.[59] Such an article surely placed the history and continuation of salvational surgeries in plain view. The bishop wrote, "We must utilize every manner of pursuing the serious obligation of liberating souls from damnation, which our lord God put in our trust."

Echoing the language of his eighteenth-century predecessors, Becerra y Jiménez continued, "today we must call your attention to the miserable condition of children that remain in their mother's wombs after those women have died . . . it is of the utmost importance that nobody let the opportunity to practice surgery pass by." To demonstrate his point, the priest copied several paragraphs from Joaquín Castellot's translation of Cangiamila's *Sacred Embryology*. Bishop Becerra y Jiménez ended the piece with a note on the utility of confession in the application of the surgery. He proposed that the use of a curtain in the confessional booth would encourage the woman to "admit to anything—or anything possible—even, perhaps, how advanced [a pregnancy] might be."[60]

One incident provides particularly strong evidence of religious and state medical cooperation during this era. Dr. Antonio Suñol was employed as a resident surgeon at the Santa Clara mission in 1841, and on December 28 that year he collaborated with the priest Jesús María Vásquez del Mercado to produce an infant by means of the caesarean operation. The child—whom the priest named María Juana—emerged deceased and received a conditional baptism. Other missionaries continued to do surgeries as well. In 1845, priest Juan María del Refugio undertook surgery in the San José mission in Alta California. His subject was Guadalupe Moraga, a woman of unstated religion and ethnicity. Guadalupe Moraga apparently "died as a consequence of the operation that they performed after her unsuccessful birth" and did not receive the last rites before her death. Given that one of the officiants characterizes the woman's death "as a result of" the operation, this must mean that Juan María del Refugio did not wait until her death to commence surgery. Here we see a real difference between the first caesarean operation—in New Spain, 1766—and the last, in Republican Mexico in 1845. The first operation was done only when Agueda was certain to be dead, and the child survived (for a short time, at least); in 1845, the operation appeared to have been a contributing factor in Guadalupe's death.

As Chapters One and Two have shown, theologians, physicians, parish priests, bishops, archbishops, and reform-minded Bourbon officials deliberated the utility of the caesarean operation in late eighteenth century and early nineteenth century, invoking a variety of motives and ideologies. Charles III invoked reason and science to combat a black legend that proclaimed Catholicism and absolutism had mired Iberia in backwardness after the Protestant reformation. Jesuit missionaries opposed the secularization of parish administration but were eager to further investigations in the natural and biological sciences. Franciscan missionaries embraced the operation, in part to underscore their corporate relationship with Indigenous Mexicans and their own loyalty to the Crown. American theologians differed from their European counterparts in interpretating the salvational caesarean. Reformers in New Spain tailored mandates to the political and social climate of the region, just as they did in the viceroyalty of Peru.

For all colonial authorities, a scientific reform of infant baptism was a desirable outcome of the rationalization and restructuration of parish administration, for it offered a more straightforward—if coercive—means of evangelizing Indigenous peoples. While the interventionist Bourbon state dismantled the privileges of the nobility and the Catholic Church, they attempted to create a more direct, unmediated relationship between the State and its subjects. Reformers not only wished to incorporate Indigenous groups as culturally assimilated subjects of the Crown by dismantling the parish system that kept Indigenous peoples separate from mestizos and Spanish; they also sought to create a uniform group of political subjects.

Some missionary priests believed that forced coercion was preferable to outright warfare with rebellious groups such as the Apache. In this context especially, the surgery became a means with which to threaten Indigenous women. It suggested that refusal to comply with Christian mandates would result in death of the mother, the carrier of Indigenous traits, to save the unborn, who would then be successfully converted into a Christian vassal. Some believed that the subjugation of Indigenous groups called for war, and scientific Christianization was the only path to success. This bolstered the colonial government's "reconquest" of Indigenous peoples via the assertion of new forms of corporal dominance and religious hegemony. While some priests resented the obligation to become surgeons, others viewed it as a powerful way to persuade Indigenous people that children were created in God's image and that their souls would be eternally damned if not baptized.

Surgical salvation also represented new heights in the scientific reform of priestly duties, which was part of the subordination of priests in general and the regular clergy in particular. Bourbon reformers obligated regular clergy to bureaucratize childbirth, punish parishioners' sexual promiscuity, perfect the baptismal sacrament, and promote radical theological interpretations of the fetal soul. This was part of the endeavor to create modern—and even, enlightened—political subjects, whose spiritual relationship with God rested on the individuality of their own soul, even in its embryonic state. These two ideological trends—surgery as a means of waging a spiritualized reconquest of Indigenous and socially marginal groups, and the Enlightenment focus on the individuated fetal soul—shaped the paternalistic and racialized roots of obstetric health care in modern Mexico. The remaining chapters will track the legacies of these epistemological origins and explore how they have endured for centuries.

Part II
Surgery and Postcolonial Salvation

CHAPTER THREE

The Moral Perfection of the Individual and the Species

Ovariotomy and the Medicalization of Hysteria, 1840s–70s

While the cesarean operation in colonial Latin America was most closely tied to the politics of Indigenous evangelization, hysteria seemed to affect women of all groups and classes in postcolonial Mexico. Underscoring the range of women apparently vulnerable to uterine ailments, this chapter begins with three vignettes featuring hysteria diagnoses in distinct times: 1840, 1861, and 1876. Though relatively close in years, their cases highlight the rapid medicalization of therapeutic approaches to obstetrics and gynecology. While the first patient found relief with opium poultices, by the third instance surgeons insisted that the young woman's condition merited ovariotomy, the surgical extirpation of the ovaries. Together, the three cases help illuminate the politics of women's health care within the dramatic political context of mid-nineteenth-century Mexico.

In 1841, an unmarried twenty-seven-year-old woman fell victim to hysteria while residing in an affluent home in Mexico City. Although little is known about this señorita's life, she clearly enjoyed economic privilege, as her comforts included beautiful gardens and a staff of domestic workers to tend to her needs. Yet one could say that she was a social prisoner of this compound: she very rarely left her residence due to the frequent attacks that embarrassed and worried her loved ones. Well-connected in Mexico City's elite class, her family arranged for her to receive medical attention from some of central Mexico's most prominent health care providers. These physicians, Jeeker and Espejo, had been alerted by colleagues to the señorita's curious situation, in which her hysterical attacks manifested as pelvic convulsions and caused her to faint. The fits occurred several times a day, in both private and public locations, and seemed unrelenting.

When Jeeker and Espejo were unable to cure the woman's hysteria with hydrotherapy (long baths) or pessaries (weights placed inside the vagina), their final recourse was to provide opium patches on her lower back to calm the muscles. Unlimited oral doses of opium likely meant that the girl began to pass her time in a euphoric daze. Though she may have acquired an addiction, the physicians seemed happy to accommodate her with a life of bed rest and substance use. Their writings portrayed her condition as a source of entertainment, not as evidence of moral degeneration or biological weakness.[1] Nor did they attribute her hysteria to demonic possession, as Nora Jaffary tells us that doctors would have done prior to the eighteenth century.[2]

Twenty years later in 1861, a nun named Guadalupe toiled long hours in a convent called Los Cinco Señores in Mexico City. Perhaps her days began early and required her to be on her feet without rest. At some point Guadalupe experienced symptoms of hysteria severe enough to prompt her to seek medical attention. Her nervous attacks and episodes were concerning to the head sister and administrator, a nun named Reverenda Madre Presidenta de Regina, who granted permission for Guadalupe to receive within the establishment galvanic baths administered by a clinician.[3]

These baths involved the use of a low electric current, and they likely required Guadalupe to immerse herself for hours at a time. Although some found the treatment effective for nervous symptoms, others complained about scalding water.[4] Galvanic baths, which involved a combination of hydrotherapy and electricity, were first used in 1836 in a London hospital. The approach was based on the theory that conscious and reflexive actions alike are related to neural processes, meaning that electromagnetic currents could stimulate the nerves and alleviate hysterical symptoms such as paralysis and convulsions. Thus, Guadalupe's doctors employed the most modern medical techniques for hysteria, even in a convent and even under the supervision of religious women. Whereas physicians treated the 1841 case as behavioral and sexual, their 1861 use of galvanic baths represented a more medicalized, but only slightly more interventionist, approach. Guadalupe's 1861 care transpired under medico-religious collaboration inasmuch as religious women controlled the medical space. They welcomed a clinician to offer a medical cure, but only under the authority of the head sister.

By the 1870s, doctors had embraced a much more medicalized view of hysteria, associating the condition with problems during childbirth as well as behavioral and neurological pathologies. Many believed ovariotomy (the surgical extirpation of the ovaries) to be an ideal cure for hysteria and a range of other behavioral and moral concerns. First practiced by English physician Spencer Wells in 1859, ovariotomy became the first major abdominal surgery to be widely implemented in the nineteenth century.

Surgery was appealing because when done early enough it allowed surgeons to extirpate two ailments: cystic ovaries before they ruptured, and ovarian tumors before they metastasized. One problem was that obstetricians almost never knew when a woman had an ovarian cyst or tumor unless those became so large that they were palpable through the abdominal wall. By the 1870s, physicians theorized that the pressure of such growths would constrict or excite the ovaries, provoking immoral, irrational, or pathological behavior. Ovariotomy promised moral correction, and surgeons in Mexico were eager to have it: after all, a new republic required an improved, reformed, and more useful kind of citizen. Not just popular in Mexico, ovariotomy spread rapidly throughout the world. Yet, it remained extremely controversial: by 1891 Wells himself decried the overtly racialized practice of "extirpating women's ovaries like the 'aboriginal spayers of New Zealand.'"[5]

The third case of hysteria, observed in 1876 and documented by Manuel Ramos in 1880, initially appears similar to that of the wealthy señorita from 1841. But this time the young woman under observation was four months pregnant, and she was a patient in la Casa de Maternidad. Apparently she experienced extensive convulsions, explosions of laughter, and libidinous movements of the pelvis. Though she still had a grasp of her senses, both intellectual and sensorial, "her face displayed an expression of self-satisfied voluptuosity."[6] Ramos postulated that she was experiencing a kind of eclampsia resulting from hysteria, likely caused by compression or agitation of her ovaries. This caused a "cerebral commotion" resembling the euphoria of drunkenness. Ramos insisted that this made her an excellent candidate for ovariotomy, although his records do not clarify whether she underwent the surgery.

By exploring the onset of a surgical approach to hysteria, this chapter contributes to Frida Gorbach's analysis of the condition's particular salience within nineteenth-century gendered discourses.[7] It is inspired by Jan Goldstein's study of the secularization of French hospitals during the same time period, a process that shifted the national approach to reproductive science.[8] Led by the Parisian psychiatrist Jean-Martin Charcot, late nineteenth-century psychiatrists undertook a typologization of hysteria, dividing it into four stages. Psychiatrists emphasized that demonic possession and mystical ecstasies were not religious experiences; rather, nuns and religious figures who experienced corporal possession must be suffering from insanity, not devotion. Goldstein insists that this epistemological shift, the "political construction of hysteria," was laicizing at its core. She explains, "Clearly this redefinition of the supernatural as the natural was secularizing in impact and in intent. . . . If, at the *fin-de-siècle*, more Frenchwomen than ever before fell sick with a condition called hysteria, their illness was in part a political construction."[9]

Whereas the previous two chapters explored theologically inflected surgeries, this chapter shows that medical efforts to enact salvation through surgery did not vanish with nineteenth-century state secularization. Instead, ideas about women's bodies and minds were reconfigured: moralized and medicalized in new ways. The chapter proceeds chronologically, with its main focus on the decades-long period of liberal constitutional reform known as *la reforma* (1854–76). *La reforma* followed Mexico's independence from Spain in 1821 and was a key time for national medical training and hospital administration.

Another important component of nineteenth-century medicine, explored at length here, was the establishment of a religious health care regime in the 1840s, followed by the expulsion of those health care providers in the 1870s. This discussion provides insight into the institutional culture of Mexico's hospitals and clinics, which underwent significant shifts. Nineteenth century establishments transformed from religiously administered spaces of refuge and spiritual care to, in one case, a lock hospital that collaborated with the Sanitary Police to detain and castigate social outcasts and unruly women, including sex workers. An analysis of how women medical authorities came to be seen as irrational—and even hysterical—sheds light on gendered aspects of national debates about religion, citizenship, and medical authority during Mexico's monumental liberal reforms.

Postcolonial Independence and the Religious Modernization of Mexican Hospitals

Like most other Latin American countries, Mexico entered postcolonial statehood following an armed War of Independence. By 1821, the leading insurrectionist, an Afro-Mexican man named Vicente Guerrero, brokered peace with the royal officer Augustín de Irturbide. The blueprint for independence, the Plan de Iguala, preserved the Catholic Church's status and authority in Mexico and proscribed governance by constitutional monarchy.

The postcolonial nation soon abolished the enslavement of Africans, African-descendants, and Indigenous people and extended citizenship to all. In fact, state-builders eliminated racial categorization itself; the classification of people by color, language, or indigeneity was now prohibited in legal, state-based, and census records. During colonialism the Spanish caste system had forced enslaved and Indigenous Mexicans to the bottom of the social hierarchy, while the colonial judicial system had paternalistically made Indigenous people a protected class of their own, exploited for labor. Following independence, colonial racial categorizations collapsed into each other; yet even while race melted away from national nomenclature, Indigenous and African-descendent communities continued to confront deeply rooted inequities and prejudices.

Although religious hospitaler orders had largely maintained stable hospitals and care facilities throughout the colonial period, administering these institutions became complex in the decades immediately following independence.[10] Emperor Augustín de Iturbide, Mexico's first post-independence head of state, expelled the last of the hospitaler orders during the Revolution of Independence. Meanwhile, one of the country's early Republican leaders, President Anastasio Bustamante, sought to establish a new era in public health in 1831. In that year he oversaw the creation of the Facultad Médica, which was replaced in 1841 by the Consejo Superior de Salubridad (Superior Sanitation Council); still, state-sponsored medical education remained spotty for the next several decades, during which the United States usurped half of Mexico's territory via the Mexican-American War and the Treaty of Guadalupe Hidalgo.[11] Whereas religious orders had previously maintained *colegios* within which to train and house elite physicians, apothecaries, and barber surgeons, most were defunct by 1840. When physicians treated patients, they did so in one of two places: in the patients' private homes, as we saw in the case of the convulsing señorita, or in the convents that attended to their spiritual needs. Religious administrators carefully guarded convent doors and sometimes insisted on approving medical treatments before allowing doctors to enter and practice medicine within.[12]

The Superior Sanitation Council was to assume the tasks of the defunct Protomedicato, which had until that time coordinated public health, granted and renewed medical degrees, and oversaw hospital administration in the colonies. Owing to the relative dearth of national medical schooling in the 1840s and 1850s, elite students like Jeeker and Espejo commonly traveled to Paris or Edinburgh for clinical education. This was the case for Manuel Andrade, who studied in Paris in the 1830s and witnessed the successful efforts of las Hermanas de la Caridad, who offered health care in France and twenty-eight countries throughout the world.

Las Hermanas de la Caridad belonged to a volunteer association that had originated in seventeenth-century France and was supervised by the Society of Saint Vincent de Paul. The organization offered a new form of religious practice for women. Instead of committing to a cloistered and contemplative lifestyle, the sisters served the poor and marginalized in hospitals, orphanages, schools, and prisons. Perhaps they had some true solidarity because many Hermanas were themselves impoverished, having been allowed to join the society without the payment of a dowry.[13] Their success revolutionized French bishops' view of women's religious congregations and sparked a novel kind of modernized religious medical practice. Although their admissions process was distinct from that of other Church orders, state authorities still generally saw las Hermanas as having the same qualities as nuns of a religious institution.[14]

Las Hermanas collaborated intensely with another Vicentian order in Mexico, las Señoras de la Caridad, a volunteer association of women who performed charitable duties for the public. For example, whereas las Hermanas de la Caridad toiled long hours to prepare pharmaceutical remedies, las Señoras de la Caridad often delivered those concoctions to other hospitals as well as to prisons and private residencies. Despite their important auxiliary role, las Señoras de la Caridad were distinct from las Hermanas. Las Señoras were generally married, elite women who resided in their own homes and routinely offered assistance to the sick and poor, whereas las Hermanas were unmarried women who took up residence in the institutions where they worked. Both groups show that Mexico City's burgeoning public health system was one of marked collaboration between religious, state, governmental, and even imperial authorities. This too was salvational medicine.

Upon returning to Mexico from Paris in 1842, Andrade advocated for bringing the Vincentian organizations to Mexico. In 1844 the Society of St. Vincent de Paul successfully petitioned the government to authorize the congregation. Las Hermanas de la Caridad quickly established a broad philanthropic network in Mexico City, and for the next three decades they would be the only religious organization authorized to offer hospital care in Mexico City.[15] From 1844 through the late 1860s, the sisters were pivotal in modernizing Mexican hospitals, often converting centuries-old and defunct hospital buildings into functioning clinics.[16] By the 1850s las Hermanas staffed and administered eight of the thirteen clinics in Mexico City; they additionally maintained an orphanage, a poor house, a school for girls, and three *colegios:* San Vicente, San José, and el Sagrado Corazón.[17] The women also worked as apothecaries and prepared 8,000 free remedies per month; by the early 1870s, the sisters controlled more than one-third of Mexico City's thirty-eight pharmacies.[18]

The mid-nineteenth century thus witnessed the religious modernization of the national health care system, which would persist even in the context of drastic state reform efforts. As mentioned previously, Mexico's prodigious liberal reform began during this time, in 1854. The reforma is closely associated with Mexico's liberal and Indigenous Zapotec President Benito Juárez, who served five terms: 1858–61 as interim, then 1861–65, 1865–67, 1867–71, and 1871–72. The reforma sought, among other things, to limit clerical power and Church property holding, to gradually secularize state functions, and to establish a federalist system. Some interpreted this as an attack on the entrenched authority of the Church. Such conflicts contributed to mid-century civil wars, many of which were led by Indigenous people who demanded state-based rights, thereby shaping the meaning of liberalism and citizenship.

In the context of rising liberalism and its discontents, some questioned whether a religious group like the Hermanas should possess medical power and authority. Members of the Superior Sanitation Council raised questions about the sisters' ability to prepare complicated medicines as early as 1852, citing that it was not legal for women to practice medicine or manage apothecaries. Yet still they allowed the sisters to offer the remedies, and common people clearly trusted their qualifications.[19] One Catholic journalist railed against the prejudices implicit in gendered prohibitions: "Why should we consider a woman more inept than an untrained male assistant? Why are women prevented from being pharmacists? Just because a woman is a Hermana de la Caridad, is she incapable of weighing a gram of strychnine, brucine, or arsenic, and mixing it with an ounce of fat?"[20]

The only official set of regulations regarding the sisters' role in hospitals was published in 1852, when the local government issued a thirty-four-article set of bylaws governing them. These affirmed the sisters' important clinical role and upheld las Hermanas' religious organizational model, for example, by maintaining the sister's right to elect the *superiora*, or head sister.[21] Modeled on the power structures of the convent systems, the head sister enjoyed virtually absolute authority over the hospital's staff. Even clinicians were sometimes limited in their ability to question her decisions. For example, the head sister divided responsibilities among the sisters as she saw fit, and medical officials were prohibited from interfering with this process.[22]

The bylaws explained that the sisters' main therapeutic responsibilities included administering medication and providing patient care. They also participated in examinations by doctors and medical students. When the sisters accompanied students to the bedside, they did so as supervisors, ensuring that the students dispensed the correct amount of medicine and that they did not alter the physician's orders. They accompanied fully licensed physicians, but in this case it was to familiarize themselves with medical routines so that they could complete the duties at night and in the absence of doctors.[23]

By all scenarios, las Hermanas guarded patients carefully and were integrally involved in clinical procedures, especially pharmaceutical therapies. They exerted real influence over other medical practitioners, to the point that they alone possessed the keys to hospital establishments and even conducted tacit surveillance of male medics. Further proof of the sisters' influence is found in stipulations that the head sister alone controlled the hospital keys, and that she had the right to fire any employee of the hospital at her own discretion, male or female, with the exception of ecclesiastics and physicians.

Benito Juárez enshrined his support for religious health care in law during his first presidential term. With the "Law Secularizing Hospitals and Welfare Establishments" of February 2, 1861, Juárez officially expropriated hospitals owned by ecclesiastical corporations. Yet his measures allowed flexibility in secularization by granting local government authority to arrange hospital administrations, meaning that religious health care fell into a regime of municipal exceptionalism. Importantly, Juárez's 1861 decree classified las Hermanas de la Caridad as a "civil group," not a religious corporation.[24] This exception, which was reiterated in the 1863 legislation that officially banned religious communities, affirmed, "The suppression of existing religious communities does not, and should not, include las Hermanas de la Caridad, because they do not live monastically, and because they are dedicated to caring for the sick and suffering."[25] Despite his dedication to secularizing the nation, Juárez intended to make las Hermanas de la Caridad a permanent fixture in Mexican hospitals. This was a spiritualized kind of health care indeed.

Yet clinicians began to complain that the sisters prevented them from performing medical treatments with which they disagreed. Medical students first voiced this grievance in 1861, when two practitioners wrote, "in our time as residents, we have witnessed the following: when a Hermana de la Caridad disagrees with a medicine that has been prescribed by a physician, she will refuse to administer it, even though we know that their opinion in medicine does not merit much consideration." The students' denunciation also hinted at moments of cooperation between medical professionals and the women. As they mentioned, "if a doctor befriends the women, they will refrain from calling him in the middle of the night, therefore damning the patient to continue suffering."[26] Of course, it is also possible that the sisters simply chose to administer the treatments themselves. This accusation was duplicitous, suggesting that the sisters were both too autonomous as practitioners and simultaneously too selfish; they allegedly disrespected practitioner's wishes but also neglected patients when they wanted to favor some practitioners by relieving them of work. As we will see, the students themselves were grappling with the meanings of the reforma while reflecting on how Mexico's health care system could be repurposed for various kinds of social regeneration.

Medicine during the Restored Republic, 1868–76: Expelling las Hermanas de la Caridad

Public health and medical training began to undergo broad institutional and epistemological shifts in the second half of the 1860s, especially following France's imperial invasion of Mexico and occupation of the nation from 1861 to 1867. The term "restored republic" refers to Mexico's re-establishment of a republican government following their defeat of the French in 1867. The now-even-more-heroic president Benito Juárez regained the presidency after fighting in the battle against the French in Puebla, and in 1868 he established the Escuela Nacional Preparatoria (National Preparatory School), or ENP.

The national school offered broad training to students in philosophy, letters, law, and medicine. It was an enormous endeavor, with the first class enrolling at least 700 students.[27] This allowed students to receive their medical training in Mexico whereas they previously would have studied medicine internationally, likely in France, Scotland, or the United States. For example, Santiago Zambrana y Vásquez attended the University of Havana for his medical training in the mid-1860s, but when he came back to Mexico he excitedly filed his thesis with the ENP and started to practice medicine in Mexico.[28]

One of these students, Alberto Salinas y Rivera, attended the ENP from 1868 to 1871, and published a medical thesis as part of one of the school's first graduating classes.[29] His thesis, entitled *Medical Morality*, provides a fascinating glimpse into his discussions with other students and lectures from professors. He emphasized the principles, values, and norms that he believed should govern doctors in the course of their practice, which would in turn shape Mexican culture and society. Salinas y Rivera also used the word "moral" in an introspective sense to refer to the morale among his medical cohort. The student first focused on the importance of a nationalistic school of medicine and medical ideological approach to social issues. Because other countries had distinct climates and traditions, for Salinas y Rivera it was "disgraceful" that Mexican health care providers understood their people through international scientific ideologies.[30]

Salinas y Rivera also believed that a "medical corporation" or "medical corps" should replace the religious corporations that controlled the hospital establishment. In his view, religious hospital administration was a self-serving or dishonest form of philanthropy that was more interested in maintaining religious authority than making medical progress.[31] It was for that reason that the young student advocated a stronger system of governmental support for medical students and recent graduates. Funding for their studies and an adequate professional salary would help to distinguish proper providers from other medical practitioners, including las Hermanas de la Caridad. As he explained, "in today's society, people always look for reasons to ridicule and condemn science, even though, by nature, it is exempt from such attacks; the scientific conduct of a physician, no matter how justifiable, is never acceptable in the eyes of the public, because the public is always willing to attribute doctor's motives to sinister causes, and to represent state of the art practitioners as more criminal than the bandits that seethe and swarm in the streets."[32] Salinas y Rivera concluded that clinical practice in Mexican hospitals was excessively polarized, or "of two extremes." While popular practitioners displayed an "exaggerated distrust of science," medics "sometimes trusted science too much." Both extremes depreciated diagnostic and therapeutic outcomes, and allegedly put doctors in a "delicate" position. As the medical student's writing shows, Mexico's first generation of nationally trained clinicians imbibed from their lessons a certain disdain for las Hermanas' moral and medical authority, painting them as foreigners and impediments to creating a Mexican school of medical thought.

Meanwhile, the state-based infrastructure for secular medicine grew. The Superior Sanitation Council, which had become defunct during the second empire, re-formed in 1871. This group now demanded more space in which to practice than they could find in la Casa de Maternidad alone. Luckily for the Superior Sanitation Council, political alliances were made possible by shifts in local government, and especially in the new class of federal politicians who emerged after 1871.[33] The council began to agitate for the expulsion of las Hermanas de la Caridad from Mexico City's hospitals, thereby reducing religious influence in the newly established medical school. With an eye toward this larger goal, the council's immediate aim was to assume control over the administration of two institutions—the Hospital del Divino Salvador for insane women and the Monasterio del Guadalupe—and to place both facilities under the sole control of medical personnel.

Under the restored republic (1867–1871), Mexico City politicians had a contentious relationship with the Superior Sanitation Council, and the government regularly rejected its correspondence due to its allegedly "disrespectful" tone.[34] Following the election of a centralizing and anticlerical president, Sebastián Lerdo de Tejada in 1872, the Superior Sanitation Council quickly published new bylaws, which it had refused to do under Juárez. The organization expressed enthusiasm regarding plans for the creation of a sanitary police force. These actions—along with the amicable tone of correspondence—indicated that a friendlier relationship with the new executive order characterized this period. The council also made a cryptic, but suggestive, agreement to "oppose the unconstitutional elements that currently remain" in administration of the hospitals—that is, las Hermanas.[35] In response, Lerdo de Tejada issued a "presidential decree ordering that the Superior Sanitation Council assume control over the administration of all public health," a measure for which the body had been agitating since late January.[36] Lerdo de Tejada's decree indicates that he was willing to begin ceding control over the administration of public hospitals as early as 1872. The president and public health authorities likely sought to enact the measure in a gradual manner to avoid angering the public. Perhaps they intended to maintain the sisters' nursing services while usurping their administrative capacities.

Lerdo de Tejada's reforms granted the Superior Sanitation Council the power to appoint and remove physicians, superseding even the federal government's authority to do so. A sharp increase in the availability of physicians underscores the context of the president's reform: whereas the Biblioteca Nicolás León holds only seventeen theses published between 1840 and 1861, at least 193 doctors began practicing between 1862 and 1873.[37] These figures alone indicate that the expulsion of las Hermanas was inseparable from the expanding functions of the licensed medical corps, whose growing claims to scientific authority were increasingly recognized by the state.

The medical initiative to assume power over Mexico City's hospitals gained momentum near the beginning of Lerdo de Tejada's presidential term. In late 1871, the Superior Sanitation Council held a meeting to discuss the merits of seizing the Hospital del Divino Salvador for insane women and the Monasterio del Guadalupe, which at the time was also a hospital.[38] The meeting minutes, which summarized the council's discussion, revealed the following consensus: "In agreement with the intentions of the authorities, we propose to take over the administration of the Asilo de Mugeres Dementes [Hospital del Divino Salvador]. Of course, given the imperfections of the Asilo, the Monasterio de Guadalupe is preferable. However, the problematic and capricious administrators [i.e., las Hermanas] who jealously guard the Monasterio prevent us from doing so; they cling to the resources they have gathered and they plan to stay there forever, even as the reform authorities perform their inspections and attempt to exercise the necessary amount of vigilance over the women."[39] Here is evidence that some authorities were in agreement with the council's annexation objectives. Nevertheless, the council saw no hope of attempting to seize the Monasterio de Guadalupe. Although they would have preferred to assume control of both asylums, the sisters in the Monasterio presented so much resistance that physicians hesitated to encroach on that space.

Some doctors in attendance stated that it would be difficult to administer the clinics in the sisters' absence. Not only would they lack personnel with whom the patients felt comfortable, but there would also be a shortage of furniture and medicine. After debating these concerns, the council settled on the following assessment: "Surgical operations such as the ovariotomy are necessary for effective treatments. These surgeries have been successfully performed in this asylum, although they are rarely discussed. The operations are in large part possible due to the excellent hygienic standards in this establishment. The Asilo de Mujeres Dementes is in good condition, even though it is not under the heel (*bajo el pie*) of an authority that scientific progress would demand."[40] While they esteemed the cleanliness of the religious women's clinics, officials still believed that the promises of advancement outweighed the logistical disadvantages of ousting the administrators. They explained, "Even if [the government of Mexico City] orders further reform of the current administration, this will not be enough to adapt it to the aims to which it should be destined. The difficulties presented are unnecessary, and despite our best efforts we have made little to no progress; the buildings are already there, and so it is unwise to buy a new Asilo de Mugeres [*sic*]. It would lack the necessary elements, and the only problem with the existing territories is the people who control them."

The council did not simply accuse las Hermanas of "jealously guarding" their establishments but also of stymieing potential medical progress. In their view, past reform efforts had been laudable but inadequate because las Hermanas quixotically protected the clinics to prevent major changes. In particular, the physicians insisted that the sisters' presence would prevent them from performing medical treatments upon the women who were to be detained and hospitalized by the incipient sanitary police force. As the meeting minutes explained, "We must claim the ability to detain and isolate those women whose illness demands their imprisonment, as well as those whose exaggerated dishonesty and immorality prompts even their most unfortunate companions to turn their heads in disgust; and I have not even mentioned the outsiders."[41]

In other words, physicians sought to grant sanitary police the authority to detain women so that they could be forcibly treated in hospitals. Their main targets were women deemed "insane," "immoral," and "outsiders." It is unclear whether "outsiders" referred to women from other states, other countries, or both. Some members of the council voiced opposition to forcible detainment and argued that compulsory detainment was an unethical practice. Dismissing these qualms, other members insisted that the initiative would uplift Mexican medicine by allowing doctors to imitate European practices. "These proposals," the minutes read, "satisfy the requirements of even the most scrupulous hospitals in Europe. We would like to be an outstanding example and to offer a happy tale to the enlightened men from the old continent."[42] Eurocentrism inflected on the Superior Sanitation Council advocacy for fundamental shifts in the purpose of the clinics in question.

While historians have always seen the drive for las Hermanas' expulsion as a function of liberalism, the council's proposal to take control of the asylum can be interpreted as positivistic and illiberal. The writing was positivistic in that it sought to schematize people according to their presumed worth to the nation inasmuch as society, according to positivist philosophy, functioned like a biological organism that needed to be cultivated purposefully to achieve maximum productivity. Furthermore, the outlined approach was illiberal, at least in the classical sense, because it rationalized the use of force to treat citizens as prisoners while sublimating their autonomy. In subsequent chapters we will see that these became major themes in late nineteenth century reproductive health care.

Gabino Barreda and the Positivist Theory of the Soul

There were many reasons that physicians and public health officials wished to usurp the clinics administered by las Hermanas de la Caridad. While authorities broadly saw the women's labor as an appropriate stopgap during the first decades of the reforma, once the ENP was underway and the Superior Sanitation Council was fully functional, they seemed to be more of an impediment than their presence was worth. As we have seen, and as will be discussed in more detail later, at least one surgeon advocated for the expulsion of las Hermanas because he believed that their presence impeded the performance of ovariotomy surgery, given that the asylum for insane women was "not under the heel of an authority that scientific progress would demand."[43]

Not everyone agreed that ovariotomy was therapeutically necessary. Salinas y Rivera, for example, believed that the performance of ovariotomy as well as ovarian puncture led to the general public's distrust in medicine. Salinas y Rivera opined that surgeons needed to be "retrained in medical observations, so as to avoid making absurd diagnoses that damage both the health of our patients and our own reputations."[44] By that time, as few as five ovariotomies had been performed in Mexico: one in a private home, three in the Hospital San Pablo, which was administered and staffed by las Hermanas, and one in 1870 in the Hospital del Divino Salvador for insane women. The medical student who documented the surgeries theorized that the last woman, operated on in the Hospital del Divino Salvador, died of nervous exhaustion due to her hysteria.[45]

A more interventionist approach to hysteria had clearly taken root by the 1870s. This section explores these phenomena in relation to positivist philosophy, and in particular, Gabino Barreda's "positivist theory of the soul." Dr. Gabino Barreda, one of a generation of Mexican physicians who had studied medicine in Paris in the 1840s, personally knew Auguste Comte—the "father of positivist philosophy"—as early as 1848.[46] Barreda returned to Mexico eager to rebuild the nation's medical institutions with an epistemological school of medicine known to historians as Paris Medicine.[47] Barreda would echo Comte's Positivist School of Philosophy in many of his publications and public oratories, beginning in 1863. He then became the director of the ENP upon its founding and through its first decade (1868–78). It is therefore unsurprising that the ENP was founded on the basis of a strictly positivist curriculum. Because it offered the highest level of medical, jurisprudential, and philosophical training in the nation, its professors, administrators, and graduates were crucial actors in Mexican history. As Charles Hale has demonstrated, positivist doctrine became the core of all intellectual assumptions and policy decisions in Mexican higher education and political administration from the 1870s forward.[48]

The core of positivist political philosophy was the idea that society functioned according to a "positive" (real, or phenomenological) set of "true"—and biologically demonstrable—laws. Because they were universal, these could be proven by means of logical scientific inquiry, which in turn meant that only experimental research could reveal the rules that governed biology and society. At its core, positivist philosophy held that societies must undergo a progressive transformation, in which governance would transition from theological underpinnings to metaphysical ones, and finally to "positive" understandings of the world.[49] Once governments reached the positive stage, policy decisions and interpersonal relations alike would be dictated by a thoroughly scientific understanding of society.

Positivists such as Comte and Barreda were motivated by visions of a utopian future. They believed that scientific progress could lead human individuals and societies to a state of moral perfection, characterized by love, solidarity, and intelligence (empathetic, humanistic, and intellectual). Positivists described these forms of "improvement" by using the language of moral and biological "regeneration." Although positivism was meant to overcome religious and metaphysical worldviews, it shared a similarly salvational outlook. Philosophers loyal to this outlook proposed that the uniform implementation of scientific methods—in education, medicine, agriculture, economics, law, psychology, sociology, and other areas—would result in the moral and biological regeneration of individuals and societies.[50] Given this ideology, it is not surprising that Barreda's first positivist tract, published in 1863, was entitled "On Moral Education."[51]

Positivist biological theories provoked the onset of much more interventionist approaches to hysteria, inspired by scientized efforts to overlay new cultural understandings onto the concept of morality. Comtean positivism dominated scientific understandings of psychology, psychiatry, and the behavioral sciences in the 1870s and 1880s. During this time, neurologists theorized that the mind could be located throughout the nervous system, and that mental and physical "reflexes" were two interconnected components of one integral nervous system. This understanding—known as "pan reflex" and "cerebral reflex"—posited that the spinal cord had many little brains and therefore produced unconscious feelings throughout the spine and nerves.

This complemented the assertion that the soul was a material, not a metaphysical, entity. Specifically, positivists believed that the soul was an electrochemical substance—probably made of neurons—that resided in each organ and acted as the "mind" of that organ and influenced its functions. They came to the reasonable conclusion that because organs seemed to produce physiological states, scientists could build empirical data sets by measuring sensations and by attempting to control for the factors that caused or influenced these sensations. Such ideas dovetailed with the introduction of the terms "neurosis" and "psychosis" to refer, respectively, to neural processes and their associated subjective feelings. Pointing to a dialectical relationship, scientists hypothesized that mental states triggered physiological states, and that organs (such as the uterus and the ovaries) provoked mental states as well.[52]

By the early 1870s, medical students learned that hysteria resulted when "innervation and nutrition accumulate[d] in the reproductive organ and its contents."[53] Such an accumulation was, allegedly, deeply rooted, beginning early in life and becoming pathological sometime after a woman reached sexual maturity. The reference to excessive "nutrition" alluded to a problematic physical matter or material energy, conveying that the patient's organism had devoted excessive energy and growth to developing the reproductive organs. Internal examinations allegedly offered proof of this claim by demonstrating that hysterical women had excessively "veiny" and "meaty" reproductive organs. This discussion recalled the racist pathologization of African women's primary and secondary sexual characteristics as excessively enlarged and engorged, a trend epitomized by early nineteenth-century writings on Saartjie Baartman by the French naturalist Georges Cuvier and others.[54]

The racist and biologically essentialist discourses of early century polygenists had intensified by the 1870s. In students' writings on hysteria, for example, "innervation" had a more explicitly biological connotation, referring to the degree of stimulation of a muscle or organ by nerves. The suggestion, then, was that a hysterical woman's uterus dominated her neural functions and prevented her neural—electric—energy from flowing toward the other organs that required innervation. Many positivistic scientists believed that the brain, heart, stomach, eyes, lungs, and genitals all had one or many "minds of their own" (neural control centers), and that all organs—but especially the brain—needed innervation to exert the correct moral affect. In other words, Mexican students took part in a dominant intellectual trend in mid-century reproductive medicine, which considered the reproductive organs as the "sexual control centers" for women's behavior and thus as the seat of their emotional and social problems. As historian Ornella Moscucci has demonstrated, by the late nineteenth century women's destinies came to be seen as thoroughly determined by their biology. In her words, "Woman was classed with the child and the primitive, and both femininity and savagery were seen to be pathological states and an arrested stage of development of the human species."[55]

Gabino Barreda offered one of the clearest midcentury explanations of the alleged relationship between an individual's organs and his or her moral or intellectual state.[56] He wrote, "Let us recall that each organ is capable of exerting influence over the intellectual and moral state of the individual. This influence is proportional to the relative development—or, progress [*desarrollo*]—of that organ. In this, we have strong evidence of a natural solution to achieving moral perfection. The moral perfection of the individual and of the species will be achieved by developing the organs that contribute to good tendencies, and by diminishing, whenever possible, those that contribute to moral decline." He continued, "If we could produce the desired effect—that is to say, the artificial atrophy of some organs, and the development or growth of others—we would succeed in modifying the soul in a most convenient way. How could we exert influence over those organs, which appear to be outside of our reach? How can we achieve the modification of such deeply placed organs? Science is not silent in the face of these novel, grand, and interesting questions: her explanations are as categorical, precise, and clear as we could possibly desire."[57]

Barreda strongly implied that the solution for "such deeply placed organs" was surgical. He seemed to direct physicians to extirpate the ovaries of hysterical women, and those of others with so-called moral afflictions, with the goal of regenerating (and eventually perfecting) individuals' moral and intellectual tendencies. Here Barreda drew inspiration from Auguste Comte's Positive Theory of the Soul, which claimed that the perfection of organs would eventually raise the nation's collective level of development. Because positivists viewed society as a living organism, it could only advance with the regeneration of the *individual* organisms (humans, and their organs) within. Thus it was part of Barreda's philosophical worldview that organs dictated affect, and that it was therefore necessary for scientists to manipulate—or remove—the organs of those citizens with moral afflictions.

Such reasoning suggests an explanation for why the Superior Sanitation Council insisted, in late 1871, that "oophorectomies are necessary for the effective treatment of women." It explains why it was necessary to secularize Mexican hospitals, given that religious women had played a major role in modernizing Mexico City's hospitals and, throughout the 1860s, had monitored treatments by male surgeons. Those religious women apparently opposed the oophorectomies—to the degree that the doctors' intentions to practice this surgery led them to call for the expulsion of the religious hospital administrators in 1871. Thus, in some ways oophorectomies signaled the arrival of positivist medical science to Mexico City's reproductive health clinics.

Conflicts over Patient Treatment under President Lerdo de Tejada

The council's proposal to forcibly intern women in Mexico City's asylums and clinics became the the source of conflict with religious hospital administrators by 1872. This was likely because the Society of Saint Vincent de Paul emphasized "service to the poor" as a guiding principle of their organizations, and because the sisters' epistemological approach sought to evangelize people by demonstrating sympathy and concern for their well-being. This is not to say that religious health care was less coercive than secular care. Indeed, and as the first section of this book argues, conscripted evangelization entails spiritual, psychological, and corporeal violence. Nonetheless, as las Hermanas were not medical men who sought to demonstrate their cutting-edge scientific prowess, the religious women's therapeutic methods arguably entailed less trial and error. While members of las Hermanas were beholden to an evangelizing form of patient care, surgeons emphasized recruiting patients to clinics so that they could pursue treatments that would elevate Mexico's status in the eyes of the international medical community. Nineteenth-century doctors, in Mexico and elsewhere, upheld different ethical standards when medical subjects were deemed insane, when they were sex workers, or when they were part of a marginalized or vulnerable group.

The Superior Sanitation Council and Welfare eventually found success with their proposal to expel las Hermanas, but only after another three years of further agitation. Between 1872 and 1874, the council cooperated with the president on major initiatives. One of these was the establishment of a national effort to forcibly detain and administer medical treatment to women, which will be explored at greater length in chapter 6. President Lerdo de Tejada himself ordered this policy in a letter to the president of the division of health projects, and the council's meeting minutes, cited earlier, showed their early support for the program.[58]

For decades, las Hermanas and other public health officials in Mexico had adopted a so-called French approach to sex workers. This amounted to tolerating sex work, offering sanctuaries in which women could voluntarily intern themselves, and undertaking a charitable attempt to "save" so-called fallen women. Mexico's Parisian-inspired permissiveness shifted drastically in March 1872, when the Superior Sanitation Council modified the previous prostitution bylaws and, after much ado, created the Sanitary Police force. The obligatory inspection of "public women" had officially commenced, and officials were required to keep stricter records regarding their status.[59]

The new measures proved to be a source of major conflict in the Hospital San Juan de Dios, where the sisters had been administering since 1844. In late 1873, the president of the Superior Sanitation Council wrote that las Hermanas posed two problems in that clinic: "the first is a question of science, and the other, a question of authority." He elaborated, "I refer to the hospitals, and I blame those who have tried to reform the administration."[60] In his view, no amount of reform would make las Hermanas more amenable to the goals of modern science; hence, those who had tried to reform the sisters and to cooperate with their administration were also at fault. Mexico's highest public health official believed that the religious women posed a scientific and administrative threat to the hospitals, and he refused to cooperate with them.

Related complaints escalated prior to the expulsion. In 1873, the federal government ordered that all patients must remain in the hospital until they passed an inspection by the Sanitary Police. In other words, Lerdo de Tejada now insisted that physicians had the final say in a key hospital matter. This essentially signified that las Hermanas could no longer treat patients autonomously, and that a trip to their clinic meant placing oneself in the state's hands. The hospital San Juan de Dios was the main destination for these women, some of whom were infected with venereal disease. Las Hermanas referred to such patients as "*arrepentidas*," or "repentant women." Whether they were regretful or not, it is clear that many had sought repeated treatment from the sisters, who permitted them to combine at-home treatment with hospitals stays. The new sanitary regulations of 1872 sought to uproot this managerial system by decreeing that women could no longer receive venereal disease treatment in their homes, but las Hermanas seemed unwilling to relinquish their control.[61]

Dr. José Ignacio Bravo y Alegre lamented the sisters' administrative autonomy in June 1873. In a letter to the governor of Mexico City and the president of the Superior Sanitation Council, he complained that Margarita García, a "repentant woman," had allegedly been reinfected with a sexually transmitted infection in the hospital after undergoing treatment. According to the surgeon, Margarita must have been infected in the hospital, because "las Hermanas de la Caridad agreed that they would only admit patients to the 'cured' wing after they received medical clearance from a physician."[62]

This underscores that although the sisters sometimes cooperated with doctors and sanitary agents, they still oversaw the movement of patients and made decisions regarding their admission to various wings of the hospital. Bravo y Alegre's comment indicated that medical professionals were sometimes obliged to conform to the sister's administrative practices instead of vice versa.[63] His comments concerning reinfection implied that Margarita continued to sell sex while in the hospital, and thus that las Hermanas could not be trusted to protect a sterile clinical environment. For Bravo y Alegre, the women's hospitals were like brothels—if not like convents, rife with secret homosexual vices. Of course, historians now know that patients still suffered from sexually transmitted infections after treatment because antibiotics had not yet been developed for the infections. Although doctors and others experimented amply with antiseptic and rinses and mercury-based injections, these were marginally effective.

Physicians frequently voiced this concern to the Superior Sanitation Council and the governor of Mexico City. Bravo y Alegre, for his part, accused las Hermanas of permitting women to "commit barbarities amongst themselves, such as masturbation, sodomy, and who knows how many other depredations." He claimed that these actions were an additional cause of reinfection after medical treatment, and he argued that because "these women do not wish to understand verbal reprimands—and probably never will—their behaviors are not easy to extirpate. But I believe that with enough vigilance, and rigorous punishment, they might be corrected, at least." For Bravo y Alegre and his contemporaries, the hospital needed stricter, masculinized oversight and harsher punishment than the sisters were willing to provide.[64]

At the same time, it is evident that surgeons did not have the autonomy to enforce punishments, despite their desire to do so.[65] "In my humble opinion," Bravo y Alegre continued, "they will only start to respect the authorities if we issue harsh punishments, because these people are so stubborn that they do not fear anyone."[66] He suggested fining prostitutes with a hefty sum of 210 pesos for refusing to comply with the demands of modern science. The public health commission agreed to this amount, and additionally ordered that if the women or their pimps could not pay, the hospitals were to transfer their debt to the government of Mexico City. The decision implied a means to ensure that the state backed the medical elite unless it wished to assume the financial burden for las Hermanas' presumed negligence.

Public health officials employed arbitrary and nebulous definitions of prostitution, meaning that not all women imprisoned in the Hospital Morelos were sex workers, despite that institution's reputation as a health care clinic for women who sold sex. The 1873 bylaws of the Sanitary Police stated, "Any woman who has been forcibly detained and held in the hospital shall be considered an unlicensed prostitute, and she shall be submitted to the correctional penalties as decided by the governor of Mexico City."[67] This vague definition led the Sanitary Police to reach the premature conclusion that some lower-class women were prostitutes, especially when they were seen in public places conversing with men. It also encouraged the stereotype that waitresses and maids would eventually succumb to prostitution because they presumably lacked propriety and financial resources. What was more, the bylaws provided the Sanitary Police with carte blanche by guiding the state to arrest women at will and by allowing the state to absolve itself via charges of prostitution.

When the president of the Superior Sanitation Council weighed in on the issue in 1873, he formally accused the sisters of releasing hospital patients without acquiring permission from a physician. As he lamented, "the medical diagnosis does not even determine the future of the patient after she leaves the inspection wing. Her final destiny is completely in the hands of the hospital administration, which is thoroughly incompetent in this matter." The president of the council continued, "We, as doctors, do not have—nor can we have—oversight over the administration, and we cannot claim such a responsibility because it has not been granted to us: not via law, nor bylaw, nor tradition."[68] Despite some attempts to reform las Hermanas' administrative style, the clinicians felt threatened by the sisters' authority.

The religious women, for their part, resented medical encroachment so much that they frequently discharged patients before doctors authorized them to do so.[69] One newspaper defended the sisters, claiming they freed dangerous women for their own safety. "Regarding the recent denunciations of las Hermanas de la Caridad in [the hospital] San Juan de Dios," the journalist contended, "there have been valid motives behind las Hermanas' decisions to release patients early, which always causes a scandal. Police have had to defend las Hermanas when patients attack them with scissors, sticks, and whatever else they find."[70] While it is possible that las Hermanas aided patients in staging violent rebellions against the new policies, it is also conceivable that officials sought to vilify patients who rebelled against forcible internment. Either way, the newsworthy scandal provided evidence of the sisters' resistance to medical protocol, and of their refusal to conform to coercive new sanitary regulations.

The Congressional Debate and the Expulsion

Mexico's most prominent politicians gathered on December 3, 1874, to debate the decree that would expel las Hermanas de la Caridad from Mexico. Large crowds of people filled the congressional chamber as well as the plaza and streets that surrounded the building. Common Mexicans were eager to participate in the hotly contested discussion, but politicians did not tolerate their presence for long; indeed, the attendees were so loud that police officers soon forced them out of the hall.[71] These debates are instructive for understanding the patriarchal medicalization of modern health care, as well as the ways in which politicians understood concurrent salvational and secular trends in medicine.

Congress members who favored expulsion overwhelmingly invoked gendered and anticlerical justifications to support their position. Senator Robles Gil, for example, began the debate by portraying the episode as a key element of Mexico's battle against the Catholic Church. He claimed that liberals did not necessarily seek to attack religious freedoms (which were protected under the laws of Reform) but rather to amplify the individual freedoms emphasized in the constitution. In his view, the attack targeted monastic vows and communal living, not the religious women themselves.

Senator Mateos had a stronger position against the sisters; but at the same time, he sought paternalistically to "rescue" them from Church institutions. While he claimed that the sisters utilized state money to fund their hospitals—which made them self-interested practitioners instead of charity workers—he also expressed incredulity and anger at the notion that they rejected a life of motherhood. "We weep when a womb dries up," he asserted, "because we recognize that the mother is all-important." By insisting that women were aberrant or pathological if their wombs withered from lack of use, Mateos made clear that in politics as in medicine, a woman's behavioral norms intertwined with her sexual and reproductive functions.

Patriarchal medical rhetoric drew from, and contributed to, nineteenth-century ideological currents that reified womanhood and femininity as essentialized traits tied to the domestic sphere. The more women agitated for equal civic and social incorporation, the more incentivized clinicians and politicians were to disseminate repressive ideas about their proper place in society. For prominent liberal politician Enrique Cabrero Mendoza, the sisters were themselves victims of a tyrannical and immoral Catholic Church, which encouraged young women to suppress their natural and patriotic urge to reproduce—and all to line the pockets of their wealthy directors. The senator concluded by asserting that "las Hermanas are enemies of liberty,"[72] while expressing the hope that all religious orders, priests, and nuns would be expelled from Mexico in the near future.

This discourse is striking because it bears little resemblance to the evidence presented here, in which public health authorities gained authority in Mexican hospitals with the support of President Lerdo de Tejada, and finally pushed to expel the nuns when they could no longer reconcile the sisters' practices with their own goals. Most public health officials shied away from an anticlerical argument for the ousting, even while they skillfully employed the political rhetoric of reform to gain control of the institutions. On a clinical level, however, their proposals aimed to discipline the sisters' patients so that they might become respectable citizens of a forward-thinking, liberal nation. Las Hermanas became intolerable when they blocked these efforts. This suggests that the sisters were acceptable as health care workers, and especially as nurses, but only when they acquiesced to patriarchal medical agendas. Some liberal politicians echoed this masculinist rhetoric by advancing the socially conservative notion that women were biologically and culturally predestined to be "angels of the home," and so that the Catholic Church was depriving Mexico of wives and daughters when it made them useful in the public sector.[73]

Other legislators opposed the expulsion. Congressman Rosas Moreno decried as absurd the allegation that las Hermanas had "strangled infants to death."[74] He disputed the accusation that they distributed "8,000 wretched pharmaceuticals per month," arguing instead, as another journalist did as well, that without them 10,000 people would be left without medical treatment and care.[75] Yet another writer suggested that their approach was humanitarian and confronted legislators with the following proviso: "You no longer support las Hermanas de la Caridad? Then kick them out. But we demand substitutes just as humanitarian, and no one is more humane than they."[76]

Martínes de la Torre, a congressman who opposed the expulsion of the sisters, disagreed that all religious instruction was monastic and recalled Benito Juárez's declaration that "the society of Hermanas should exist, because they are solely dedicated to charity. They themselves have said that their convent is the street, and the hospital room is their cell."[77] De la Torre emphasized that because the exception granted to las Hermanas was written into the constitution, neither the special commission nor congress were legally empowered to propose or decree their expulsion. Furthermore, the measure needed two-thirds of the vote, which it lacked by one ballot.[78] A lawful degree would have needed the approval of the legislatures of the states outside the Federal District, a measure that congress left unpursued.

In the aftermath of the expulsion, many speculated that Lerdo de Tejada failed to provide a tangible rationale for the eviction or that his true motive was occluded. Politicians' accusations against the sisters were vague—and sometimes nonsensical—with references to "frightful plots" and "perverse mysteries" concocted inside of "hellish conclaves."[79] In response, one journalist declared in exasperation, "We would like to see just *one* shred of evidence against las Hermanas de la Caridad!" This journalist was not particularly sympathetic to the sisters, given that his critique of them contradicted most depictions of their charitable work. "They fill a gap left by the government," he said, "even though they do not do so with a particular emphasis on solidarity. Whether they are here or not is a purely legislative question. But we demand to know: Why now, and only now? And if they are useful, why are they being expelled?"[80]

With this emphasis on "useful citizens," the journalist (who was quoting a senator) echoed the sentiment of *juarista* liberals, for whom secularization was a kind of constitutional Enlightenment that was compatible with

Catholicism. These liberals were more concerned with removing juridical and social obstacles associated with religion that prevented the creation of useful citizens. They aimed to move religious influence back to more tolerable levels, but not eradicate it from society. This explains why local and federal authorities jumped to their defense when the sisters first came under attack during the early 1860s.

There was also an epistemological clash driving the expulsion. On the one hand, for the patriarchal medical establishment, medicine bolstered moral and corporal policing; on the other, las Hermanas adhered to an evangelizing style, hoping to save people's souls while soothing their ailments. In the closing days of 1874 when the sisters surrendered the Hospital de San Juan de Dios—one of their most populous and establishments—large groups gathered to block the streets surrounding the clinic, and the crowd erupted in "shouts, laments, and expressions of sadness and pain." As a Mexico City newspaper reported, the "poor patients, enclosed in the hospital, banged on the windows and called out to their 'mothers' in the most shameful way." Among those "unhappy patients" were "women who hung from the windows of the establishment in true desperation."[81] Even journalists recurred to stereotypes about pitiable patients in need of salvation and viewed the expulsion as a battle between religious evangelization and scientific medicine.

On December 14, 1874, President Lerdo de Tejada issued a decree declaring that the state no longer recognized monastic orders or permitted their existence. He informed the governors of all Mexican territories that las Hermanas had been suppressed by executive order, and that they were to be deported if they did not abandon their institutions within thirty days. When 410 sisters were expelled from the port of Veracruz in January 1875, the public was scandalized by reports claiming that most of the deported women had Mexican citizenship.[82] While a liberal government might profess to take citizenship claims seriously, these stateswomens' loyalties fell on the wrong side of Lerdo de Tejada's regime.

As Jan Goldstein found in her research, nineteenth century French hospitals witnessed concurrent developments. By the 1870s French physicians vociferously protested religious influence in hospitals and alleged that las Hermanas de la Caridad were insubordinate to doctors. They agitated for the secularization of French hospitals, a process that was complete by the end of 1883. The laicization program "was justified by its advocates on several grounds: as tangible support for the 'scientific method' against the 'metaphysical spirit.'"[83]

Strikingly, then, in both Mexico and France, the expulsion of las Hermanas de la Caridad dovetailed with the politicization of the hysteria diagnosis; the creation of a positivist republican state; male medical authorities' desire to exert increasing authority over reproductive health care the paternalistic idea that women were incapable of practicing scientific medicine, and the political attempt to link reproductive health to high-level anticlerical politics. Notably, the process occurred in Mexico ten years earlier than in France, illustrating that Latin American nations often inspire European scientific trends instead of parroting them as is commonly assumed. Furthermore, it was in this context that postcolonial Mexico emerged as an important site of clinical practice, as reforma surgeons sought salvation through surgery, sometimes by addressing women's moral turpitudes via experimental ovariotomy and the medicalization of gendered behavioral norms.

CHAPTER FOUR

The Salvation That Only Medicine Can Provide

Therapeutic Abortion and Artificial Premature Birth, 1850s–70s

In 1871, an unmarried twenty-five-year-old woman in Mexico City sat alone, unsure to whom she could confide her predicament. Her parents knew that she had had a suitor several months earlier, but they did not know why she had stopped speaking with him. They were unaware that she had become pregnant unintendedly and faced a situation encountered by countless women throughout history who have sought to terminate an unwanted pregnancy. Historians of Mexico have pointed to a wide variety of means for this end. For example, in 1794 in Yahualica, Jalisco, a priest named Bartolomé Veles Escalante had impregnated a twenty-year-old mestiza, María Bustos. Wishing to terminate the pregnancy, Bustos's mother contacted an Afro-Mexican midwife named Barbara Morales and requested that she supply "remedies to bring [María's] cycle back."[1]

Almost eighty years later, in 1871, many Mexican women still used herbal remedies for menstrual regulation. But these were certainly not guaranteed to end a pregnancy, especially those of advanced gestation. Perhaps the young elite señorita had already tried herbs, or perhaps she lacked access to them. Maybe she was too embarrassed to ask her family for that kind of assistance. She knew that in earlier decades she could have left her child in an orphanage run by religious women, having seen the cradle-sized turnstiles in crechés throughout the city. Things were different now; some of the religious orphanages had been shuttered, and some had been converted into hospitals. Women's issues were national issues: the liberal reform laws had passed, and women were attending public school in higher numbers as well as spending more time in public life around the city.

The young woman was not sure where she fit in all of these changes, perhaps due to the degree with which she had been sheltered within the confines of her families' elite social world. Yet she could no longer deny that she had a problem, and she assented when her mother insisted that she confide in a trusted and confidential physician. She had fallen "prisoner to moral sufferings, which drowned her in a state of indescribable distress." Disturbed by the onset of this "nervous hysteria," the young woman's family requested medical treatment from Mexico's National Medical School.

For her house visit the school's professors elected Eduardo Navarro y Cardona, who had been studying obstetrics for one year. When he spoke with the young woman in her home, he discovered that she had "become a fallen woman" when her pregnancy began approximately seven months prior. Navarro y Cardona's sanctimonious narration belittled a woman of her class for falling pregnant without the economic backing of marriage. Apparently, in his words, her "seductor had abandoned her, after offering to tie himself to her with the sacred bonds of marriage." Perhaps the young woman did not know that the medical student was judging her while extracting information from her and that he would write a portion of his thesis about their conversation. Carrying a pregnancy was intimate knowledge for the girl, and she guarded the secret carefully before finally divulging her quandary "during a moment of intimate dialogue."[2] The young surgeon seemed to be her benevolent confessor.

Navarro y Cardona proposed that the pregnancy was "unnatural" because it had caused the woman intense moral suffering. He insisted that surgeons should force the expulsion of the seven-month-old fetus. Only by performing this procedure, "artificial premature birth," would they solve the "moral crisis" caused by childbearing. The young woman needed to be saved from her circumstances, Navarro y Cardona insisted, and this was a "salvation that only medicine could provide."[3]

The young woman had a therapeutic abortion, even though her doctors staunchly refused to refer to it as such. Instead, they called it "artificial premature birth," a term that blurred the lines between therapeutic abortion and the provocation of premature labor. Although Mexican surgeons referred to therapeutic abortions done in other countries by that name, they used coded language when it came to their own operations.[4] On one hand, surely they did not want to lose their licenses for having performed abortions. On the other hand, perhaps doctors referred to the surgery as "premature birth" because they truly did not perceive themselves to be performing abortions and hoped that the fetuses they extracted would miraculously survive. Perhaps that was what they told their patients and their patients' families as well.

Addressing this space of historical ambiguity and productive silence, this chapter highlights medical efforts to reconcile Catholic beliefs with the salvific termination of pregnancy. It argues that therapeutic abortion was spiritualized surgery as well, because it was a "salvation" for some pregnant women; indeed, as Navarro y Cardona wrote, it was one "that only medicine could provide." Physicians steadily asserted the benefits of secular medicine during Mexico's reforma while politicians sought to exert social and cultural authority over women. In previous decades the señorita likely would have confessed to a priest and left her child in the care of her family or religious women. Now her confession to an obstetrician meant that surgery influenced her fate.

THIS SEÑORITA JOINED DOZENS of other women in the late 1860s and early 1870s who underwent therapeutic abortions and artificial preterm births. Though Dr. Francisco Flores Troncoso noted that Mexican doctors provided surgical abortions as early as 1853, it has been the topic of very little historical analysis. The operation had many indications: pregnancy termination protected a woman in case of life-threatening conditions like eclampsia, and it safeguarded her social reputation in case of illegitimate pregnancy. Artificial premature birth was contentious because it seemed to always entail the death of the fetus and because it almost always ended in death for the childbearing person as well.

Abortions performed by other health care providers had similar outcomes in the nineteenth century. When herbal tinctures and teas failed to restore women's menses, pregnant people sometimes recurred to midwives, butcher-surgeons, other healers, or doctors to intervene in more invasive ways to remove fetuses. A range of cavity-opening, puncturing, and scraping devices allowed practitioners to empty the uterus, sometimes causing pain, hemorrhaging, and infection or sepsis. Wealthier and well-connected women could pay for more cautious and confidential care. Therefore it was not new for doctors to participate in the termination of pregnancy, although elite university-employed physicians carefully protected their reputations and therefore were not likely to write about offering abortion care.

Over the course of the nineteenth century obstetrics morphed from midwifery (and "male midwifery") into a branch of scientific medicine, affording practitioners increasingly intimate knowledge of public and private patients. Because physicians were often elites, they enjoyed connections with modern state builders who participated in the construction of social, cultural, and political institutions of surveillance and control. Political and social developments influenced the information that obstetricians gathered about their patients' sexual and reproductive habits, and vice versa. In the United States, the first anti-abortion campaign occurred in the 1850s and was led by a Harvard-trained physician, Horatio Robinson Storer. Storer gained the support of the fledging American Medical Association, and by the 1870s most US states had passed anti-abortion legislation. By the 1890s the Comstock Act criminalized the sale of contraceptive medications and devices, further heightening the criminalization of women's efforts to manage their fertility.[5]

In contrast, I have seen no evidence of a physician-led anti-abortion movement in nineteenth century Mexico. Instead there appears to have been a tacit acceptance of, and participation in, fertility control that was couched in a social-salvational rhetoric that alternately heeded, reformed, or rejected Catholic reproductive doctrines. Elite, privileged women had access to confidential in-home care, while marginalized and unruly women's reproductive decisions were much more likely to be made under duress or coercion from male authorities.

Meanwhile, the medicalization of reproductive health care and the visibility of abortion care appeared to influence Church doctrine. In 1869, Pope Pius IX (1792–1878) removed the long-held distinction between "animated" and "unanimated" fetuses, officializing the intellectual movement catalyzed by Cangiamila's *Sacred Embryology*. Pius IX's papal bull, published in *Apostolicae Sedis Moderationi*, declared that all products of conception were animated with a rational soul, and that abortion merited excommunication. The timing of Pius IX's insistence can also be viewed as a reaction to midcentury intellectual trends—including Darwinism and positivism—which had revolutionized inquiries into the biological and natural sciences. Pope Pius IX insisted on ideological coherence about the meaning of fetal life, and his message was clear: although some procedures and theories presented a threat to religious claims about the unborn, authorities should protect them at all costs.[6]

Just as with ovariotomy, medical notions about hysterical women and unnatural pregnancies cannot be understood outside of the context of Mexico's midcentury political climate, in which liberals aimed to laicize and liberalize state functions while curbing the influence of the Catholic Church on politics and society.[7] Nor can they be understood outside the heightening of papal authority over the Church—the force field in which debates over abortion took place. After the midcentury, the tenor of these debates had dramatically changed. The previous chapter examined the effects of state secularization on the management of hospitals and clinics in Mexico City. Building on that analysis, this chapter explores how salvational surgery shifted and persisted in the context of state secularization and medical modernization.

Following Hannah Arendt's definition, secularization here refers to shifts in medical epistemology within the context of an institutional separation of church and state, with a rise of a secular state that assumes the educational and welfare functions once performed by religious corporations.[8] There was also a decline in previously accepted symbols and doctrines associated with fetal life, meaning that Cangiamila's "spiritualized" idea of the fetus lost some of its influence because medical authorities de-emphasized and demythologized the mystical and supernatural elements of embryology. Though complicated, secularization evokes a rising interest in rationalization and observation by modern and state-based modes of inquiry, as well as a turn away from the metaphysical and toward more tangible (and especially legal) understandings of personhood.[9]

Complementing the last chapter's focus on the gendered dynamics of hospital administration during the reforma, this chapter contemplates medical epistemologies, medico-cultural training, and attitudes toward the role of "fallen women" in a liberal society. What this reveals is a transformation of the state's approach to managing women's social lives. Many liberal politicians and doctors believed that women had become morally downtrodden as a result of their subordination and exploitation at the hands of men and the Church. Some blamed women's continued subjugation on their exclusion from productive economic labor as well as the moral burdens and stresses of childbearing. For this reason, reforma physicians asserted scientific reconceptualizations of morality and moral authority. They envisaged morality as both an affective and biological quality, and as something that not only influenced sexual reproduction but also the status of the nation as a whole. Therapeutic abortion was salvational in the context of Mexico's reforma, but the politics of this salvation were complex.

This new approach to pregnancy termination was biologically deterministic inasmuch as it proposed that morality or lack thereof could be traced to the functions of specific organs. We have already seen the roots of these ideas in the previous chapter, in which Gabino Barreda put forward a Comptean positivist theory of the soul to explain hysteria and encourage ovariotomy. According to this school of thought, Mexico could only be improved with adequate amounts of investigation on—and reform of—those organs, as well as the fetuses that sometimes acted as organic lesions within.

Biological regeneration would complement social efforts to uplift women as reformed and productive members of the republic, curing them of the promiscuity or hysteria that made them idle, irrational, or pathological. There was an important class element at play, too: during the provenance of reproductive health care, middle-class and elite women seemed to receive more social, emotional, and spiritual counseling than their lower-class counterparts. They also had more ready access to the surgical termination of pregnancy, as is the case today. Doctors certainly emphasized their cautious treatment of elite women, even if this was an accident of the historical record because these women were overrepresented in obstetric writings from the era.

Women who underwent therapeutic abortions or medically induced premature labor in the early 1870s were very likely to find themselves in la Casa de Maternidad. In 1861 Benito Juárez re-established the institution, which had been founded during the late eighteenth-century as a confidential place in which illegitimately pregnant women could have a "secret birth." Although the majority of patients in la Casa came from the working class, the clinic became a place where women of varied social classes sought health care before, during, and after pregnancy.

Writing in 1888, the physician and medical historian Francisco de Asís Flores y Troncoso explained the state division between public and private clients: "When the hospital for the poor was recently founded," he wrote, "a wing was designated for those who made prior reservations, and only Spanish women were received there." Patients with reservations were permitted to occupy bed space in the facility up to one month before giving birth. In addition, a hospital regulation directed nurses to escort those with prior reservations through a separate entrance of the clinic and make their stay as comfortable as possible.[10] In its 1860s iteration, la Casa de Maternidad encouraged women to surrender their newborns to la Casa de Cuna, an orphanage for illegitimate offspring. The establishment and re-establishment of la Casa de Maternidad dovetailed with moralized efforts to reform women who had committed sexual transgressions.[11]

Authorities took particular measures to attract elite clientele to the new institution and to maintain their patronage. The clinic provided patients with clothes, diapers, pillows, blankets, sheets, and mattresses. The clients ate large amounts of bread, meat, cheese, tortillas, eggs, rice, and beans, and the cooks prepared their meals with salt, lard, and sugar. In fact, until 1886, la Casa spent more money every month on meat alone than on medications and equipment. Occupants of the clinic also consumed large amounts of chocolate, coffee, tea, wine, and even liquor.[12]

A state commitment to clientelism had the effect of convincing women to place themselves in surgeons' hands, to some degree at least. During the same time period in which Juárez had supported las Hermanas de la Caridad, the revamped Casa de Maternidad offered an alternative, nonreligious space for medical practice. This signaled an expansion of the state's interest in reproductive health care, as well as the growth of a professional medical corps. In this vein, it also demarcated the creation of two distinct "camps" of reproductive health care: religious, on the one hand, and state-run, on the other. Support for la Casa was particularly strong during Maximilian of Austria's Empire (1863–67). Maximilian's wife, Carlota, was especially influential in this trend because she was the head of the newly reinstated Junta Directiva de Beneficencia. She is rumored to suffer from hysteria, though archival evidence of this is sparse. Political influences in the clinic were thus varied, ranging from colonial, to imperial, to reforma-inspired.

Midcentury Miscarriage and Abortion, in Medical Theory and in Mexican Legislation

The interplay between mind, body, nerves, and pregnancy captivated midcentury obstetricians, prompting new speculation on centuries-old ideas associating women's emotional and sensorial experiences with their pregnancy outcomes. Many believed that embodied phenomena imprinted themselves onto reproductive trajectories, such that a woman who was burned might give birth to a baby with birthmark in the place of her injury; likewise, experiencing a strong or unpleasant emotion might interrupt pregnancy and provoke the birth of a "monster." In this vein, the previous chapter explored related ideas by delving into theories about the moral influence organs were understood to exert onto their host bodies.

Similarly, some midcentury physicians believed that emotional or moral disturbances could occasion an "accidental abortion," or in contemporary nomenclature a miscarriage. This was a common position influenced by humoralism. Evidence of its prevalence can be found in Francisco Menocal's 1869 thesis, which was entitled *El aborto en México* and was the first book-length study on miscarriage in modern Mexico. For his doctoral study Menocal interviewed sixty-eight women, finding that the majority of them had experienced some form of miscarriage. He insisted that it was an extremely common occurrence among Mexicans of all classes. As proof, he cited one interview subject who claimed that seven of her twenty pregnancies had ended in accidental abortion, though she had not elected to terminate any of the pregnancies. "It is difficult," he claimed, "to find a mother who has many children and who has not had an abortion [miscarriage]."[13]

Menocal explained that abortions were divided into two categories: they were either unpredictable accidents, or they resulted from a woman's emotional or physical predispositions or weaknesses. The "accidental" causes included those caused by food, drink, odors, and the effect of physical acts as small as yawning. Of sixty-eight women interviewed, Menocal claimed that twenty-three of their reported miscarriages could be attributed to such "unfortunate coincidences." Other accidents, in his view, were best classified as the result of negligent actions, such as excessive intercourse during pregnancy.[14] Even so, pregnancies were most frequently lost due to a woman's "physical and moral" deficiencies or her "predisposition." Menocal's examples of physical inadequacies were vague; in this category, he simply mentioned that his professors, Drs. Barreda and Jiménez, believed that "in Mexico, the most common cause of miscarriage is women's weak organization."[15]

For his part, Menocal seemed to believe that emotional suffering was a much more common cause of pregnancy loss. Explaining that accidental abortion of a pregnancy was often occasioned by "a strong emotion which is violent or unexpected, because it often provokes uterine contractions," he postulated that "other emotions might also influence a woman's soul, such as happiness, fear, rage, surprise, and extreme sadness." He continued, "We can attribute these causes to the considerable number of miscarriages that our capital city is sadly witnessing in this era. Above all, it seems likely that we can add hunger and misery to the list of moral emotions that afflict our unfortunate people."[16]

Although Menocal described many paths to pregnancy loss, medical publications saw little discussion of women who chose to terminate pregnancies, and surgeons very rarely wrote about surgical abortions. Reforma doctors in Mexico City even seemed to refrain from accusing midwives and other healers of providing abortion care, though it had been, and would be, a common accusation in the prior (colonial) and subsequent (Porfirian) eras. For Menocal and his colleagues, elected abortion did not seem to be a cause for concern, and medical or surgical abortion was not worthy of discussion. His only firm claim was that the success or failure of a pregnancy was related, above all else, to a woman's emotional and biological state. Although he declined to make social judgments or recommendations, Menocal implied that the nation would only attain happy and successful reproduction if its women were biologically sound, without any hysterical tendencies or other forms of moral weakness.

Mexican legislators seemed to agree with the implication of Menocal's work, which downplayed intentional or surgical abortion. In 1871, the criminal code of the Federal District treated the topic.[17] Article 569 (chapter 9) defined abortion as "the extraction of the product of conception, and the unnecessary provocation of its expulsion by any means." Article 571 stipulated that an *attempted* abortion could not be punished, and that only *completed* acts deserved punishment.

For the abortion of legitimate children, the criminal code proposed a two-year prison sentence both if the termination had been practiced intentionally and if the mother was an "honorable" woman who had also hidden evidence of her pregnancy. Prison time increased to three years if the woman was "dishonorable" or "had not hidden her pregnancy." The recommended punishment for abortion was five years in prison if the product had been conceived during marriage. However, this time was reduced by half if authorities proved that the fetus had already died before the termination of pregnancy. There was little emphasis on the spiritual life of the child—in fact, the 1871 penal code made no mention of fetal baptism, which was of extreme emphasis in colonial obstetrics. The 1871 penal code did not define "product of conception" or take a stance on when the unborn were ensouled. In opposition to the colonial preoccupation for fetal life, the focus had shifted toward adults, with a marked concern for the pregnant woman's social reputation.

There was an emphasis on affect, as seen in the clause that stipulated that abortion was a more serious crime when it occasioned emotional or physical harm. In cases in which a person caused an abortion by morally coercive or physically violent means, the penal code called for them to withstand a 25 percent increase in the prison sentence. Indeed, abortion was only "criminal" and punishable by a prison sentence when it had been brought about in a violent manner, unless the violent agent was the child's mother. In other words intentional abortion was not criminal unless the mother herself had terminated the pregnancy. In addition to decriminalizing "harmless" or "gentle" medical terminations of pregnancy, this clause emphasized that women had a moral responsibility to avoid harming their offspring with their own hands. The penal code's emphasis on gendered behavioral expectations corroborates Nora Jaffary's argument that late nineteenth century state officials became more fixated on infanticide than abortion.

Finally, this clause was important because it seemed to create a loophole within which doctors, pharmacists, barber-surgeons, and midwives could continue to provide abortions via the administration of herbal tinctures and by means of bloodletting as they had done in previous eras. In fact, the penal code explicitly declared physicians, surgeons, and midwives exempt from the clause that sought jail time for those found to be guilty of terminating a pregnancy by so-called violent means, although the legislation left "violence" undefined. If found to be guilty of "provoking a violent abortion," health care providers would lose their license for one year. Though they would not face legal prosecution, this might occasion the loss of their livelihoods or careers.

Although the 1871 code penalized abortion, it simultaneously marked the beginning of a liberalizing approach to the issue. As Alicia Márquez Murrieta has noted, because the 1871 law codified conditions under which abortion was acceptable, it initiated a trend by which physicians, lawmakers, and the public would "accept the practice of abortion in certain circumstances."[18] In many ways this positioned the 1871 penal code (and thereby the liberalizing Mexican state) in opposition to Pius IX's stance on the matter. Because papal authorities assumed that all products of conception were alive and ensouled from the moment of conception, they insisted that *any* kind of abortion—at any stage—would be a criminal act.[19] The papal declaration used a broad definition of abortion: it described the act as a termination of pregnancy whether it had been brought about by medicines, poisons, violence, or other forms of planned procedures, or by overbearing physical stress or labor. As we shall see, some Mexican doctors' surgeries seemed to challenge this stance, although they believed themselves to be delivering redemption in the process.

Hysteria and Artificial Premature Birth, 1870–74

The 1871 Legislative Code of the Federal District made several conflicting statements on the termination of advanced pregnancies. On the one hand, the law stated that termination of pregnancy was not allowed "at any stage of gestation." On the other hand, it stipulated that after the eighth month of pregnancy had commenced, "the procedure may also be called 'artificial premature birth.'" Article 570 clarified that artificial premature birth "should only be viewed as necessary when the continuation of pregnancy pose[d] the risk of death, and when two or more surgeons agreed that the procedure could save the woman." If practiced unnecessarily, artificial premature birth "should be punished under the same terms as abortion." However, as mentioned previously this became less consequential because obstetricians appeared exempt from these punishments. Although artificial premature birth does not appear to have received any scholarly attention in the historiography of Mexico, it comprises an important part of abortion history. Not only did legislators mention it specifically, but it also left some of the most provocative medical records in nineteenth century reproductive health care.

In 1873, Eduardo Navarro y Cardona published postcolonial Mexico's first writing on the topic. The report, an eighty-one-page doctoral thesis, described extensive clinical research on the subject and drew on the examples of more than one dozen such operations. Navarro y Cardona began his study by offering a definition of the procedure. "Artificial preterm childbirth," he explained, "involves the removal of a human egg when the product is already viable, both legally and physiologically, but before the natural end of pregnancy." In other words, the purpose of the procedure was to force the birth of a live child. Key to this definition was that the child was "legally viable," meaning that it was of such advanced gestational age that it could potentially survive outside of the womb. Although fetuses over six or seven months of gestation might be able to survive outside the womb, in practice they very rarely survived. Whereas abortions fell into two categories (intentional and unintentional), "artificial premature birth" was always considered "artificial," or "provoked," because it was always due to human action.

Obstetricians evoked three reasons for inducing premature labor. First, as Navarro y Cardona explained, the surgery became indicated when disease threatened the mother's life; because maternal disease could cause the fetus to perish, the logic went, it followed that a rational course of action was to remove a viable product before it too died of disease. The second rationale, rather vaguely described, comprised "any serious maternal condition during pregnancy." Finally, the third included "any obstacle or circumstance that could, at some point, prevent the *natural* progression and termination of the pregnancy." Tellingly, emotional disturbances were considered as harmful as disease or illness to the natural progression of a pregnancy.

It is notable that Navarro y Cardona and his colleagues reframed "natural" as a social and not scientific concept. The young medical student discussed this topic, explaining that his position was based on the views of Juan María Rodríguez, the head instructor of obstetrics and the director of la Casa de Maternidad. Navarro y Cardona wrote, "In obstetrics, we had always categorized preterm labor in two ways: natural and artificial. Yet, for Sr. Rodríguez, professor at our medical school, that manner of classification is flawed. He believes that no birth should be seen as "natural" (in the lexicological sense of the word, at least) when the child is born affected by some kind of illness or an uncommon provision."[20]

Rodríguez's radical new definition implied that a child incapable of surviving preterm birth may not have been so natural, after all. In this way he contested Enlightenment era writers who had focused extensively on the miracles of God and nature. For them, generally, so-called natural phenomena were both rational and miraculous. They obeyed the laws of nature, but humans possessed an obfuscated view of laws that were best understood by supernatural or Godly forces. Rodríguez and his students sought to shift both the meaning of natural childbirth and the meaning of natural reproduction itself. If diseased and unhealthy mothers and fetuses were unnatural or pathological, they should be exempt from the norms that governed normative pregnancy and childbirth.

Artificial preterm birth was a lengthy procedure, beginning with the ablation of the cervix via incisions with razors or knives. Subsequently, surgeons generally broke the amniotic sac, causing the uterus to begin to contract. A continuous stream of water in the uterus then augmented the contractions and flushed the child out of the womb. The procedure was generally combined with simultaneous bloodletting via the patient's ankles. This upset the woman's humoral balance, making childbearing inconvenient for the body and increasing the chances of a preterm birth. During the introduction of water, most doctors injected a syringe of holy water into the uterus to provide the unborn with a conditional baptism.[21]

Navarro y Cardona's text narrates nine cases of forced preterm childbirth. Perhaps the most dramatic and lengthily narrated story was that of twenty-six-year-old "Señorita X," whose identity was protected in medical writings. The student's concern for her public honor suggests that she was an elite woman. Yet his writing did not protect all aspects of her identity; he made clear, for example, that she was unmarried and had taken refuge in la Casa de Maternidad in 1870 at six months of pregnancy.

Señorita X disappeared from her parent's home without leaving any notice of her future whereabouts. For two months she remained in the hospital where she was hidden from her family. On July 21, the visiting day for "debt collectors, friends, and family of patients in the maternity hospital," her "disgraced mother suddenly arrived." As Navarro y Cardona commented, "it is easy to imagine what transpired during their conversation: the unfortunate mother had found her daughter in that refuge after looking for months. The waves of her justified anger reached their peak, and this caused her daughter to have a grave headache." Señorita X reportedly could not eat her afternoon meal, nor could she sleep well that night.[22]

The next morning, the medical students noticed that the patient's bed was in disarray. Furthermore, "she suddenly took on the appearance of an imbecile. Her gaze was vague and uncertain, and her eyes flitted around nervously. Her pupils were enormously dilated, and the muscles of her face twitched. She was indifferent to questioning, her nostrils flared, and she grasped her thumbs in her hands. The vaginal examination, which we decided to practice at this time, only seemed to increase her suffering."[23]

The students called in Dr. Ortega y Aniceto, who arrived shortly and noticed that the señorita's fetus seemed to be moving excessively.[24] They "catheterized the patient to examine her urine, which seemed to exacerbate her suffering as much as the vaginal examination." Although the doctors' mention of the young woman's discomfort seemed to indicate her resistance to the procedures, she was unable to refuse them. Perhaps she had not paid for her room in the clinic since she could no longer access her parents' money. Perhaps if she had been a paying patient she could have exerted more agency over her participation in the invasive examinations that disconcerted her. Although she was afforded some privacy in terms of her identity, her dishonorable behavior threatened the agency and privilege usually wrought by high-class patients. Having been disowned by her parents, this señorita seemed closer to being a ward of the state.

A urine analysis convinced the obstetricians that Señorita X did not have traces of metal or high sugar in her urine, nor was she displaying edema in the face or limbs. Nonetheless, Dr. Ortega y Aniceto proposed that she might have eclampsia and prescribed a purgative to induce vomiting. He also ordered eight ounces of bloodletting from her left arm.[25] Ortega y Aniceto then invited Dr. Eduardo Liceaga, head of the Superior Sanitation Counsel (Consejo Superior de Salubridad), and another prominent public health official, Dr. Casasola, to the hospital to discuss therapeutic options. "At this precise moment," Navarro y Cardona reported, "our own Sr. Rodríguez arrived at the clinic to study one of the patients, and he altered his plans to assist us with this case, instead." Rodriguez suggested administering a high dose of potassium bromate as a purgative, but Liceaga wished to provoke labor before giving the medicine: "He suggested that only after we emptied the womb could we turn to a more conventional method for these circumstances."[26] Ortega y Aniceto proposed to combine both methods by administering potassium bromate while dilating the cervix.[27]

When Señorita X was placed on a bed, covered in a thick cloth that "could not be penetrated by our gazes," the medical team began to introduce continuous currents of water through the vaginal canal and into the uterus to provoke labor.[28] They simutaneously pursued other interventions, as Navarro y Cardona explained: "The moment arrived when the surgeons believed that it was indispensable to extract more blood; following the bloodletting, Dr. Casasola did not waste time in applying chloroform." Because the fetal heartbeats had become almost imperceptible, the team of doctors "broke the amniotic sac and baptized the product," presumably, via the use of an intrauterine syringe. Then they "cut through the cervix by making incisions of six to seven millimeters, which permitted [them] to introduce the tongs of the forceps."[29] "Rodriguez, using incredible force, managed to extract a dead fetus."[30] Señorita X hemorrhaged, and, as Navarro y Cardona poetically described,

> In the midst of the fog of fatigue that enveloped us all, the angel of death beat its black wings in our place of refuge. Prisoners of an indescribable weariness (*desaliento*), we contemplated the last moments of this unfortunate woman, who succumbed to her destination without uttering a single complaint. Her tongue, torn to pieces, offered blood that mixed with froth, which spewed forth violently. Her eyes, seemingly fixed, were frightening. Her face, craned excessively to the left, twitched under the skin, and her limbs, splayed haphazardly about her body, did not respond even to the most intense of stimulations, including electric shocks.[31]

He continued, "All of our efforts were in vain. When we were all convinced of this fact, and when we knew that the terrible spectacle of death had forever wounded our pride, we silently prayed to the heavens for the soul we had seen suffer so. The clock marked ten hours and fifteen minutes of the night."[32] Navarro y Cardona's narration evinced a strong emotional response to the señorita's suffering and death. He and the other doctors seemed to soothe their own remorse and horror by engaging in meaning-making rituals like offering prayer, praising her bravery, recognizing that their self-conception as healers had been damaged, and rationalizing the cause of her death as unavoidable. Given that the señorita could have remained pregnant without being killed during surgery, it seems fair to surmise that her doctors were creating medical knowledge at the expense of her life. It is striking that the surgeons collectively emphasized her uncomplaining resignation to the fate of death. Although the circumstance was vastly disparate, their celebration of her sacrifice recalls Cangiamila's insistence that mothers be willing to die in order to protect or save their unborn children's souls. Both cases implied corporeally based castigation and the devaluation of pregnant people's survival.

Although Navarro y Cardona had opposed the induction of labor in this case, he denied that the course of treatment had caused the patient's death. Instead, he insisted that the "fatal conversation she had with her mother had provoked strong emotions, shame, and perhaps regret." This had "violently incited her nervous system," making her "hysterical."[33] He maintained that the bleedings were "justly recommended" in the circumstances, and that "inhalations of chloroform have saved the lives of many women in Mexico and abroad." In the end, he insisted, "None of our heroic and rational measures deserve anything less than applause,"[34] and he postured defensively with the following conclusion: "Perhaps our actions will not appease those who blindly follow the French school, but our national clinical procedures justify this operation, and before this evidence, all further discussion is unnecessary."[35] While it is unclear what Navarro y Cardona meant by "the French school," it is possible that he may have been referencing to las Hermanas de la Caridad because they were trained in France.

Although the next case had some elements in common with that of Señorita X, it also provided a strong indication that nonelite women received even more discriminatory care, in part because the obstetricians seemed unconcerned about protecting their public honor. This patient was also an unmarried woman who sought refuge in la Casa de Maternidad; however, the doctors did not use honorifics to reference her. Instead of calling her "señorita," they chose a more generic phrasing: "the woman." Not only was she unmarried, but she was so unfortunate in her personal circumstances that she arrived at the clinic alone, without any friends or family to assist her. Though she was reportedly quite young, her age was unspecified.

Navarro y Cardona's colleagues believed that this girl was experiencing "deception, fear, and shame" that resulted from her hysterical condition and "combined to eventually produce grave physical effects." It appears that her doctors did not approach her with much patience. Indeed, when she developed a nightly fever they rather hastily decided to provoke premature labor. In contradistinction to the previously discussed señorita, their decision did not require a debate among the highest public health officials in Mexico City. Surgeons bled eight ounces from the patient, applied chloroform, and brought on the expulsion of her fetus by lacerating her cervix and flushing the uterus with warm water. At this point they were able to extract the infant with forceps. Afterward, and as Navarro y Cardona mentioned flatly, "both were dead and the patient hemorrhaged profusely." Here, obstetricians appear to have declined to perform an intrauterine emergency baptism; similarly, there was no mention, as previously, of praying for the mother's and infant's souls while lamenting the patient's pain and suffering.[36] This is suggestive evidence that the patient's socioeconomic class and public reputation affected her treatment in several ways; it very likely influenced the ease with which doctors made the decision to intervene, and it may have influenced the spiritual care offered to the maternal/infant dyad. At the very least, social status certainly influenced the tone with which the young surgeon memorialized patients in his thesis.

While the previous two women sought refuge in la Casa de Maternidad to avoid their parents, some women underwent treatment in their homes. One such case was that of the twenty-five-year-old featured at the beginning of the chapter, for whom therapeutic abortion was the "salvation that only medicine can provide." Of this woman, Navarro y Cardona wrote, "La señorita ***, twenty-five years old and of a nervous constitution, became a fallen woman in February of 1871." Although she admitted her pregnancy to the medical student, her parents remained unaware of her condition. Interestingly, Navarro y Cardona maintained complicity in guarding her "medical secret." He believed it important to hide the pregnancy from the señorita's mother "so as to avoid prolonging the damage to the unhappy patient's mindset."[37] This student of surgery clearly understood unwanted pregnancy to be the source or cause of severe mental health disturbances for women. On the one hand, he overlaid his understanding with a biologized discourse about hysteria that denied patient's agency over their own health. On the other hand, he may have been ventriloquizing women's own words about the distress they experienced as well as their desire to end their unwanted pregnancies by any means possible.

Navarro y Cardona was willing to keep the elite 25-year old's medical secret, but he became increasingly nervous about the idea of intervening in her pregnancy. His trepidation, he said, owed to the unfortunate fate of Señorita X. This can be interpreted as additional evidence that a patient's social status influenced their treatment; perhaps it was because Señorita X was an elite woman that her providers were perturbed and dismayed by her agitation. In fact, their sympathy seemingly made them want to remove the product that caused her so much emotional distress. It seems likely that because Señorita X's parents had abandoned her at la Casa de Maternidad, obstetricians felt a certain amount of liberty in performing a surgery likely to result in death.

By contrast, Navarro y Cardona's trepidation accelerated in this case because the patient's family was monitoring his actions. Her parents were clearly invested in the outcome of the treatment, underscoring that this señorita was not an ideal candidate for an experimental surgery. Finally, her parents apparently did not know (or did not wish to admit) that she was pregnant, a fact that would make explaining the surgical induction of labor difficult.

With these factors in mind, Navarro y Cardona entered into a debate over several days with Dr. Rodríguez and other leading obstetricians at la Casa de

Maternidad. The physicians finally decided that they would provoke the señorita's preterm childbirth at the beginning of her seventh month of pregnancy.[38] They believed that this delay would not only give them time to explain to her parents that she was pregnant, but it would also increase the infant's chances of survival.

In the end, however, no operation was necessary because the baby was born prematurely and without intervention; both mother and child survived. Since labor is rare before the seventh month of pregnancy, one wonders if the young woman was taking oxytocic herbs or exploring other ways to induce contractions. This "happy case" prompted Navarro y Cardona to declare, "Anytime functional disorders embitter the life of a patient (when they should, ordinarily, be fleeting, tolerable, or remediable), that patient should consider undergoing forced premature childbirth after 210 days [6.9 months] of pregnancy. If we proceed with this understanding, we may save the lives of many mothers and children."[39]

The examined cases thus far have been those in which the woman's emotional or social circumstances were the only cited cause for the unnatural state of their pregnancies. Another group of women appeared in Navarro y Cardona's research. These patients, who suffered from physical disabilities and illness, complicate the nexus between artificially induced premature labor and therapeutic abortion. They also show that, even in the case of physical ailments, doctors sometimes viewed a woman's social or emotional health as a determining factor of her ability to give birth to a child. This is exemplified by the story of a thirty-eight-year-old woman who came to la Casa de Maternidad at eight months pregnant. Eclampsia was quickly threatening her life, as her blood pressure was so high that she had gone blind. Sadly, blindness was not the only problem she had faced that day: the pregnant patient had been present that morning when her young niece died in an accident. Doctors theorized that this trauma had caused a kind of hysterical shock and that her eyes had transmitted the moral affect to the rest of her body. Such mind-body disturbances meant that the continuation of natural pregnancy was impossible.

The medical team decided to let blood from the patient, but her family "stubbornly refused" to allow this and demanded a consultation with another doctor. That doctor "not only approved the bloodletting that had been ordered but declared that it should be repeated if necessary." The clinicians extracted ten ounces of blood from each of the woman's ankles, but several hours later she was comatose and nonresponsive.[40] When physicians proposed inducing premature labor in order to extract the infant, her husband, "Señor P," refused to consent to the operation. Eventually, however, they persuaded him to agree.[41] After debriding the patient's cervix with a razor blade, doctors flushed her uterus with a current of warm water; meanwhile, her family steadied her legs and watched as the medical team inserted forceps into her uterus and removed the infant. The "product," one medical student reported in his clinical observation, "arrived in an apparent state of death. I baptized it, and then I cut and tied the umbilical cord." The patient survived her stay in the hospital, but the student ended his case report with the dejected admission that he never knew how her health progressed because "the P. family did not call for [him] again."[42]

Another case involved a twenty-eight-year-old woman who Navarro y Cardona described as a housewife. She had "sufficient wit" to assist her husband with his multiple business negotiations, which had blessed them with substantial economic privilege.[43] Three miscarriages had plagued their marriage; perhaps, according to her surgeon, this was due to a "lack of space in the uterine cavity." One of Navarro y Cardona's professors explained to the woman's husband that due to her "poor structural build" she would "be exposed to grave risks if she did not undergo artificially induced labor."[44] Her family was reportedly alarmed, and they resisted the idea of an operation, demanding a second opinion. As such, the patient was transferred to Mexico City, where she was examined by five professors of medicine (Hernández, Licea, Iñigo, Olmedo, and Espejo y Larrea), who then gathered to discuss her in another doctor's home in Toluca. Once again, when it came to operating on wealthy women, the nation's leading surgeons deliberated at length; in this case their conversation even appeared to become a social event. Although most of them agreed that the procedure was indicated, two abstained. Eventually they decided to terminate the gestation of the then seven-month-old fetus.

On the morning of August 28, 1870, they began to fill the woman's cervical cavity with sponges of increasing size, which was meant to dilate the orifice and provoke premature labor. This task was not complete until the night of August 30, which indicates both the difficulty of accelerating that process, and the additional caution that they displayed in caring for the patient in question. Once the doctors were able to break the amniotic sac, they reportedly "encountered the opportunity to apply the forceps." "Even after the instrument was in place, it did not begin to work until, after many difficulties and much tractions," the medical team "succeeded in extracting the child." As

Navarro y Cardona wrote, although the fetus was born alive, "he bled profusely from the mouth and then died."[45] The patient also experienced a hemorrhage, but ultimately she survived the ordeal.

In 1871 this patient was in search of pregnancy care again. She and her husband met with Navarro y Cardona and explained to him what had happened during her previous pregnancy. By the end of the conversation, the woman and her husband decided to trust Navarro y Cardona, and they asked for his assistance during this pregnancy. When the young doctor examined the *señora,* he declared that her "slow movements and weary demeanor revealed the interior of a person accustomed to suffering—a person with a Christ-like resignation to her sad fate." Perhaps this comparison to Christ was a conscientious effort by Navarro y Cardona to inflect religious overtones onto her therapeutic regime. Upon "placing the patient on the edge of the bed and practicing the vaginal examination," the medical student reported, "I noticed that although her vaginal-uterine canal did not present any abnormalities, it was true that her pelvis had a deformity which demanded the provocation of premature labor." "However," Navarro y Cardona reflected, "I was fearful of committing a lamentable error, and so I solicited the advice of my mentor, Dr. Rodríguez."[46] With the permission of this patient and her husband, the medical student brought Dr. Rodríguez to their home.

Dr. Rodríguez noted that the woman had a considerable number of osteopathic or bone-related deficiencies, including osteomalacia or softening of the bones, which typically occurs due to a vitamin D or calcium deficiency. The condition tends to cause luxation or dislocation of the femur bones, benign outgrowths of cartilaginous tissue on a bone, and pelvic osteosarcomas, or cancerous tumors of the bones. The patient certainly had significant health ailments. The medical student and his mentor concluded that "the poor patient's health problems were deemed to be considerable obstacles to the natural progression of the pregnancy."[47]

As with other women, Navarro y Cardona and Rodríguez initiated surgery by injecting warm water into the patient's uterus. This was advantageous, Navarro y Cardona explained, because it was "as simple as it was inoffensive."[48] Once the chloroform had "taken effect to the degree that they could operate," they began to employ forceps in their efforts to extract the fetus.[49] Dr. Rodríguez made an "enormous effort" to introduce his hand into the depths of the patient's uterus, at which point he was able to grab one of the feet. "Pulling this as far out as he could, he baptized the infant as soon as possible. After a great deal of difficulty we finally had the child in our arms, although it had apparently deceased by that point."[50]

Although the provocation of premature birth clearly had poor outcomes for mother and child, Navarro y Cardona cited the above case to underscore the therapeutic necessity of the procedure. He also made the following statement, which cast dissenters as outsiders and traitors to the national tradition: "Those who do not approve of an operation that intends to save the lives of mothers in circumstances that endanger their lives and those of their children, must, from this day forward, explain and justify their negligence as practitioners of medicine in Mexico."[51]

In contrast to medical sources from previous and subsequent time periods, writings about therapeutic abortion highlighted important moments of dissent from patients. For example, Navarro y Cardona insisted, "We must not consider the patient's reservations, which should have dissipated in light of countless wise suggestions that could have been made to dissuade her from her fatal end, and not the least of these were the conclusions that we knew of—that the most eminent doctors from London concluded that artificially induced labor is ethical, moral, safe, and useful."[52] He continued, "We can definitely affirm that we have secured the right to perform this operation, and that it has been employed almost every time it has been necessary."[53] Perhaps it was a Freudian slip when he referenced patients' own misbehavior as causing their "fatal end." Finally, it is interesting that the doctor phrased the medical prerogative to operate in rights-based language.

Doctor's efforts to address some women's moral distress and disreputable behavior required them to argue that women's "unnatural" emotional, physical, or social status transformed their pregnant bodies into an "unnatural" state. Only by removing the product of conception, doctors argued, would these women again be able to again enjoy natural levels of emotional and physiological health. In this way, proponents of the operation went against a major point that undergirded the earlier, religious use of the caesarean operation—namely, the idea that saving the spiritual life of the fetus was more important than the corporal life of the mother. An insistence that ensoulment occurred at conception—and that the spiritual and corporal salvation of the unborn should be prioritized over the life of its mother—was no longer obviously epistemologically embedded in rationales for reproductive surgery in the 1870s. Although postcolonial doctors assumed the roles previously occupied by priest-surgeons and began to extract and baptize infants, their focus was no longer on this ritual alone. Whereas priests sought to extract preterm infants explicitly for the purpose of baptism, reforma doctors endeavored to extract preterm infants to alleviate their mothers of the alleged "emotional stress" of pregnancy, thereby allowing them the opportunity to become respectable, reformed, and useful citizens of the republic.

Experimental reproductive medicine gave physicians the chance to prove that morality could be defined and improved by scientific inquiry. Because obstetricians saw sociology as a science that could be influenced by biology, reforma doctors argued that the performance of oophorectomy could improve the moral (mental) status of individual Mexican women, and thus of the nation. Likewise, the premature removal of a product of conception could restore a woman's moral state. Interestingly, the Mexican secularization of reproductive science did not stem from European scientific discourse. Much of it was internally generated, was a response to prior Catholic understandings of those topics, and both responded to—and was bolstered by—political developments during Mexico's reforma.

Resultingly, these discourses gained particular strength in applicability: all women, regardless of racial, class, or social standing, could be too hysterical for pregnancy. So emotionally or morally weak that they were unable to support a pregnancy, the termination of their pregnancy seemed foretold, whether by accidental or intentional means. A range of women fell under the purview of this new science, from elite and impoverished patients, to señoritas (women with honorable or virginal public reputations), and sex workers. Modern obstetrics staked claim over the reproductive potential of women who hid illegitimate births to protect their honor, much like religious authorities had done in the eighteenth century. Surgical termination must have been a welcome option for some women. Nonetheless, the operation buttressed paternalism in reproductive medicine when realized under salvational dictums. When pregnancy termination was a choice, it was a constrained one.

It is important to underscore that the re-branding of abortion as artificial premature birth took place within the context of heightened masculine influence over fertility control options. Women had traditionally recurred to midwives, barber-surgeons, apothecaries, and female relatives for abortions. Those requesting pregnancy termination from university-trained physicians were much more likely to be elites receiving treatment in their homes. Complicated, difficult, or intrusive abortions had always carried the risk of death; sadly, even the most qualified surgeons had dismal survival rates for artificial premature birth, perhaps worsened by their zealous use of razors and forceps. The cases in this chapter show the persistence of some class-based surgical agency. But most patients could not exercise such agency: doctors decided when to end their pregnancies, and under what rationales. Sometimes they held long deliberations among themselves before agreeing on an intervention, but they generally did not document consulting their patients in the course of those conversations. When physicians did seek approval to pursue surgery, they often requested permission from a patient's husband or family, underscoring that a woman's social status depended in part on her guardians' resources and advocacy. Women who were alone or abandoned by their families became particularly vulnerable to aggressive intervention. When doctors requested male family members' acceptance of procedures such as bloodletting and pregnancy interruption, those family members often initially refused. Sometimes families exerted agency by choosing to withhold their future business from elite surgeons. Even upon a family member's reluctance, however, medics seemed to always proceed with further treatments. This represented an epistemological shift consistent with heightened patriarchal state and scientific interest in women's reproductive lives. As the next chapters will show, late nineteenth-century iterations of salvational surgery would no longer so forthrightly pit mothers and fetuses against each other, but instead together against the state.

Part III

Racial Science and Surgical Salvation

CHAPTER FIVE

A Uterus in Our Hands

Obstetric Racism, 1869–1910s

A fetus, in the hands of science, is possibility manifest. It is now up to doctors to influence politicians—and all other authorities—to rise up like Moses and Mohammed in support of the doctrine of science: first, with the goal of punishing the sinful; and then, toward the moralization, progress, and unity of the masses.[1]

—Ramón Estrada, medical student of the Escuela Nacional Preparatoria

In April 1911, a heated debate took place in Mexico City's Academy of Medicine.[2] *El Imparcial* reported on the incident in an article entitled "Elongated Head Shape Predominates in Mexican Children." The newspaper relayed that a foreign Dr. Landa delivered a talk about the problem of small cranial measurements among Mexican children, claiming they signaled racial degeneration. Dr. Nicolás León, one of Mexico's most prominent obstetricians, answered that Landa's conclusions were "perfectly useless." Two others agreed with Dr. León's denunciation of Landa's cranial measurements. One, Dr. Mejía, suggested that small cranial capacity in Mexico did not indicate subnormal intelligence among the population.

According to Mejía, the problem lay elsewhere. Mexican skulls were not inherently small, he said, but they were forced to elongate during birth because "the pressure of a small pelvis obliges the head to take a certain shape." Dr. Landa conceded that "that he has very little experience in the area, but in general, the idea seems accurate." Craniometry figured prominently in this scene in which a U.S. doctor challenged Mexicans on how their youth measured up to international standards. In response, Mexican obstetricians emphasized the extent to which they believed that insufficient maternal structure was harming and deforming Mexico's prospects. Such claims stemmed from, and took part in, the transnational practice of evolutionary anthropology, a conceptual apparatus that systemized dominion and dehumanization by typologizing the modern world according to hierarchies of races, nations, cultures, genders, and abilities. This chapter offers an intellectual history of how racial science affected Mexican obstetric care in the late nineteenth century. The next chapter will turn to an examination of patients, with emphasis on how they came to be interned in Mexico City's clinics, and how their health care changed over time.

Drs. Landa, León, and Mejía's sentiments were also inspired by national and transnational politics. In the early decades of independence, the postcolonial state initially maintained a commitment to monarchy and institutional Church privileges such as property holding. As described in chapters three and four, liberalism swept the nation by the 1850s, in part due to Indigenous and other marginalized communities' demands for state-based rights. The liberal reforma prevailed. Yet liberalism transformed over the course of the last two decades of the nineteenth century; we already saw the origins of this transformation with President Sebastián Lerdo de Tejada's approach to women suspected of sex work and others imprisoned in asylums. As historian Charles Hale has shown, the ideological tension between the classic, rights-based liberalism of the reforma and the authoritarian-style positivism of Díaz's cabinet of elite technocrats (*los científicos*) became a major source of conflict between scientific autocrats and the late nineteenth century Porfirian regime.[3] This period, which coincided with the Gilded Age in the United States, was a time of massive industrialization and capitalist exploitation of people of color and marginalized classes.

In Mexico this time period was the Porfiriato: the highly centralized dictatorship of Porfirio Díaz, which spanned 1876–1911. Like President Benito Juárez, Díaz was also of Indigenous descent, and he was also a war hero who had fought in Mexico's liberal reforma. But unlike Juárez, Díaz's brand of liberalism morphed into authoritarianism. A certain amount of authoritarianism was necessary, he believed, to maintain his dictatorship via the manipulation of electoral results which allowed him to stay in power. Díaz needed a strong government in order to attract and keep the foreign investment that would allow him to build Mexico's technological, educational, and infrastructural potential. He simultaneously sought to whiten Mexico's cultural and biological makeup by incentivizing European and American immigration via "colonization" schemes, which offered foreigners land to own and cultivate. Crops like henequen and coffee began to boom with additional investment, and some mining efforts redoubled. Forced into debt peonage, Indigenous and Black Mexicans did not receive a fair share of the wealth they were creating. Targeted wars against certain Indigenous groups persisted, too. Just one example can be found in the Porfirian state's incessant warring with the Yaquis in the north, which led to the deportation of some rebel Yaquis to the Yucatán peninsula on the Gulf Coast.[4]

Some of the progress gained by marginalized communities during the reforma receded as large multinational corporations usurped their land. Díaz fixated on another kind of evolvement: development, made possible by scientific rule as a path to modernity. Colossal investment made Mexico City a dazzling metropolis and a playground for the elite investors who came for business. A robust economy of sex work arose, in which the city had no shortage of brothels, bars, and entertainment for wealthy and powerful men.[5] This meant that the lower classes needed to be theorized, understood, dominated, and controlled in the name of progress. Reproductive health care formed a core part of these research efforts.

Medical racism in Mexico intensified in the 1880s, as President Díaz increasingly influenced the ENP's curriculum and personnel. Díaz was apparently preoccupied with reproductive politics, with particular emphasis on whether Mexican women's pelvic capacities were normal or pathological. This was partly because his wife, Carmen Romero Rubio, had fertility problems and never had birthed live children. It thus sadly suggestive that when a student wrote his thesis about stillbirths, he dedicated it to president Díaz himself. Carmen and the president's relationship suffered and allegedly led Díaz to fixate on the idea that her pelvis was deficient, malformed, and incompatible with childbearing. To make matters worse, his first wife and true love (who was also his niece Delfina) had died in childbirth after she had successfully borne seven children.

As the Porfiriato progressed, scientific politics effectively reshaped higher education and led doctors to conclusions like those expressed in public in April 1911. This chapter and the next track how elite preconceptions of race, class, and gender influenced medical practices in public hospitals during this time, and how positivist thought impacted state relations with marginalized groups by embedding racial and social prejudices in purportedly neutral bodies of scientific knowledge.[6] It is widely acknowledged that positivism, as a philosophy of governance, provided the theoretical core of policy assumptions for the Díaz dictatorship, and that policy-makers in his regime held increasingly deterministic and prejudicial views over the course of the regime.[7] Díaz's científicos worked to place themselves at the core of the modern Mexican elite, and they were able to occupy the political offices they had long sought by the 1890s.[8] The científicos believed that political regimes paralleled stages of human evolution and that Mexico, as a matter of positivistic fact, required a strong state to impose modernization on degenerate communities in order for democracy to function eventually. To bolster social and political agendas, los científicos turned to comparative anatomy, and especially phrenology and pelvimetry, to classify human groups.[9]

Porfirian obstetricians constructed a scientific ideology they called pelviology (*pelviología*), which used comparative biometrics—pelvimetrics (*pelvimetría*)—to suggest that racialized Mexicans and their descendants had "defectively organized" bodies that harmed their reproductive potential.[10] This claim was measured through the following lines of continuity. First was the growing acceptance of the idea of racial and class hierarchies. Second was the belief that such deficiencies could be remedied by scientific knowledge and technical interventions. And third was the strengthening of masculine medical epistemology couched in the rhetoric of national progress. A main argument is that "organization" became a catchphrase with which to diagnose cultural and biological forms of "backwardness," and that doctors' fixation with the concept of "organization" allowed them to map Catholic metaphysical claims onto a positivist framework that viewed the body as the base of material and moral functions.[11] Like during the reforma, behaviorally regenerative surgery was inspired by the impulse to replace religion with science. Even as medical literature became secularized, obstetric racism retained its claim to moralized dogma.

As writings about pregnancy shifted from religious to racialized in the late nineteenth century, cultural claims over reproduction took on stark new formations. Ramón Estrada, the doctor who introduced this chapter, conveyed this sentiment most perfectly in his unsettling proclamation that "a fetus, in the hands of science, is possibility manifest." He urged doctors to influence politicians in the service of two goals: "punishing the sinful" and achieving "moralization, progress, and unity of the masses."[12] Couched in the rhetoric of progress, a moralization crusade played out on the bodies of some of Mexico City's most vulnerable women. The themes in this chapter appear in some fifty medical studies published between 1877 and 1911. The studies were rich not just in number, but for how they documented clinical practice and patient volume. Professor Nicolás San Juan, for example, reported in his 1880 study that he had personally examined and collected notes on an average of more than 2,500 patients per year for three years. He totaled 8,612 examinations in all.[13] If these numbers are accurate, he must have examined six to ten patients per day during his time in the clinic. This is important because it means that the forms of therapeutic trialing that will be discussed here affected tens of thousands of patients over the course of the Porfiriato.

From "Happy Births" to Monstrosity and Deficiency

In 1869, Juan María Rodríguez wrote *Brief Notes on Obstetrics in Mexico* because he aspired to become director of the Escuela Nacional Preparatoria (ENP) obstetric clinic.[14] Unlike the student dissertations I will discuss later,

Rodríguez did not write about one specific area of obstetric research and practice. Rather, he described his experiences with rare and challenging cases involving tumors, cysts, and hemorrhages that interfered with childbirth. Of the seventeen cases Rodríguez described, he only once mentioned the use of chloroform and forceps. The fact that within just twenty years these two medical interventions came to be widely employed—and became sources of intense contention and debate—reveals the degree to which obstetric practices changed over the course of the Porfiriato.

Rodríguez's publication was historically significant due to his discussion of dystocia, which refers to difficulty in labor and birthing. Subsequent clinicians would argue that dystocia was a common problem among Mexican women due to their small pelvic measurements, yet Rodríguez, in contrast, affirmed that the great majority of births in Mexico were "natural and happy."[15] Likewise, his publication did not attribute biological differences to nationality, class, or anatomy (as many that followed would), although his discussion of midwives certainly contained a moral rhetoric indicative of nineteenth-century politics. Declaring that midwives were "incapable women, without education, and possibly devoid of morality," he claimed that, naturally, they "degraded and corrupted" the "art" of attending childbirth.[16] Midwives knew they were marginalized; as Jaffary tells us, in 1892 midwives "protested against the regulation that the Consejo Superior de Salubridad has imposed on them, which they [saw] as tyrannical.[17]

As a last note, Rodríguez's eleven-year employment as head of the ENP's obstetric clinic demonstrates how limited the medical elite was in nineteenth century Mexico. One individual could vastly impact the discourse of medical practice and training. Through the 1870s, obstetric discourse was only marginally shaped by explicitly racist rhetoric. Although Rodríguez may have exhibited the elitist, gendered prejudices of the Porfiriato, he had not yet developed a positivist method of measuring anatomical deficiencies, as students of the ENP's obstetric clinic in the 1880s would.

Rodríguez's influential writing shows that theories about race and degeneracy were not just fixated on women's ability to birth fetuses but also their ability to gestate them. The doctor contributed extensively to medical discourses about monstrosity, which reflected and reified bio-social theories about personhood, race, heredity, and evolution. Historians Nora Jaffary and Frida Gorbach have extensively analyzed the science and culture of theories about monstrosity in Mexico, demarcating how the pathologization of reproduction occurred in tandem with heightened popular scrutiny of women's reproductive choices. By the 1890s, doctors and the press described monstrous fetuses in clearly racialized terms: as animal-like, degenerate, and so horrific that mothers needed to be protected from seeing them. This was a marked change from the pride, wonder, and curiosity that late Bourbon creoles had displayed toward abnormal fetuses.[18]

Jaffary shows that Juan María Rodríguez, writing in the 1870s, viewed monstrosity under a Lamarckian rubric: as an acquired condition that was environmentally driven and thus potentially within a "spectrum of normalcy" and regenerable.[19] By the 1890s, the medical view of monstrosity was exemplified by doctors Ramón Ramírez, who participated in the construction of the national *salón de teratología,* and who "adopted as a central premise the examination of whether the country's production of monstrosities demonstrated that the nation belonged to the racially normal stock of Europe or whether such monstrosities represented a pathological variety of the species."[20] Writing about the twentieth century, historian Frida Gorbach considers obstetricians who believed to have found evidence that Mexicans were a monstrous race as a whole.

This section analyzes monstrosity's shifting relationship between racialization and concepts of personhood. It does so by examining Juan María Rodríguez's writing about the birth of a monstrous fetus in 1869, with particular attention to debates about fetal personhood as well as Mexican women's anatomical structure and womb-based pathologies. Gabino Barreda had asked Rodríguez to write the treatise; once finished in 1870, Rodríguez read it aloud before the entire medical school. Although the subject of Rodríguez's treaty was a "monstrous" fetus, born in Durango in 1868, his real intervention was to propose a Mexican school of embryological thought. His lecture argued that the weakest Mexican products of conception perished in the womb and that some even disappeared entirely, or "regressed" to nonhuman matter.

The product of conception born in Durango was quite distinctive in form, as it appeared to have a humanlike head and appendages. The epidermis, apparently incomplete, opened to reveal an assortment of growths attached to the main body; the protrusions appeared to be four additional fetuses. The fetus was so "monstrous" that it attracted the attention of foreign doctors, including two from the United States who reportedly "made a concerted effort to purchase" them. Rodríguez rejected their offer, citing the monsters' patrimonial value.[21] He wrote: "calculating that my country was also worthy of possessing such an interesting monstrosity, I resolved to prevent them from doing so. In the end, I made them agree to only take with them a dozen photographs, which they paid for." For Mexico's foremost obstetrician, the fetus was particularly instructive because the "monsters" "offer[ed] a fantastic opportunity to contemplate the prolongation of an anomalous embryonic state." The state was "anomalous" due to its lack of humanistic development. Rodríguez explained, "It is undeniable that one of the headless monsters was reduced almost to the condition of a crustacean or an insect. Even if this is not a novel finding, it certainly proves that the use of reason among organized beings is dependent upon the stage of development that they are able to reach."[22] The phrase "organized beings," presumably meant to convey "beings with a human organization."

Rodríguez believed that an unborn product was only human when its cells divided into five distinct regions of bone development: cranial, neck, thorax, lumbar, and sacrum/coccyx. He explained, "Immediately following [the development of those bone structures] the organs begin to develop. These [organs] correspond not only with bone structure, but also with the senses, respiration, circulation, digestion, and reproductive function." The anomalous products of conception showed no sign of this bone development. They were originally destined to become human, Rodríguez explained, but instead underwent a "regressive" process of degeneration that transformed them into "parasites" (*parásitos*), "mullosks" (*moluscos*), and "shells" (*conchas*).[23]

The above discussion exemplifies Rodríguez's continued focus on the skeleton as the key marker of human development—in his words, "regressive development is notable, above all else, in the skeletal system." The doctor believed that monstruous fetuses underwent transformations in which the bones in their head shrank in size, altered in form, or disappeared. "On some occasions," he argued, "the entire product [*producto*] disappears entirely, and in its place is left just a bit of serous liquid. This—most extreme—form of fetal regression is called liquefaction of the product."[24] Those lacking the evolutionary potential to become a "monster" disappeared entirely. In contrast, multiple factors affected the monstruous fetuses from Durango. According to Rodríguez: "a lack of nutrition, a compression of the uterus, or both at once, provoked the retrogression that modified the fetuses under examination."[25]

Heavily influential here was the Meckel-Serres theory of recapitulation, which had its origins in the 1820s and posited that the embryos and fetuses of mammals assumed the appearance of that species' past evolutionary forms. Accordingly, the unborn proceeded through chronological replays of the species' history during various stages of in-womb development. Recapitulation theory is commonly summarized as "ontogeny recapitulates phylogeny." Ontogeny refers to the development of an organism, and phylogeny refers to the development of a group, or species. This became known as the biogenetic law, which held that researchers could study evolutionary relationships between taxa by comparing the developmental stages of embryos of organisms from those taxa. Evidence from biogenetic law supported the theory that all species on Earth share a common ancestor, and that one could explain fetal development (in particular, the early similarity between embryos of different species) by examining fetuses as representations of evolution by natural selection.

Rodríguez's interpretation echoed most closely the German scientist Ernst Haeckel's 1866 take on the Meckel-Serres theory.[26] Because Haeckel argued that evolution was progressive, he also endorsed Jean Baptiste Lamarck's theory of acquired characteristics. Lamarck (1744–1829) theorized that organisms could acquire or alter traits based on the use or disuse of their anatomical parts, and that parents could transmit acquired or altered features to their offspring. Lamarck's ideas competed with Darwin's theory of natural selection as the mechanism for evolution. Haeckel, for his part, incorporated both notions into his theory of biogenetic law. He lent credence to the idea that higher order organisms had progressed through the "lower life form" phases during normal embryological and fetal development.[27]

Haeckel proposed that fetal deformities result when development prematurely stops, and that such deformities characterized lower life-forms. Although many mid-nineteenth-century biologists were intrigued by the notion that ontogeny recapitulates phylogeny—and the vast majority believed this to be true—Haeckel's beliefs fell on the outer extreme of this intellectual current. Haeckel, who was born in 1834 and who died in 1919, was one of Germany's most famous Darwinists. He was also infamous for his stark racism. While most mid-nineteenth-century scientists believed that *Homo sapiens* belonged to one species, Haeckel proposed that human groups belonged to twelve species and four separate genera. He believed that the "inferior" races would ultimately be exterminated in the struggle for existence among humans—by colonialism, war, or natural selection.[28]

Rodríguez apparently found Haeckel's racist theories convincing. However, Frida Gorbach points out that it was not until the twentieth century that obstetricians would extend racist theories about Mexicans to assert that the Mexican "race" was monstruous as a whole.[29] Though Rodríguez was working earlier, at the start of the Darwinian turn, he emphasized that some Mexican children were losing the battle to natural selection. The doctor asserted that the transformation of the unborn, from a simple-celled organism into a complex animal or human, did not just mirror an evolutionary process; rather, in-womb transformation was an evolutionary process, and fetal degeneration represented evolutionary failure. According to Rodríguez, this degeneration could be identified when fetuses that should have progressed and become human regressed and became "monstrous" or "crustacean" creatures instead. Whereas Enlightenment Catholics had insisted that monstrous fetuses were unequivocally human, Rodríguez disagreed. For him, monstrous forms of regression seemed to nullify the potential humanity of some unborn products of conception.

For Rodríguez, the successful "evolution" of embryonic cells depended on their growing conditions. He insisted that when the unborn became monsters in Mexico, it was due to excessive uterine compression. He wrote that compression was a likely influence in the "development of the three parasites." In one passage, the doctor referred to the products of conception as "parasites" and then, in the next sentence, called them "embryos." He gendered the embryos as female, seeming to underscore their alleged weakness. He suggested that "because the embryo was enclosed in an egg that could not widen freely, it became impossible to overcome the obstacles around her." It was this compression that prompted "the moment in which monstrosity began."

Rodríguez viewed the products of conception as if they were stuck in conflicting forces of development. He theorized that uterine compression acted as a centripetal force that directed energy toward the center of the organism, while fetal growth exerted a simultaneous but oppositive centrifugal force. He wrote, "At each step, these competing forces exerted conflicting influences: at the same time that some influences interrupted the evolutionary process, others provoked the retrogression of development."[30] By theorizing that uterine compression interrupted developmental and evolutionary processes, Rodríguez presented a racialized version of the medieval notion that monstrosity resulted from a mixing of centripetal and centrifugal forces.

Apart from this, Rodríguez's revision of Aristotelian terminology is noteworthy. The doctor referred to a "vegetative, or nutrition-seeking" fetus, and asserted that the monsters in question were this type of "creature."[31] However, unlike Aristotle, Aquinas, and other pre-nineteenth-century embryologists, Rodríguez did not believe that the "vegetative" phase was limited to the first weeks or months of gestation. Instead, he proposed that a fetus could shift between vegetative and other states of existence. This was allegedly a novel notion, and one that he claimed was a significant Mexican intervention in embryological science.

Whereas pre-Enlightenment thinkers saw the heart as containing the essence of humanity, and whereas Enlightenment thinkers proposed that this essence was contained in the rational brain, by the late nineteenth century scientists such as Rodríguez conversely preferred to see human traits in bone structure, which was hard, easily defined, and rationally organized—in a word, positive. Without the skeleton, they believed, no other organs would be possible—indeed, where would they sit in a body that was devoid of its structural organization? As such, the product of conception was not alive, nor did it possess human life if it lacked proper bone structure.

This was what Rodríguez meant when he referred to the "rational organization" of fetuses, in which the human senses and human functions (respiration, circulation, reproductive functions) only followed the development of bones (first) and organs (second). The human traits came last, a point that he repeatedly emphasized. He insisted, "None of this [bone and organ development] occurs in crustaceans, in headless many-legged creatures, or in insects." Therefore, "this [discrepancy] is only explained by the zoological ladder, in which some creatures are ultimately reduced to the simple condition of an embryo."[32] Here, the human embryo was indistinguishable from the simplest organisms.

Rodríguez's proposal necessarily probed the concept of personhood because it was difficult to argue that a human product of conception could lose its personhood and regress to a simpler state. Like Darwin, Rodríguez completely avoided the topic of ensoulment; in effect, even if not in intent, his definition of "human" was unrelated to the presence or absence of a prebirth fetal soul. He also did not mention of the use of baptism to save those souls. Rather, his definition of personhood seemed to rest on the potential of the child to survive outside the womb. This left the question of fetal "regression" into monstrosity unanswered: Did monstrous fetuses "regress" from human to parasite, or did they "evolve" from crustacean to human? The answer was unclear, a fact that Rodríguez himself admitted. Even so, it is clear that fetal ensoulment, a matter that had historically been at the heart of Mexican embryology, was incompatible with Rodríguez's embryology.

Rodríguez's embryological proposals thus constituted a departure from previous Catholic and Mexican embryological epistemologies. Although he did not mention Pope Pius IX's 1869 declaration that life began at conception and should be preserved as such, Rodríguez did acknowledge the difficulty of proving any metaphysical claims, including his own. Given that he had "not been able to penetrate the invisible world [of the womb]," he recognized a limited capacity to understand "the mysterious phenomena that make human organization possible, and other beings that surprise us." As such, he explained, "I utilized all the information available to my eyes and my sense of reason; even so, I fear that my hypothesis might not even simulate the truth."[33]

Medical student Carlos Esparza, who dedicated his 1881 thesis to Gabino Barreda, offered a less equivocating statement on embryology. He wrote, "As the French positivist school has taught us, human life is nothing more than organized matter in a dynamic state." He continued, "Every function of life can be observed, even by studying something as simple as cells."[34] Esparza further insisted that that the human soul is made constantly by the electric (neural) energy that flowed from the brain to the organs and, as such, the soul only exists because the human body exists. In other words, his was a materialist approach which overtly argued that the soul is not a divine endowment.

Rodríguez's discussion further supported Darwin's theories of natural selection. He argued that the weakest Mexican fetuses perished in the womb, and that some even disappeared entirely, in an ultra-"natural" manifestation of "natural selection." If natural selection was working as a mechanism of evolutionary change in Mexico, Mexican women's unnaturally small wombs were liquefying the unborn before they could evolve into humans. As in other countries, in Mexico embryology slowly ceased to be a topic of overt investigation. Rodríguez's approach became the standard line throughout the late nineteenth century, especially because, as Frida Gorbach, Ana Maria Carillo, and Nora Jaffary have shown, he exerted an enormous amount of influence over obstetric training.

A New National Science: Mexican Pelvimetry

The preceding section explored Juan María Rodríguez's theory that women's stunted wombs sometimes squeezed products of conception so tightly that they did not develop into fetuses. The rest of the chapter will focus on the science of pelvimetry, which came to propose that structural imperfections negatively affected Mexican women's entire reproductive system. This was facilitated by the racialized framework through which Porfirian doctors' research questions, methodology, and results were framed and interpreted—a framework that claimed, as its underlying assumption, that Indigenous Mexicans were underdeveloped and less evolved.

Mexico's first scientific treatise on pelvimetry was published in 1881 by a student named Florencio Flores.[35] The work, entitled *Comparative Pelvic Measurements,* sought to produce the first study comparing how Mexican women's pelvises literally measured up with those of European women. He intended this foundational study to offer "precise knowledge" about what he called "the pelvic canal," and he proposed that this knowledge, in turn, would become "the only rational base upon which to justify intervention in childbirth."[36] Flores based his study on the cadavers of twenty-six women who had perished in Mexico City's hospital system. "Cadavers," he wrote, "are the only books that I have consulted, because it was only there that I could see reality manifest."

Of the twenty-six cadavers from which Flores derived knowledge, seven had belonged to Indigenous women and the rest were, according to him, "Indigenous mixed with European." Flores used the telling phrase "of the Indigenous race." Because his education had been so steeped in debates about speciation and race, this was likely a purposeful statement, intended to suggest that Indigenous Mexicans were biologically distinct. Because more than a quarter of patients in this sample were Indigenous, it is possible that approximately the same percentage of reproductive surgery patients were Indigenous as well.[37]

Flores described the methods he used for measuring pelvises in women who were alive, as well as those who had died. "Digital pelvimetry" was the main examination performed on live women, consisting of the insertion of a doctor's fingers into the vaginal canal in order to estimate its inner width, located at the end and the bottom of the pelvic cavity. Even before performing the digital exam, Flores claimed that there was an easy visual and tactile clue to help in identifying the "structural deficiency." He explained, "Among the women with the structural deficiency that I refer to, the majority have a vulva that is placed far back, and which is facing directly downward."[38] This hypothesis led Flores to suggest that women with small pelvises should receive a preventative incision in the labia to facilitate childbirth. Thus, the historical origins of the episiotomy, incisions into the perineum during childbirth, were partially based on racialized ideas about marginalized women's peculiar sexual anatomy and pelvic deficiency.[39]

Flores next set out to map the mechanics of Mexican childbirth. He derived a standardized analysis by placing a dry pelvic bone on a large sheet of paper then turning it in different directions to trace the angles that it formed. He was also interested in measuring the angle of the inner and outer pelvic bones, as well as approximating the slant of the pubic symphysis, which is the cartilaginous part where the two pelvis halves join at the front. Finally, Flores sought to measure the angle of the pelvis as a whole, which he accomplished by hanging recently deceased bodies and skeletons from fishhooks connected to the ceiling.[40]

Flores laid out some preliminary conclusions toward the end of his study. He claimed to have demonstrated "how to characterize and perfectly distinguish the distinct problem that affects the interior of the Mexican pelvis."

Like Rodríguez, he insisted that this had nothing to do with a lack of vitamin D (which causes both osteomalacia, a softening of the bones, and rickets, which makes bones brittle). Rather, Flores insisted that these conditions were "so rare as to be true novelties in Mexico." "I believe," Flores wrote, "instead, that Mexican pelvises simply have a structure that is completely distinctive. This seems to be caused by the alterations that were stamped into the pelvis when the primitive race mixed with the conquerors."

Even so, Flores admitted some uncertainty in the matter. "For me," he wrote, "it is difficult to say exactly how this occurred." A final note in Flores's thesis has to do with the acceptance of his ideas by his professor, Juan María Rodríguez. As Flores reported, "Each day Professor Rodríguez becomes more convinced that there is a particular condition affecting the angle of the pelvic canal in Mexico." "As a result," the student wrote, "Rodríguez has established wise guidelines regarding vaginal inspections, the use of the speculum, and the insertion of the hand and the forceps in the vagina."[41] This burgeoning school of thought clearly influenced doctors' use of obstetric interventions throughout the course of the Porfiriato.

The pelvic deficiency thesis continued to develop in coming years and was even summarized in the massive (2,300 page), three-volume *The History of Medicine in Mexico*, written by doctor-cum-historian Francisco de Asís Flores y Troncoso in 1888. He dedicated a large portion of the third volume to Mexican obstetrics and gynecology, describing the most influential doctors, theories, and practices of his era. The doctor discussed pelvimetry several times, and in the third volume he theorized that the future of Mexican medicine would revolve around the practice of "racial identification via skeleton structure." Accordingly, "the identification of the Indigenous race by means of their skeleton is another point that has captured the attention of our studies." Flores y Troncoso alleged that Juan María Rodríguez had "observed that natural birth presents some difficulties in Mexico, and so he has supposed that the pelvic configuration and the birthing canal of Mexican women must be somehow defective."[42]

Asserting that Indigenous women exhibited flawed reproduction, he added, "Upon further investigation, we discovered that the pubis of Indigenous women is higher than in the women of any other race, and it is characterized by a notable downward and backward inclination." Flores y Troncoso characterized Indigenous women's pelvic cavities and their birth canals as inadequately sized and erroneously shaped. It is particularly significant that he used the freighted words "downward" and "backward," because the terminology implied that Indigenous people exhibited biological signs of failure in the evolutionary race. As Indigenous communities ostensibly hindered modernization efforts by means of their "cultural backwardness," the medical establishment theorized that Indigenous women's "backward" bodies rebelled against progress as well.

Flores y Troncoso theorized that mestizaje was the process through which Indigenous people had "contaminated" the "Spanish race" with a faulty pelvic structure. Conflating race, nation, and indigeneity, he wrote, "Now, as we have observed the same problem in Mexican women, it must result from the mixing of the Spanish race with the natives of this country. In the first group we do not encounter anything to explain the cause of the modification of the pelvis, so it is natural to suppose that in the second group we find the faulty trait, one that has without a doubt been passed down hereditarily since the conquest, and in its remains we still find these particularities."[43]

Flores y Troncoso referred to the Indigenous "race" as one monolithic group, distinct from the "Mexican race." Yet the term itself was a misnomer, given that people spoke (and speak) hundreds of distinct Indigenous languages in Mexico, and their identities cannot be collapsed into one category. At the time, more than one-third of the nation's population spoke an Indigenous language. Thus, Flores y Troncoso extended "race" to mean both nationality (Mexican) and ethnicity (Spanish or Indigenous). He proposed that scientific medicine was a tool with which to define the racial boundaries of the imagined national community, to conceptualize a racial definition of Mexicans, and to show that (mixed group) "Mexicans" were, supposedly, less biologically deficient, and therefore perhaps more redeemable, than Indigenous Mexicans.

Flores y Troncoso simultaneously used race as an ambiguous term and as an exact one, as a cultural and national identity and also a biological category. Along the same vein, the doctor did not offer cultural or geographic descriptions of Indigenous people. By referencing the hereditary "remains" of native groups, he asserted that they were vestiges of the past instead of part of the nation's social fabric. Even if he was purposefully ambiguous about the political definition of indigeneity, he wished to determine which inhabitants of the Federal District qualified as "pure" Indigenous people. It is worth noting that Flores y Troncoso was not an obstetrician but a general practitioner and historian. He proposed, however, that pelvimetry was the paramount tool for racial taxonomy, and he mentioned phrenology only as a last aside.

Flores y Troncoso voiced anxiety about the extent to which Mexicans exhibited Indigenous traits, and he proposed that scientific medicine could identify an allegedly weaker hereditary strain. He continued, "At any rate, we can amass the data we have collected so far to identify the skeletons of the Mexican women who have extraordinarily high pubic bones and pelvic cavities with pronounced downward and backward inclinations. These characteristics, along with the molars, will perfectly identify a woman of the pure Indigenous race. Another useful manner of identifying this race is the configuration of their cranium and their facial angle."[44] In this passage the physician suggested that some Mexican skeletons could be classified as "of the pure Indigenous race." He was clearly preoccupied about the effect of miscegenation on the hereditary makeup of Mexican women, who were allegedly becoming contaminated by Indigenous traits to the point where distinguishing between the groups had become difficult. The doctor essentially proposed that the medical establishment should assume responsibility for identifying the problematic portion of the nation to make the whole stronger. Ultimately, however, he was unclear as to whether he sought to improve Indigenous Mexicans via miscegenation or to protect non-Indians from further contamination. In Flores y Troncoso's view, the seeds of racial degeneracy were present at the beginning of life, and the uterus and pelvic cavity represented much more than anatomical pieces of a larger whole. Not only were they the most intimate hollows of the body, but women's reproductive organs were essential to the state because national and racial strength began with generation and incubation, and the inheritance of a "faulty trait" could have broad social consequences.

Pelvimetry continued to develop for decades after Flores y Troncoso's assessment of the field. José de Jesús Sánchez Gómez published the next important text on the topic in 1891. Sánchez Gómez articulated the existence of a new paradigm in Mexico, which proposed that "the pelvis is at the root of all the great phenomena having to do with conception, gestation [pregnancy], and birth—all are rooted in its enclosure." When physiological problems interfered, he proposed, this converted human reproduction into a "pathological process."[45] This, apparently, marks the first use of the concept of "pathological birth" in Mexican reproductive science, which is not surprising in the context of the 1890s, marked by ascedant scientific ideologies about racial pathologies, racial hygiene, and atavism.

Sánchez Gómez interviewed women in the Hospital de San Andrés, asking them questions about their place of birth, source of income, and reproductive history. Sánchez Gómez also utilized ropes to approximate pelvic measurements. He did this both during autopsies by approximating the distance between the ischium (commonly known as the pelvic bones) with a piece of string. Like Flores, Sánchez Gómez used an internal method of approximating the width in the pelvic cavity, although his manner of describing the process was more detailed than Flores's 1881 description. Sánchez Gómez's process was to insert the hand into the vagina and extend the fingers downward in search of the pubic bones. After touching each ischium, clinicians would withdraw their hands and estimate the distance they had felt. While the pelvimetric processes were all compromising in some way, Sánchez Gómez's was invasive in a more intimate manner.[46]

Sánchez Gómez became influential due to his promotion of pelvic measuring devices known as pelvimeters, which in many ways represented a generalization of pelvimetric science. With a new external method for performing pelvic measurements, scientists no longer had to perform invasive digital examinations or wait for a living patient to become a corpse and then a skeleton. The focus on interior angles lessened as pelvic width became a visual manifestation that could be quantified with just one piece of technology. Sánchez Gómez did not include drawings to depict pelvimeters, but the devices are still on display in the medical museum attached to the Biblioteca Dr. Nicolás León, where the Escuela de Medicina's dissertations are archived.

Pelvimetric research gained considerable momentum at the end of the Porfiriato. Between 1897 and 1919, the professor of medicine Juan Duque de Estrada published at least nine studies on the topic, totaling over 300 pages of work. Duque de Estrada's research began in a maternity clinic in Mexico City, where he first worked as a student intern; he continued to work there as a practitioner in the clinic after earning his degree. His findings eventually formed a central part of the medical school's curriculum, and as a result he became the head professor of the obstetric clinic and oversaw student training there for thirty years.

When Dr. Antonio Sordo Noriega eulogized Estrada's life and work in 1955, he emphasized Estrada's contributions to the topic of study. He wrote that over the course of Estrada's time at la Casa de Maternidad, the influential clinical director had developed the "belief that, in plebeian patients (*el sector social*), the pelvis of Mexican women presents some peculiar characteristics. In many cases, he was able to study the anomalies and defects that explained the clinical phenomena that characterized these women's inability to give birth."[47]

Duque de Estrada's own writing spoke to these themes. He wrote, "The difficulties that I have seen and experienced have convinced me that the Mexican pelvis is, as a rule, deformed." He did not believe it would "be accurate to call these mere pathological rarities." Instead, he insisted that the "deformed

Mexican pelvis" was "a national trend." Upon observing women with "infantile pelvises" and "retarded pelvic development," Duque de Estrada wrote that he "took advantage of [his] position at la Casa de Maternidad to collect narrow pelvises, and whenever possible, to autopsy and deconstruct the cadavers." Sometimes it was these efforts—taking advantage of his position to collect cadavers—that ended the lives of people like the young woman who was found in the Devil's Alley and brought into la Casa (as described in the introduction to this book).

Duque de Estrada was particularly convinced that Mexican pelvises were "imperfectly developed" and displayed "a lack of—or retardation in—development." "Some of these," he wrote, "maintained an infantile build," while others "were stretched backward, with small all-around dimensions." He defined "infantile" as a "general lack of physical development, and appearing like the pelvis of an eight-year-old child."[48] Estrada's use of the word "infantile," new to Mexican pelvimetry at the time of his writing in the early twentieth, strongly echoed theories of atavism and racial inferiority. Duque de Estrada also repeatedly described patients and midwives as "disgusting" and "dirty." Both groups of women, in his view, were consumers and distributers of marijuana and other illicit herbal remedies, such as those derived from plants known as *zihuatlpatl, cuernecillo de centeno,* and sarsaparilla, which is made from the *Smilax ornata* plant and is a natural painkiller.[49]

Dr. Juan Duque de Estrada's work magnified the conceptual link between the angle of the pelvic bones and the space within the cavity. As opposed to measuring three overlapping triangles, as previous researchers had done, Estrada simply proposed that as the slope of the pelvic bones increased, the internal diameters of the cavity decreased. His study's semantics also affirmed the institutionalization of pelvimetry as a distinct field of study in Mexico. Even Estrada's terminology reflected this epistemological shift: he referred to his work as "pelviology" (*pelviología*) rather than "pelvimetry." This was an ideology, not just a set of metrics, and it was an ideology that biologized and racialized Mexican women's national worth as mothers and citizens.

Duque de Estrada presented three additional conclusions regarding his subject of study. First, he said, "difficulties in birth (dystocia) are due to excessive length of the pubis and its abnormal backward inclination." Second, "this deformation is very frequent, and is the principal—if not, the only—cause of dystocia in Mexico." Third, this condition is "so frequent that it can be said to characterize and distinguish Mexican pelvises." Thus, the bodies of women imprisoned in state hospitals were codified and typologized according to the preconceptions of pelviology, the grand scientific ideology of

Porfirian reproductive science. These arguments were facilitated by the racialized framework through which doctors' research questions, methodology, and results were framed and interpreted—the framework that claimed, as its underlying assumption, that Indigenous Mexicans were underdeveloped and less evolved, at least on an "organizational" level.

Porfirian Reproductive Science: Positivism, Hereditarianism, Darwinism, and Spencerian Thought

Historians of science have demonstrated that Mexican medicine was profoundly influenced by Lamarckism and neo-Lamarckism, which emphasized the inheritance of acquired characteristics and the environmental determinants of health.[50] However, as others have pointed out, neo-Lamarckism developed in dialogue with Spencerian, Malthusian, and Darwinian thought.[51] This was especially the case from 1880 on, when Mexican physicians began to focus more intensively on the intergenerational transmission of hereditary traits. Intellectual currents intermingled with biologically deterministic state-building theory, in which physicians argued that because biological defects were transmitted via heredity, these shortcomings affected the intellectual and moral development of individual Mexican citizens and the polity as a whole. Moreover, in large part because of their belief that scientists were the most fit members of society to direct that change, advocates of positivism sought to elevate the sciences to the status of a religion—an organizing ideology upon which to base all state functions.[52]

What follows is an examination of these themes as applied to theories of racial heredity in works by Gustavo Ruiz (1877), Carlos Orozco (1880), and Manuel Flores (1880), with particular attention to how obstetricians linked gender, anatomy, behavior, and vital force. With his 1877 book, *Heredity and Its Medico-Legal Applications,* Professor Gustavo Ruiz became the first Mexican scientist to write extensively about Darwinian and Spencerian ideas, and to present them to an audience of Mexican scientists. Even while Ruiz discussed these foreign thinkers, he was careful to cite his closest influences, particularly doctors Gabino Barreda and Juan María Rodríguez. Prior to Ruiz's study of heredity, he had worked as a surgeon in the Hospital Juárez and as a professor of philosophy, veterinary science, and medicine in the ENP. He had also been the director of the Ángel González y Echeverría Hospital, as well as the head of the gynecology clinic in that institution. Ruiz aimed to create a specifically Mexican school of thought on race and heredity, albeit one heavily influenced by other thinkers. As a professor in the medical school of the ENP, Ruiz had enormous influence over how students learned about these topics. Indeed, it is more than likely that his textbook was assigned to all students of the ENP.

In his text Ruiz developed a nuanced theorization of heredity, though he began by acknowledging the difficulty of defining and analyzing the topic. Ruiz offered an accurate overview of Mendel's plant studies of the 1860s, though those were not the subject of much international attention at that point.[53] He sought to convince the "evolution-deniers" that all species were capable of changing over time, and that heredity was a key part of these transformations. His starting point was a discussion of artificial selection and natural selection.

Ruiz insisted on three main points. In his words, "first: heredity is the point of departure for every improvement; second, it is the origin of all degeneration; and third, it is the mechanism through which we can perfect and conserve good races."[54] Here Ruiz twice declared his loyalty to Darwin's ideas, emphasizing that heredity was the most important potential source of human improvement, instead of climate, culture, morals, or salvation. By this schema, however, heredity also represented the potential downfall of the Mexican "race(s)." The tenor of such debate illustrates that some still doubted hereditarian theory, or the idea that a person inherited their organization and constitution from their parents. By this time, scientists were convinced that animals slowly inherited different characteristics, but there existed little agreement about exactly what sparked speciation or transformative evolutionary mechanisms.

Ruiz, for his part, made explicit his concept of race. He explained, "I use race with the same liberty as zoologists, and without sticking too closely to the narrow, naturalist definition."[55] This was another way of affirming his allegiance to a Darwinian view of race. That is, he believed that races had branched off a common zoological tree as a result of natural and artificial selection. Lamarck, on the other hand, was a naturalist who believed that all groups, species, and "races" would naturally improve over time, but without branching off into other species. Thus, when Ruiz declared that he was "not a naturalist," he was essentially disavowing Lamarck's theories of inheritance.

Ruiz believed that males alone created the spermatic "germ" of heredity. This theory posited that although women bore children, women's heredity was not actually transmitted to the children. Ruiz explained that this was due to the "supremacy of the creation of men."[56] Strong men, Ruiz suggested, would only create sperm to father a boy. By contrast, a man who was effeminate, degenerate, or temporarily weakened, even as a result of illness, would create a girl.

Constructing men as the authors of human heredity was widespread and not unique to Mexico. However, its articulation in Mexico during the Porfiriato is of particular interest due to its unique social implications. Namely, it seemed to open a rhetorical space that facilitated the targeting of women for reproductive controls, not just because of the racial degeneracy that could result from their cramped wombs but also because of the question of paternity. Hypothetically—in the case of, say, a light-skinned woman, a European immigrant to Mexico City, for instance—hereditary traits might be inconsequential, especially if a woman birthed a child who carried its father's "degenerate" traits. But in the case of a dark-skinned Indigenous woman, the racial consequences might be grave. This line of reasoning strengthened the rationale behind influencing the fertility of all "unruly" women, not just those who allegedly showed signs of hereditary weakness.

Ruiz fretted in particular about racial degeneration in Mexico. "In my view," he wrote in 1877, "we cannot deny the tendency of the races to degenerate. This is known as atavism, and is the best proof we have of the powerful influence of heredity."[57] Like many Lamarckian thinkers, Ruiz left discursive space for the degenerative influence of the environment. He spoke to the potentially degenerative effects of social conditions, explaining "the poor conditions of the proletariat class become an inexhaustible source of degeneration for the children of families who are as miserable as they are numerous."[58] At the time Ruiz was writing, there existed no consensus about the degenerative formation of Mexican women's biology. His theories were doubtlessly formative for later ideas about atavistic organization.

Ruiz finished his treatise with two firm conclusions. Regarding heredity, he argued that physicians "must use observation to establish the cases in which there is ample evidence to prove that any natural, pathological, or monstrous trait before us might be hereditary." Second, he proposed that theorists "must pay particularly close attention to the hereditary influence that links diverse mental defects with the absence of morality." This was a novel use of the concept "moral" and of "morality," and it seems to have been the first time that a nineteenth century Mexican physician linked morality and heredity. The second half of Ruiz's statement gestured toward the utility of selective efforts at population control. In his words, "in this way [after identifying the links between hereditary conditions and morality], we will be able to eradicate the roots of many irresponsible families who deserve to be enclosed in an asylum, and who disturb society with their unprecedented crimes."[59]

Criminality, Ruiz proposed, was inherited from sick, mentally ill, alcoholic, and criminal parents. He insisted that such heredity resulted in an "ill organization, which almost forces the subject to do its will."[60] Here, "organization" appears again as a representation of a person's mind or spirit—almost as a comment on their essence as a rationally organized being. It is therefore ironic that although late nineteenth century scientists had pivoted away from inquiries into the meaning of personhood, they seemed to inevitably circle back to that core set of moralized and salvational questions.

For Ruiz, "organization" comprised a woman's uterus and mental state as well as the organization of her skeleton. Although Ruiz's thesis was mainly theoretical and not anatomical, he was apparently the first Mexican scientist to argue that "structural deficiencies" were hereditary. He seemed to be the first Mexican doctor to use the term "structural vices," which became one of the most important issues in clinical practice.

In addition to discussing heredity and structural flaws, Ruiz focused extensively on mental state, intelligence, and morality. Citing the aphorism "like produces like," he insisted that an adult's intelligence was transmitted to its offspring, such that, for example, a well-studied man would automatically father intelligent children due to this form of hereditary transmission.[61] Because most individuals could not be trusted to anticipate the potentially deleterious effects of their heredity, however, Ruiz emphasized that such "vigilance" should consist of a collaboration between the state and scientific authorities.[62] This reflected Malthusian attitudes, which insisted that the individual is beholden to society and not vice versa. Furthermore, this approach literally made the state into a kind of pseudo-biological father to the nation's children, not merely the symbolic liberal patriarch of the patria.

With the publication of the first treatise on heredity in late nineteenth-century Mexico, Gustavo Ruiz started a trend that would influence many future students. Among these was Carlos Orozco, who in 1880 earned his medical degree with a study entitled "A Comparison of Medical Practice and Hygiene, from a Social Perspective."[63] Orozco, for his part, emphasized the importance of preventative medicine. As he put it, "a true doctor is not he who limits himself to correcting the deviations of the body, but rather, he who corrects them in anticipation." This, Orozco insisted, was the only way to ensure the "improvement of humanity."[64]

Orozco's discussion clarified some of Ruiz's comments on heredity and "organization." He opened his first chapter with a related point: "The study of human physiology offers firm proof of the relationship between the different organisms and apparatuses that make up an individual. Nobody doubts the veracity of this principle." Like Rodríguez and Ruiz, however, Orozco had an explicitly metaphysical argument in mind, which he expressed with the following hypothetical question: "This ensemble of functions—which some might call 'spirit'—is it connected in some way to organized material?" This reference to the "ensemble" of organs and bones as both "spirit" and "organized material" is telling. His interest in the connection between human consciousness and the organization of bodies notwithstanding, Orozco admitted that while the latter was clearly the purview of doctors, perhaps the former should be left to ethologists. (Ethology refers to the study of human and animal behavior and social organization from a biological perspective.) Then, citing Spencer on the relationship between organization and personality, Orozco argued that "human character is a sum of the units comprised within." Not only was this an expression of positivist materialism, but it was simultaneously a clear and explicit expression of biological determinism.[65]

Orozco then combined these Spencerian beliefs with a strong statement in support of positivist governance. In his words, "all societies have exactly the government that they deserve."[66] This was because the "organization" of the population's mind and body dictated the level of progress that that society could attain. After *knowing* these biological laws, Orozco insisted, it would be possible for doctors to "achieve their duty, which is to seek the improvement of individuals, which is indispensable for the improvement of societies."[67] Utilizing Darwinian terms, Orozco then went on to explain that by using medicine as a selective mechanism, doctors could encourage "survival of the fittest" and thereby participate in the "improvement of the species."[68] Of course, there was some irony in his insistence on a purely biological understanding of the body in light of his simultaneous assertion that unevolved body-spirits rationalized state-sponsored selective breeding.

Orozco made an explicit connection between the Mexican reforma, Catholicism, and social progress. In his words, "we can find an example of useful moral and intellectual variations by comparing communities." Those communities, he continued, "that were quick to adopt the Reforma—and those individuals who have abandoned Catholicism—have reached a higher state of progress." Orozco's concluding thought on this topic intended to provide a scientized and biologized diagnosis of why Catholicism was backward and retrogressive. He wrote, "The Catholic regime closes the sphere of influence of these [moral and intellectual] functions." He continued, "The conservation of the physiological state of each and every organ depends on the proper use of those organs. Without variety in the sphere of intellectual functions, these will regress. It is for this reason that the ascetics had such below-average levels of intelligence." His suggestion was that religion retards mental and physical progress with superstition, fanaticism, and a belief in miracles.[69]

Orozco ended his thesis with a Malthusian proclamation. He believed that while the human species was growing exponentially, food production was not. "The food supplies will not be enough," he insisted, "and the struggle for existence will put pressure on those who are useless to society—those who only consume food, and do not produce it."[70] There was irony in this statement as well, given how little time most doctors spent working in agricultural fields.

Less than a decade after Salinas y Rivera's 1871 publication on "medical morality," student Manuel Flores wrote his own book on medical mores and medical education, entitled *On Medical Education.*[71] Flores was a professor at the national secondary school for girls in Mexico City, as well as an aspiring member of the sanitary unit of the military. He was also a member of the philosophical society dedicated to Gabino Barreda, and was strongly influenced by Barreda's 1863 work on the same topic. In fact, Flores dedicated his thesis in the now-familiar way: "To Gabino Barreda, the eminent father and proponent of positivism in Mexico."[72]

At 356 pages, Flores's impressive dissertation was as long as it was dense. In agreement with his colleagues on the topic of heredity, he stated, "All of our investigations assume that the concept of heredity is correct."[73] Like other early Porfirian doctors, Flores simultaneously drew from Darwinian, Spencerian, Lamarckian, and Comtean thought. (He wrote that he thought Spencer's theories "explained everything."). Clear racial prejudice can be seen in his blunt affirmation that "different races have different biological functions and abilities."[74]

For Flores, science was of utmost importance because it was the only path toward progress. He continued, "This progress has been so great that it has led to our conviction that physical organization is the base of science, and moral organization is the path to its success."[75] This was a new iteration of the kind of emphasis on morality that Gabino Barreda had offered in 1877—one that emphasized structural organization and not just organs—as intimately intertwined with the scientific moralization of society. Throughout his dissertation, Flores insisted that the study was, and should be read as being, "strictly scientific, and an exploration of the science of human organization—physical, intellectual, and moral organization."[76] In this vein, the young student particularly emphasized the importance of experimentation, referring to "the clinic as the only educational means we need."[77]

Like Orozco and Ruiz, Flores offered a new definition of "organization." Previous scientists had drawn a clear distinction between organization and vital force. Organization, for them, was simply the arrangement of molecules, and, as such, it only determined structure, whereas "vital force" was the source of life.[78] Early Porfirians, by contrast, seemed to view "organization" as a matter of how a person's organs related to each other to create life, sensations, and moral feelings, as well as both conscious and unconscious movement. For Flores, the organs were a key part of understanding the concept of organization, and he emphasized the utility of surgery in this realm of scientific inquiry. He wrote, "The study of anatomy through dissection should focus on the relationship among anatomy, locomotive faculties, and intelligence." Dissection was clearly the path forward in this inquiry. In Flores's words, it was "the easiest and surest" way.[79]

There was a larger purpose, too. Flores insisted that "it [was] possible to perfect some organs by means of achieving the integrity and perfection of the other biological functions." This, Flores explained, was because "the perfection that it is possible for an organ to achieve does not just depend upon that organ, but also the state of all other organs."[80] Despite the presumed difficulty of "perfecting" an organ, Porfirian doctors believed that the mind was a synergistic function generated by the relationship between the organs. Some obstetricians adjusted their experimental practices according to this notion.

Yet at the same time Flores expressed doubt that experimentation would create "moral types" in a straightforward manner. As he wrote, "the relative power of some emotions over others is determined by the organization of the animal . . . it is for this reason that in each race and in every era, the moral type will remain constant." Thus, according to Flores, although organs might be "perfected," it was much harder to perfect an individual's "moral" state. Yet he also wrote, "Despite the obvious limits to the moral perfection of an individual, there is no limit to the gradual perfection of the group as a whole." How could such perfection be achieved? "The latest scientific advancements," Flores explained, "tend to demonstrate that perfection—in the physical sense, as much as in the intellectual and moral sense—is hereditary, and that it can accumulate in the species."[81] In other words, this was a Lamarckian-inspired long-term project in which science perfects organs, bit by bit, and heredity concentrates the effects over time.

AS FLORES'S WRITINGS DEMONSTRATE, positivist understandings of the body had undergone significant shifts by 1880. In the 1860s and 1870s, reforma physicians had believed that morality, as manifested through hysterical behavior, was to be blamed on one organ (the uterus) and could therefore be eliminated by the removal of the reproductive organs or the product of conception. By 1880, the relationship between morality and biology had shifted significantly. Physicians now saw morality as the result of a person's anatomy and "organization," and as one of the many biological factors that influenced a person's character, function, and intellect. Although the conceptual link between organization and heredity has received very little attention from historians, it is meaningful for understanding dialectical relationships between biology, heredity, evolution, and personhood under positivism.

This chapter explored a major intellectual shift: that is, a new insistence that the aforementioned characteristics were hereditary and race based, and that alterations to a person's organs or systems would not just improve their behavior but also influence the evolutionary trajectory of the species. In Flores's words, "this causal connection is complicated, but it is as certain as any other causal connection in the physical order."[82] As the 1880s progressed, doctors began to apply these theoretical foundations to their clinical research. Clinicians turned to women's bodies as valuable sites for the creation of knowledge about such difficult concepts as organization and moral type. Many even set about influencing the trajectory of Mexican heredity by means of experimental obstetric procedures.

Obstetricians voiced and embodied an allegiance to positivist philosophical trends in many ways. As this chapter has emphasized, clinicians performed anatomical measurements in their search for data to prove racist and anti-Indigenous scientific prejudice—to prove that Mexico City's impoverished classes were biologically inferior, and that the poor were downtrodden, in part, due to their faulty "moral organization." This was a moralized salvational project that treated compteam positivism as a modern scientific religion crucial for mind-body regeneration.

Positivism in obstetrics was a racial project because it reified essentialized typologies and sought to delineate racial categories based on biometric data. The contemporary implications of Mexican pelvimetry are stark, considering the contemporary use of a racial correction factor in the vaginal birth after cesarean (VBAC) calculator, which has embedded into clinical practice the incorrect assumption that African American and Latin women have a lesser probability of successful vaginal birth after caesarean solely because of their racial classification.[83] As the next chapter will explore, doctors not only performed surgeries in search of knowledge about Mexicans' racial heredity, so too did they remove some women's reproductive organs, thereby deleting them from the nation's racial future.

CHAPTER SIX

Free to Walk Wherever She Damn Well Pleased

Obstetric Violence in Policy and Practice, 1870s–1910s

In 1891, 300 women in the Hospital Morelos burst from their rooms in unison at 8:30 P.M. Charging the entry hall of the clinic where they were imprisoned, they yelled and chanted that the hospital was on fire, and that they intended to flee. Unfortunately, their efforts were futile. Apparently unconcerned by the patient-prisoners' arson, the guards barricaded the front gates before any of the women could escape. The windows were already barred shut, so the women remained trapped, and the fire was soon extinguished. When the director of the hospital reported the incident to the Secretary of State, he lamented that overcrowding and unrest in the hospital would inevitably result in another escape attempt. "It might be necessary," he wrote, "to empty the establishment."[1]

Who were these women, and why were they so aggrieved that they risked burning to death to flee their hospital imprisonment? Although it is impossible to know what motivated the patients to rebel, one example sheds light on what some may have experienced. In 1892, a Sanitary Police inspector reported that he had found a woman near the Zócalo at 9:30 P.M. Perhaps she was even toiling near Devil's Alley. Suspecting that she was a clandestine sex worker, the Sanitary Police officer arrested and detained her. The woman, whose full name was unfortunately not recorded in the archive, angrily refused to go with the officer. Because protest became the only weapon she had, she forcefully insisted "that she was free to walk—alone or not—wherever she damn well pleased." She also refused to submit to a medical examination and encouraged her friends to do the same. "In this case, like others," the head of the Sanitary Police wrote, "because the woman refused to submit to inspection, we forced her into the hospital to verify the state of her health."[2] Even in the hospital, she did not submit to vaginal inspection [*no se deja reconocer*]. On the third day of her internment, the authorities forced her into a straitjacket so that they could carry out the inspection of her insides. Perhaps the detainee interpreted this as medical rape, given the focus of her complaints.[3]

After the sanitary inspectors had found her to be healthy, they released her from the hospital at the insistence of her husband, Alfredo Sánchez, who declared his intent to challenge her internment before the law. Sánchez and his wife sought a civil hearing against the Sanitary Police, presenting a certificate of marriage and reiterating that she was not a sex worker. Still, authorities countered that she and her husband looked to recruit women to work in brothels.[4] The judge sympathized with the detainee and denounced the officers for their "immodesty and abuse of authority." Although the report did not explain why the judge reprimanded the officers for "immodesty," it appeared to be a euphemism for the violation of her bodily integrity. The judge added that officers should have used a "more convenient manner" of verifying whether their detainees sold sex for money.

This anecdote speaks to the conflicting attitudes around the rise in state surveillance over women's sexual behavior and suggests that prison-hospitals were crucial for the state's efforts to effect disciplinary control and identify potential candidates for medical research, especially related to sexually transmitted infections (STIs) and pregnancy. Combining biometric data with social Darwinist rhetoric, authorities rationalized a racialized "war on crime" that targeted the nation's poor and disenfranchised, including many women.[5] Several historians including Laura Cházaro, Cristina Rivera Garza, and Beatriz Urías Horcasitas have critically examined the topic of reproduction in relation to scientific politics in the late nineteenth century. Their studies have demonstrated that the Porfirian state authorized, and even encouraged, surgery of the most invasive kind for the poor, while elite women were exempt from experimental treatments. [6]

Using records from the Secretary of Health, this chapter addresses a key shift in the scale of Sanitary Police surveillance in the 1870s, regarding the state-sanctioned detention and inspection of tens of thousands of women. As the story about the Sánchez couple suggests, Porfirio Díaz's dictatorship saw a massive increase in the number of women detained, imprisoned, and treated in hospitals and clinics throughout Mexico City. Many patients were imprisoned in hospitals for months, where doctors subjected some to a range of medical treatments and surgeries.[7] Indeed, more than 100,000 patients passed through the doors of the Hospital Morelos over the course of the Porfiriato, making the clinic a site of extensive medical research and complaints from patients. For these reasons, the Hospital Morelos left the most extensive archival trail of the Porfirian clinics. Yet, a close focus on Porfirian medical imprisonment also complicates the picture of medical coercion during the Porfiriato: as is shown here, multiple groups—physicians, Sanitary Police, sanitary inspectors, and judges—came into conflict regarding hospital detention.

An examination of policy and practice reveals that surgery became more than a mechanism through which state authorities could manipulate the boundaries of marginalized groups' incorporation into the state while enacting racial discrimination. It also became a site of race-making in and of itself. A key component of this argument is that shifts in women's clinical treatment were integral to the racialization of obstetrics. This is explored through a discussion of how discourses about pain and neurasthenia were refracted through the particularly Mexican politics of indigeneity, gender, and social difference. Women's bodies were at the core of medical knowledge production; their agency, their choices, and their reproductive labor all affected the ways in which that knowledge was constructed and contested. Relatedly, the Sanitary Police were necessary for the making of modern gynecology as well as the creation of a state disciplinary apparatus that surveilled and repressed poor and non-white women. All of this shows the centrality of women, their bodies, and their oppression in the making of the sanitary state. Finally, because the Sanitary Police traversed the neighborhoods of Mexico City, going door-to-door like the religious orders and philanthropic groups that had done so before, their work took on a symbolic, ritualistic, and hegemonic kind of power.

The Sanitary Police and Making a State Apparatus for Gynecological Experimentation

In 1903, novelist Federico Gamboa published *Santa,* a novel about a beautiful young girl who moved from the countryside to Mexico City. There she lived a briefly glamorous life as a prostitute before developing uterine cancer and dying during a hysterectomy. Gamboa worked in the Porfirian government as a clerk, journalist, statesman, and diplomat, meaning that he had unusual access to information regarding the state's treatment of sex workers; evidently he drew on these insights for the novel.

"The Sanitary Police," Gamboa wrote, "intended to safeguard the health of the community's male citizens" by ensuring that sex workers complied with the city's regulations. However, because the Sanitary Police were on the "bottom rung on the city's administrative ladder," they often accepted bribes from pimps and sex workers. According to Gamboa, this meant that "even major infractions commonly passed unremarked." But even if some used bribes to avoid detention and inspection, the Sanitary Police were infamous for their tendency to "exercise their authority arbitrarily and commit countless abuses, even a few scurrilous ones, like intentionally hauling in helpless,

TABLE 6.1 Sex worker registrations, 1868–1879

	1868	*1869*	*1870*	*1871*	*1872*	*1873*	*1874*	*1875*	*1876*	*1877*	*1878*	*1879*	*Total*
Voluntary	2	178	151	98	82	114	85	80	92	112	87	177	1,258
Forced	3	52	33	10	26	18	68	35	33	44	23	63	408
Total	5	230	184	108	108	132	153	115	125	156	110	240	1,666

Source: Montenegro, *Breves apuntes* (1880).

poorly dressed girls, who turn out not to be prostitutes at all, and whom they finally release with a smirk and an 'excuse us, ma'am.'"[8] Gamboa implied that the Sanitary Police sexually abused the young girls they "hauled in," or at least, that their vaginal inspections were immodest and could have been the source of pleasure for some officers.

When Federico Gamboa wrote the dedication to *Santa,* he included an affective plea to a sculptor, Jesús Contreras. Here, Gamboa briefly assumed the voice of his novel's protagonist, Santa, although the novel itself is written in third-person narrative. Santa's haunting message began with the words "don't think of me as a saint just because that is my name." She then offered a saddening narrative of how she was exploited and disgraced: on public streets, in bedrooms, and in the office of the Sanitary Police. "Not even in death did I find rest," Santa's voice continued, "for some doctors chopped up my body, without curing it—my poor body, bruised and withered from the animal lust of a vicious metropolis."[9] Although the literary imagination of *Santa* is fictitious, it speaks to a core theme: that is, the rise in state surveillance over women as part of the commodification of their bodies for medical science.

Although Gamboa's story was fictional, his claims about the Sanitary Police are supported by an abundance of archival evidence. As a result of the detentions and widely publicized registration requirements, 1,661 women registered as sex workers in Mexico City between 1868 and 1879. Although 1,256 apparently did so "voluntarily," 405 were forced to register after having been detained and interned by the Sanitary Police (table 6.1). In his dissertation on the topic, medical student Francisco Montenegro narrated how they came to be detained: "As soon as we find one of these sick women, we detain and isolate her to imprison her in the hospital until she is completely cured."[10] Thus, even the so-called voluntary registrations may have been from women who had been confined involuntarily.

Some women tried to avoid registering as sex workers by refusing to confirm their identities or by attempting to alter their appearance with fake

TABLE 6.2 Sanitary Police inspections performed, 1868–1879

1868	*1869*	*1870*	*1871*	*1872*	*1873*	*1874*	*1875*	*1876*	*1877*	*1878*	*1879*	*Total*
1,122	11,596	6,001	10,623	8,263	7,249	7,149	7,199	8,560	10,016	9,557	11,246	98,581

Source: Montenegro, *Breves apuntes* (1880).

tattoos, cosmetics, different hairstyles, and changes of clothing. These practices were so pervasive that they gave way to a new realm of professional study by the late 1870s—that of identity concealment and of the signs that a woman was concealing her identity.[11] While 1,666 women registered as sex workers between 1868 and 1879, many more women underwent inspection by doctors during that period. During those years, doctors performed 98,581 vaginal inspections on women who had been detained by the Sanitary Police (table 6.2).

To be clear, it is the case that many women performed sex work during the Porfiriato, and that this work could sometimes contribute to the transmission of infections, especially given that this was the pre-antibiotic era. Porfirian Mexico City was a "city of sin": many wealthy national and international businessmen reveled in luxurious bars, brothels, and parties during their visits to the city. Women flocked from other states, nations, and colonies to make some money in sex work. Some saw very little financial gain, while others found the profession extremely lucrative. Some may have had to say goodbye to their families and communities forever. But others came from cultures that did not stigmatize sex with multiple partners and arguably did not romanticize the construct of virginity that Nora Jaffary has traced.[12] Women came from other regions too, including Europe, North America, and Asia; travel for sexual commerce gave way to much handwringing about so-called white slavery. Sometimes Mexican sex workers resented the foreign brothel employees and accused them of monopolizing their clientele.[13]

It is simultaneously clear that many Mexican women fell into the clutches of the state even though they were not selling sex for money. Perhaps they worked in dishonorable professions, such as in public markets, food stalls, pulque-breweries, or hotels. As we can see by comparing tables 6.1 and 6.2, in 1879 only 177 women were registered as sex workers, but doctors performed 11,246 vaginal inspections of alleged sex workers. It would be impossible for doctors to only have inspected the women who were registered as sex workers because they would have had to have inspected each woman on average 63.5 times per year, or more than once per week, while the maximum number of inspections recommended for sex workers was once per month. Thus, it is

TABLE 6.3 Women with sexually transmitted infections, 1868–1879

1868	*1869*	*1870*	*1871*	*1872*	*1873*	*1874*	*1875*	*1876*	*1877*	*1878*	*1879*	*Total*
78	190	219	218	219	185	212	207	232	362	289	648	3,059

Source: Montenegro, *Breves apuntes* (1880).

highly likely that doctors and the Sanitary Police inspected women who were not performing sex work. It seems probable that part of their goal was increase the population of women imprisoned in hospital clinics, where they were useful for a range of experimental procedures. For example, doctors experimented with inoculating women with attenuated STIs (likely chlamydia and gonorrhea which they did not differentiate at the time).[14]

This was a different kind of salvific surgery because it sought to redeem and regenerate the body politic through scientific advancements that drew on recent developments in germ theory and inoculation. As is observed in 6.2, however, few of the women were found to be infected with venereal disease. Of 98,581 examinations performed (table 6.2), only 3,059 uncovered any sign of infection (table 6.3). This represents 3.2 percent of the total.

Additional evidence of unnecessary detention appears in the logbooks of the Hospital Morelos. In 1882, for example, records show that an average of eleven women were admitted to the hospital each day, and up to eight women were discharged on a daily basis. This means that between 168 and 205 were held in the sanitary ward at any time.[15]

By 1881, the detentions were so numerous that the director of the Hospital Morelos wrote to the director of the Junta Directiva de Beneficencia about the matter. He complained that he did not have room to contain all the women that the Sanitary Police brought to the hospital and that the Sanitary Inspection Office, not the hospital, should pay for the women's breakfast and dinner. Apparently newcomers were often hungry due to a lack of food supplies in the hospital.[16] One hospital sanitary inspector called the situation "disgraceful." He explained, "The women are forced to use filthy sheets and smocks that have not been washed in at least three days due a lack of soap." One nurse who had been bringing soap to the hospital said that she could no longer afford to do so. Even though the Superior Sanitation Council had expanded rapidly, it remained difficult for the state to coordinate and perform the necessary functions of hospital administration. Perhaps this was because of the administrative and clinical chasm left after the expulsion of las Hermanas de la Caridad.[17]

In the 1880s the doctors who wrote about sex work became more focused on identifying the biological roots of "degenerate" behavior. They were in conversation with prominent public health thinkers and criminologists such as Edwin Chadwick in London and Cesare Lombroso in Italy, who inscribed behavioral stereotypes onto class, racial, and ethnic categories. Chadwick, in particular, claimed that filth and sloth affected one's inner moral compass and predestined individuals and families to commit antisocial behavior.[18] Writing several decades later, Lombroso biologized these ideas to the extreme. A leading positivist criminologist, Lombroso insisted that degeneracy was not only hereditary but also more prevalent in some racial and ethnic groups. Dr. Montenegro adopted many of these views in Mexico's first national study of prostitution. He asserted that sex workers "go around planting the seeds of immorality while carrying sicknesses that result in the degeneration of races and traditions."[19] Montenegro and others writing in the 1880s displayed stronger cultural prejudice than their counterparts from prior generations. They viewed sexual promiscuity as a trait of the entire lower class instead of just a few "fallen women."

Montenegro called on the Porfirian government to bolster the strength of industry, the law, and sanitary inspection and punishment, which he believed would "favor morality and national progress."[20] Like Edwin Chadwick, who argued that the poor should be interned in workhouses in order to strengthen their inner morality, Montenegro believed that foreign capital investment would improve the Mexican race. Ironically, it was the conditions of rapid industrialization and urbanization that had created both a robust sex work industry in Mexico City and the throngs of urban poor who struggled to secure housing and sanitary facilities.[21]

Montenegro blamed Catholicism for a cultural "plague" of ignorance, fanaticism, and misery. He asserted that medical authorities needed to assume control over "moral and physical education and instruction."[22] Thus, sex workers' alleged immorality and backwardness began to be associated with racial degeneration as well as a kind of Black Legend about the effects of Catholicism on Latin Americans. These associations gathered strength over the end of the nineteenth century. Yet because physicians now believed that women's deficiencies were biologically based, some saw redemption as unlikely. Due to the "insubordinate spirit that these women have," Montenegro explained, "we must submit them to the most severe regulatory methods possible, and we must threaten them with severe punishments to ensure their obedience."[23]

Montenegro insisted that "medical experimentation could serve to force these women under the cloak of scientific authority," and he underscored the importance of a "no exceptions" policy to this approach.[24] Montenegro advocated for vague definitions of infection, so as to expand the number of women who might be included in experimental STI treatments. As he explained, "Without entertaining even a shadow of a doubt, we must declare any woman who has a strange discharge to be infected with disease."[25] "Strange discharge" could have resulted from any number of conditions, including women's frequent practice of postcoital irrigation of the sexual organs, which was intended to prevent pregnancy as well as infection.[26]

The pattern of arrest, detainment, and experimental treatment continued throughout the 1880s and increased in the 1890s. By 1891, even the director of the Hospital Morelos claimed that the Sanitary Police force was "overzealous in its persecution of women." He also accused them of corruption and extortion. When the governor of Mexico City learned of the director's concerns, he responded by sending the secretary of the interior to visit the institution and conduct an inspection. Emphasizing that the visiting secretary "was unhappy with what he saw," the report portrayed "many women on the floor, or on inadequate mats, and covered only dirty sheets." Apparently eighty women in the Hospital Morelos were without beds, bedding, or meals.[27]

The interior minister worried about the use of solitary confinement as a punishment. When administrators responded to his complaint, they explained that they placed women in solitary confinement when they "engaged in immoral acts, and when they disrespected the establishment." Hospital Morelos's director wrote, "In the hospital under my direction, we treat women who have been imprisoned and who are held here against their will. We need a better way to restrain them, both to keep order and discipline, and to ensure that they receive medical treatment. Without these elements—order, discipline, and medical treatment—these women commit grave infractions. The authorities of president Lerdo's administration were in agreement with this principle."[28] The director emphasized that when women were "not controlled," they "destroyed the facilities" and "caused riots in the hospital wings."[29] Thus, when onlookers wrung their hands about conditions in the hospital, the director evoked the legacy of Lerdo de Tejada's iron-fist approach.

Meanwhile the Sanitary Police continued to bring more detainees. From the 1870s to the 1890s, Hospital Morelos had maintained a fairly steady population of approximately 200 patients. Although there were 207 steel beds for those patients, only fifty-eight of the beds had mattresses. June 1891, however, witnessed a surge in admissions: the number of patients grew to between 220 and 245 people, and the Sanitary Police brought in fifteen new women each day. By August, the hospital had between 263 and 307 patients in residence per day.[30] Food became particularly scarce; women reportedly endured weeks without consuming beans, which were previously their main source of protein. Meanwhile, the milk was adulterated; at least half had reportedly been replaced with water, causing the containers to smell foul. The director decried these conditions to acquire more money for his hospital from the secretary of the state and the city treasurer.[31]

The ethics of patient treatment and imprisonment continued to be a source of debate among the Sanitary Police, hospital administration, and governmental authorities. These entities made claims on the bodies of hospitalized women: for example, in late 1892, the head of the Sanitary Police wrote to the director of the Hospital Morelos to complain that his team had not had the opportunity to inspect all the patients detained in that establishment.[32] The director responded by reminding him that not all prisoners of the hospital were sex workers, despite their involuntary internment.[33] He wrote, "Among the voluntary patients, there are many elderly women, as well as those with skin conditions. There are some patients with syphilis, as well. We have patients who are married, and who have been infected by their husbands, as well domestic workers who have been sent here by the families who employ them. None of these women should be considered sex workers. The chief sanitary inspector believes that this hospital is only for those women who he arrests and registers as sex workers. But that is not the case."[34]

Years of such discussion led to an 1893 revision of the bylaws of the Hospital Morelos. Article 1 stated that the institution was dedicated to women suffering from syphilis, gynecological infections, and skin afflictions, but made no mention of sex work. Other parts, especially article 5, section 1, increased state oversight of the hospital by declaring that the clinic director would henceforth be named by the secretary of the interior. The secretary would also name the doctors to be employed within. The bylaws additionally stipulated that the medical school residents or students were responsible for all minor operations. This signified that the state had a vested interest in deciding who executed operations and when they did so.[35]

Articles 66 through 82 had to do with the patients themselves. Women were strictly separated into three categories: imprisoned, free, and "privileged." They were never allowed to leave their respective wings to visit women in the other groups. Imprisoned women would need the approval of the Sanitary Police before they were discharged from the hospital. Those who were not "privileged" and not "imprisoned" but "free," were referred to as *libres*, or free women. The *libres* were only allowed to leave the hospital on parole with the permission of a doctor and the director of the hospital. Those who left and did not come back on time would not be able to leave again. The "privileged" women, who resided in the distinguished wing, paid 20 pesos per day, which afforded them "comfort, decency, clean facilities, and independence." Independence presumably allowed these women to exit and enter the hospital as they pleased.

All women were allowed to have visitors for two hours on Thursdays and Sundays. However, those who wished to do so were expected to behave with "discretion and decency." They were expected to "stay in their respective beds, to obey the orders of hospital administrators, and to avoid anything that might cause chaos or disorder in the hospital."[36] Yet some patients even received photographers in a special wing of the hospital, a fact that was disturbing for the director. He complained, in 1893, about this room where outsiders allegedly photographed prostitutes: in his view, this was highly inappropriate because it must have led to sexual activity. From a historical perspective, it is significant that the hospital contained a space where women could participate in recreational, economic, and perhaps even sexual endeavors. It is striking that nineteenth-century prison-hospitals afforded some liberties to the detained.[37]

On the other hand, there was no official channel for those who wished to voice complaints about their treatment. According to the bylaws, such women were simply encouraged to speak with the nurses, doctors, medical students, and the hospital director "so that they might resolve the issues at hand." Perhaps some did, but most probably preferred to avoid the retribution that might result from complaining to authorities.

Finally, article 82 stipulated that when women died at the Hospital Morelos, their families were not allowed to collect their bodies until after doctors had performed autopsies. After a women entered the clinic, after death she belonged to the state to play a part in advancing scientific knowledge. The article did not clarify whether this was the case for "privileged" or "free" women, or whether it only applied to those who had been imprisoned by the Sanitary Police and were being held against their will. The 1893 bylaws also made no mention of consent for surgical or other procedures.

Between December 1893 and October 1894, some powerful local and national officials intervened in the Hospital Morelos in new ways. The governor of Mexico City personally donated 707.35 pesos for surgical equipment, hospital beds, and 405 patient gowns. In 1894, Romero Rubio wrote to the hospital director stating that he had utilized funds from the Sanitary Inspection Office to buy additional equipment for the hospital. Romero Rubio was exceptionally close to President Díaz because his daughter, Carmen Romero Rubio, was married to Díaz. That such a high-level politician ensured extra surgical equipment and resources illustrates the importance of gendered medicine to the Díaz presidency and cabinet as a whole.[38]

By 1897 the director of the Hospital Morelos collaborated with the director of the Escuela Nacional de Medicina to bolster the institutional framework for medical research in the clinic.[39] A wing was reserved for experimental surgeries, and a new chair was created for a professor who wished to supervise additional research. The hospital director only requested that the Escuela Nacional de Medicina pay for the changes in construction. In exchange, he promised that the school could have complete control over the new wing and its patients.

The new wing was full by 1901, and the hospital's detainees hit a new high of 363 patients. Two hundred or more were admitted each month.[40] This brought new complaints from the director, who wrote, "The patients have been complaining ever more frequently about the food, which continues to diminish in quantity."[41] The state inspector disagreed with the hospital director about the need for nutritional improvement, and bluntly asked him to stop complaining about the matter. In 1902 another 100 beds were added to the hospital, and by mid-1902 the number of patients rose to 453.[42]

Tension escalated as the Sanitary Police persisted in detaining more women than the hospital could cope with. In 1902, several women were gravely injured during a riot in the dining area, where they smashed all the plates and then attempted to escape.[43] Others began to find success with a new escape tactic: they penned letters to the governor, insisting that they were not ill and that they were being held in the hospital without cause. In his response, the hospital director wrote, "Several patients have managed to deceive the sanitary inspection doctors, and this has prejudiced the good name of the establishment and degraded the doctors."[44]

In 1903, the director of the Hospital Morelos brought a unique proposal to the city government: converting the hospital into a productive economic space where the inmates would learn a craft or trade. The hospital would then use their skills for "remunerative and regenerative purposes." Even for those women who could not be "regenerated," work would be a "good distraction"—and presumably a deterrence from future rebellions. Physical labor would be easy for the patients, the director insisted, because "more than ninety percent of them have minor conditions."[45]

Pelvic Deficiency and Clinical Practice

In the previous discussion of Hospital Morelos, few if any of the women were nearing childbirth, although presumably some had early term pregnancies. Their experimental treatments also focused more on STIs. But, as other historians have shown, provisional clinical practices extended to the realm of childbirth. Now that the chapter has examined how women were detained by the Sanitary Police, let us look at what kind of medical treatment they received. Ana Maria Carrillo and Laura Cházaro have underscored a key example of this debate, pointing to a clinical dispute that erupted in 1880, in which faculty at the Escuela Nacional de Medicina disagreed about "how to use obstetrical instruments and in which spaces and bodies it was legitimate to do so."[46]

Spurred by complaints from several parties, on at least two occasions the Beneficencia del Ministerio de Gobernación (which had regulatory authority over Mexico City's hospitals) investigated the Escuela Nacional de Medicina concerning discretion in surgical interventions such as the use of forceps during labor and birth. After its investigation, the Beneficencia del Ministerio de Gobernación stated that doctors must "try to disturb the patients as little as possible, in the physical sense as well as the moral." A debate developed in response to their decree, and a special commission of the welfare branch of the interior ministry decided that clinicians could only practice medical interventions on "the poor of this capital," who entered the hospital as an alternative to giving birth in their own "small and unhygienic" homes. Furthermore, the body declared that elite or "decent" women and children certainly "must not be bothered." When it came to the most "unfortunate and disgraced women," however, the council declared that "the patients, upon entering la Casa de Maternidad, should know that they are obligated to repay the service they demand by suffering all of the inconveniences that a clinical Hospital carries with it."[47] Some of those women were pregnant, and the biologically essentialist politics of the national school influenced their experiences with health care.

The ideological underpinnings of pelvimetry, examined in chapter 5, exerted a strong influence on other obstetric practices. Many doctors theorized that because the Mexican pelvis was "backward-facing," the uterus must be erroneously tilted as well. This was termed "retroversion," which literally meant backward-facing. Retroversion was the topic of José Torres Ansorena's thesis, which examined "the inconveniences and dangers of uterine backwardness during pregnancy, birth, and post-partum recovery."[48]

Torres Ansorena claimed that these backward tilts were much more common during childbirth, thereby rationalizing an official diagnostic nomenclature ("tilts that occur during birth"). In his thirty months as an intern in la Casa de Maternidad, Torres Ansorena observed that such tilts were "extremely frequent." He considered these a problem because they allegedly made the child descend from the womb diagonally, delaying labor.

Twenty-first century obstetricians agree that more than one-third of women have so-called tilts of the uterus. This means that variation in uterine placement is physiologically normal and not pathological. Porfirian doctors related uterine tilts to two kinds of deficiencies: those having to do with the skeleton (pelvis), and those having to do with nutrition and vital force. Torres Ansorena theorized that pelvic insufficiency and deficient vital force resulted, first, in uterine laxity, and second, in excessive extension of the abdominal wall.

In 1886, Mexican obstetricians developed an experimental approach to curing the problem of "backward" uteruses. The procedure, called "uterine suspension," used an electric current to cauterize the tissues that connected the uterus to the abdominal walls. Doctors believed that this would shorten and strengthen the connective fibers, thereby reducing "laxity" in the organic (muscular) functions and resulting in a stronger and more vital uterus.[49]

Uterine suspension was a painful process, and so it was only to be performed on women who had been anesthetized with chloroform. The first step was a digital exploration of the vagina, which allowed surgeons to estimate the location of the uterus and pinpoint the best location for the incision. This step may have been useful for diagnosing pregnancy. Clinicians next inserted a wide, fishhook type needle, with a ring surrounding the diameter of the needle. Upon insertion, the ring lodged in the skin and created a canal through which to reinsert the hook. Physicians then applied an electric current to the closed circuit to cauterize the tissue surrounding the uterus.

Obstetricians sometimes cited the use of electric "uterine suspension" to address what they called uterine masses, though they did not specify what those masses were; speculatively, it is possible that these were early pregnancies that patients or doctors wished to terminate. Electrification of the uterus was risky, and patients did not always survive; in 1886, for example, Dr. Ricardo Fuertes related the case of a patient who was referred to him "for a grave infection that resulted from a needle introduced in her uterus, for the purpose of conducting an electrical current. Unfortunately, the needle broke, and a large part of it was left inside of the uterine cavity." The patient did not survive the infection.[50]

Theories about pelvic deficiency, uterine backwardness, and vital force deficiencies led to increased interventions with forceps during childbirth. Manuel Barreiro's 1885 dissertation, *Occasions for the Application of Forceps*, reflected this trend.[51] With his emphasis on scientific standardization, quantification, and the value of statistics, Barreiro was one of the most outspoken positivists of his cohort of students. By 1892 he was a professor of medicine, meaning that that his views were assimilated into the national curriculum.[52]

Barreiro stated three goals for his study: to patent knowledge about forceps, which he claimed had "left the shadows of science"; to identify the proper conditions for their application; and to declare that forceps granted unique opportunities for interventions in childbirth.[53] Barreiro focused on childbirth as an opportunistic time; perhaps reflecting the centralization of the national state, he used militaristic language to describe these opportunities. Women's vulvas were "the gates to the field of action," while forceps were "human hands substituted with an iron instrument." For Barreiro forceps were timely and efficient: "the pinnacle of the science," and "a gift to humanity."[54] Efficiency made good economic sense, as according to historian Ana María Carillo, obstetricians charged up to 300 pesos to attend a childbirth, although they were typically only present for one hour. Midwives, on the other hand, expected only 8 pesos for their customary thirty-six-hour stay.[55]

Forceps eventually became the technology of choice for therapeutic abortions. As chapter 3 discussed, reforma-era doctors experimented with ending pregnancies via the injection of continuous currents of warm water and the gradual dilation and debriding of the cervix. By the late 1880s, doctors used forceps instead of water to open the cervix and dislodge the fetus. Barreiro lamented this fact, reminding doctors that the instrument should not be introduced before the cervix was dilated. Doing so "exposes the mother and the baby to injuries and death, in many cases."[56] Nonetheless, Barreiro deemed forceps "a uterus in our hands,"[57] and insisted that women with "narrowed and insufficient pelvises" were most in need of their application during birth.[58]

Notions about deficiency of uterine vital force continued to reinforce the pelvic deficiency thesis. This was obvious in Alberto López Hermosa's dissertation, published in 1895 and coinciding with the ideological consolidation of Díaz's regime, which was at this point completely controlled by a scientific elite. López Hermosa's work, *Anomalies of the Expulsive Force*, underscored the need to define a "problem point" in Mexican pelvis size.[59] This, he said, would continue to transform obstetrics, "a dark and hesitant practice, into an exact science."[60] "Our Mexican women," he proclaimed, "are often deficient in this category [the pelvis]."[61]

It is quite possible that physicians' insistence on birthing in a "rational," supine, horizontal position was contraindicatory for the natural progression of labor; as Jaffary has indicated, one of the first campaigns Mexican obstetricians undertook was to eliminate midwives' "evil" and "absurd" use of the birthing chair or stool.[62] They believed that medicalized labor symbolized rational progress, and that midwives' feminized labor was weak and inefficient. Some doctors even viewed feminized and traditional birthing practices as morally vile and bankrupt. Surgeons phrased alterations to women's birthing positions and practices as racially regenerative conceptual and practical apparatuses, much like the salvation offered by the cesarean operation, ovariotomy, or therapeutic abortion in earlier decades.

Hermosa also suggested that Mexican women suffered from a lack of uterine vitality caused by weak musculature. This allegedly caused insufficient contractions and was the most common pathological cause of dystocia, or difficulty birthing. Successful contractions were energetic, well directed, regular, and made use of all muscles of the uterus. Doctors evoked mechanistic criteria to define efficient and scientized criteria for childbirth, in turn, these criteria were often invoked to argue that midwives were insufficiently modern to preside over this branch of medicine. Hermosa recognized that contractions could cease and start back up again circumstantially, citing a patient whose labor ceased when her sister-in-law arrived at her home but resumed after the visitor had left.[63]

Hermosa speculated about the biological origins of anomalies in Mexican labor, proposing that "nervous and squeamish women are predisposed to complain of labor pains; this anomaly is based on a grand cellular irritability, whose core, especially in hysterical women, appears to emanate from the uterus."[64] Echoing those who connected hysteria to death during therapeutic abortion in the 1870s, Hermosa believed that "the violent nervous shock" of intense labor pain could cause death during labor.[65] Chloroform was one way to prevent this nervous shock; removing the fetus with forceps was another.

The topic of pain control elicited racialized commentaries about culture, class, and evolutionary biology. Gonzalo Páez's 1886 dissertation examined chloroform, a vapor that depresses the central nervous system of a patient and anesthetizes them to painful procedures.[66] Physicians had recognized since the mid-eighteenth century that noxious gasses would incapacitate patients, but they were hesitant to use them during surgery until the mid-1840s, when the gas was popularized for surgical use by the Scottish physician Sir James Young Simpson. Before the mid-nineteenth century, some patients employed mesmerists and hypnotists to address their pain during excruciating operations.[67]

Mexican doctors began to use chloroform shortly after its global debut as an anesthetic. The drug had drawbacks, and was abandoned by the mid-twentieth century due to its toxicity and sometimes fatal side effects, which included cardiac arrhythmia and damage to the liver and the kidneys.[68] Vasodilation becomes pronounced during labor and birth, which contributed to chloroform's tendency to exacerbate hemorrhaging, retention of the placenta, and increased tearing of the perineum and vulva.[69] The majority of scientists Páez cited believed that the drug slowed, suspended, or even debilitated labor.[70] By the 1920s, doctors were able to rely on intravenous and spinal anesthetics instead.

Páez sought to establish a biologized rationale for chloroform's use, hypothesizing that Mexican neurological functions varied by race and "organization." Comparing childbirth to the involuntary evacuation of excrement, he theorized that as a reflexive action, it did not typically require cerebral participation.[71] "Normal labor pains," the student suggested, "can be so weak that a woman can give birth without suffering, as is the case quite regularly with lower class women."[72] On the other hand, labor pains could be intense "for middle class women, and especially for those in the upper class."[73] Citing middle-class and upper-class women's "impressionable nervous systems," Páez wrote that unconscious sensitivity occurred at a cellular level, "transmitting irritation to the central cerebral receptors," where it became pain.[74] The evolutionary state of one's nervous system transformed a reflexive act into a cerebral one.[75]

Paez's arguments were concurrent with those made by nineteenth-century Anglo-American doctors, who invoked nearly identical concepts to explain alleged differences in the pain of childbirth between so-called savage and civilized women.[76] Historian Miriam Rich locates these arguments within an increasingly explicit racialization of childbirth pain in nineteenth-century medicine, showing how physicians linked childbirth pain to social hierarchies of class and race in the nineteenth-century United States. As a result, doctors in the United States did not offer comparable pain control options to enslaved, Black, and Indigenous women in the United States during childbirth, surgery, and other emergencies. Porfirian doctors in Mexico also enlisted childbirth pain to construct differences of race, class, and indigeneity.

Páez focused on racialized, economically marginalized women, making strong overtures to class categories as racialized signifiers. Because he viewed women from the "lower class" as less evolved, their cerebral "reflexivity" did not interfere with the birthing process.[77] Utterly ignored, of course, were the cultural behavioral norms influencing the degree to which women felt comfortable expressing labor pains. Indigenous and other women would have grown up exposed to dissimilar birthing rituals involving steam baths, birthing chairs, the use of cloths to apply selective pressure on the uterus, and a range of herbal tinctures to address pain, delayed contractions, and other complications. Most women would have been unfamiliar with the presence of male medical authorities during childbirth, and this likely made them uncomfortable and limited their inclination to communicate. Language was another issue; if the student's patients did not speak Spanish, of course they did not cry out to him for help. Finally, they may have feared that openly expressing pain or resistance would provoke retribution through unnecessary medical intervention. In fact, the Grupo de Información en Reproducción Elegida (GIRE) has reported that one of the most common forms of obstetric violence today involves provider aggression, disrespect, and physical violence toward women who vocalize pain. Perhaps silence was an adaptive mechanism for Indigenous women forced to birth in culturally hostile situations. Relatedly, African American women have theorized that their vocalizations and tears sometimes help protect them from maternal death by medical neglect, inasmuch as protestations call attention to their suffering.[78]

Sometimes such pathologizing constructs affected clinical care for higher-class and lighter-skinned women. Páez, for his part, believed that a "high level of conscious sensibility" could "suspend the contractions and the uterus may become sterile as a result."[79] Such sterility apparently halted normal labor, indicating that obstetric interventions were necessary not only for Indigenous women with narrow pelvises: they were also indicated for "more highly evolved" women whose hysterical cerebral activity presented cervical and muscular resistance.[80] These ideas had broad transnational reach, although they adapted to historical contingencies: indeed, scholars Miriam Rich and Laura Briggs have explored how similar ideas were invoked to justify increased obstetric intervention for upper-class white women in the US context.[81] In Mexico, Páez claimed to have "perfectly" established the necessity of chloroform for "delicate" and "hysterical" women.[82] Once again we see the biologized construct of hysteria creating and reinforcing categories of pathology and reinscribing justifications for broad-based intervention.

Whereas earlier obstetricians described Mexican anatomy as deficient in comparison to European women, Páez's discussion focused on class status within the nation. Although Páez focused on middle- and upper-class women, calling them "completely devoid of bravery," he also stated that women of all classes required the drug when they experienced an anomaly in uterine power and vital force that was related to their "insufficient structure."[83] As during the reforma, obstetricians constructed insufficiency as a moral state as well as a physical condition. Paéz, for example, stated that chloroform was "necessary for women whose moral state is exceedingly elevated, for indocile women who move constantly in their beds, or for any woman who refuses to obey any of the doctor's orders, especially when he insists that she be quiet."

He emphasized that for "women who are completely deaf to the doctor's warnings and orders, the use of chloroform is indispensable. Not using it, in fact, can result in grave consequences."[84]

Chloroform could thus be employed as a technology to elicit cooperation or punish women who refused to accept medical authority. Paéz notably referred to women who were allegedly "completely deaf." His casual descriptor recalled Rodriguez and Anzorena's description of young woman from Devil's Alley, who they claimed was "deaf." While it is possible that some of these women were auditorily disabled, it seems highly likely that some spoke Indigenous languages and did not understand the doctors' Spanish. Notwithstanding their hearing status or language spoken, it is significant that doctors pathologized women in simultaneously ableist, racist, and patriarchal ways.

Medical student Benito Feliberto also wrote about the use of chloroform during labor in his 1884 work. Feliberto's work presented a more strictly racialized argument about the effects of the drug on different "types" of women, proposing that "material goods, comfortable living, and a culture of intelligence are all factors that contribute to a general sensitivity, especially upon the reproductive organs."[85] For this reason, he asserted, "we observe that women in Indigenous communities give birth without great suffering, for the absence of culture appears to dull the reproductive organs, and they submit to their ordinary biological functions." Within "the same community," he explained, one would find "women with a more developed nervous system, and it is still more present in the highest social classes."

Although Feliberto conflated race and geographic location, he made class differentiations within rural communities. Like Paéz, his work proposed a link between mental functions ("dull") and biological functions ("reflexive"). Feliberto's thesis embraced and helped to perpetuate the deterministic trope that Indigenous people were reduced to their biological functions and were animalistic as compared with elite women. Feliberto completed his practicum in la Casa de Maternidad, where he reportedly noticed, "the French and English women especially appear to suffer more than others, and Mexican women suffer more than outsiders."[86] Although the medical student did not specify what he meant by "outsiders," he likely referred to those from Indigenous communities, who came from outside of the Federal District. By separating them from the "Mexican women," Feliberto, like Francisco de Asís Flores y Troncoso, discursively excluded Indigenous people from the national imaginary.

Surgical Interventionism, Mortality, and Debates about Medical Ethics

As the medical research community grew in size and funding in the late nineteenth century, women of all classes increasingly received reproductive health care in clinical spaces. Some of that health care was sought out by the women themselves, and some was forced via arrest and detention by the Sanitary Police. Women of all classes became vulnerable to some forms of therapeutically unproven reproductive health care within hospitals.

Like in other nations, Mexican obstetricians contended that the science of birth needed to be modernized, standardized, medicalized, and attended by a patriarchal class of highly trained physicians. Yet the antiseptic tenets of germ theory were still not completely assimilated, and, of course, antibiotics would not be developed for decades. Nora Jaffary tells us that the increase in surgical interventionism correlated with heightened infant and maternal mortality rates in Mexico City's clinics, largely due to epidemics of puerperal fever, or bacterial infections of the womb, vagina, and soft tissue.[87] Such infections ravaged women in the delicate time after childbirth, often causing sepsis and killing them in a matter of days.

The risks posed by surgical intervention are reflected in rising mortality rates over time. Some baseline data can be found in Miguel Márquez's 1881 study, which reported the outcomes for 787 childbirths in Mexico City hospitals occurring between 1877 and 1881.[88] Of these, 695 women gave birth without any intervention. Forceps were used in only twenty-eight births; seventeen other interventions occurred when doctors used their hands in an attempt to extract the fetuses from the womb. Fourteen of the fetuses were born dead, and eight women reportedly experienced difficulty during childbirth due to small pelvic measurements. Thirty-nine mothers died, which was a 5 percent mortality rate. The fetal mortality rate was similarly low, at 8 percent. These numbers indicate that before the ascendency of the pelvic deficiency thesis, which had just begun to form in 1881, low interventionism in Mexican obstetrics correlated with low maternal and fetal mortality rates.

By 1895, maternal and fetal mortality rates had skyrocketed, as demonstrated by a large data set from Manuel Leal's thesis on stemming the hemorrhages resulting from surgical procedures in three clinics (Muller, the Clínica de Partos, and la Casa de Maternidad).[89] The three hospitals had an average maternal mortality rate of 28 percent and fetal mortality rate of 62 percent. At 49 percent, almost half of the women who hemorrhaged after undergoing a surgical procedure died; infants born to hemorrhaging women died at a rate of 82 percent.[90] These statistics underscore why obstetricians worried about the dangers of forceps, on the grounds that the technology could, and frequently did, cause hemorrhaging. Even Juan Duque de Estrada—a professor of medicine who fervently advocated for surgical intervention in obstetrics—fixated on pictures of infants whose faces had been crushed by the application of forceps. For him, the dangers of delivery by forceps confirmed that doctors should carry out more caesarean operations on narrow-hipped women.

One student, Fernando Zárraga, dedicated his 1884 thesis to the topic of medical ethics, though he did not use that term. Instead, he analyzed what he called "surgical disgraces."[91] Zárraga believed that the public's distrust of surgeons was reasonable, and that doctors needed to make sincere attempts to cure ailments before resorting to relatively untried operations. He implored his colleagues, "Is it justified to open a patient's womb without first ascertaining the diagnosis? Is it acceptable to expose her to the risk of infection for the sole purpose of executing an exploratory incision? I do not believe so. I believe that we should only operate when an operation is necessary."[92]

Zárraga offered three examples of surgeries that he viewed as "disgraceful." The first patient's reportedly "unnecessary" ovariotomy caused her to die of infection. Another's infant suffered a broken femur "due to the unnecessary application of forceps." Zárraga's third example was "one of the most disgraceful diagnostic errors [he] had witnessed." Señora G, who had been "married for several years," had been trying to conceive a child with her husband. When her menstruation ceased and she experienced "other discomforts," the patient called a doctor for an in-house examination; unfortunately he did not recognize the pregnancy and instead diagnosed her with what he called a "uterine ailment." After all, early-stage pregnancies were difficult to diagnose in the 1880s, much like they had been in the eighteenth century.

The doctor "punctured the uterus and withdrew a large amount of clear liquid." When the patient began to bleed and show early signs of labor, her husband called a midwife. Perhaps he no longer trusted the doctor and felt more confidence in the woman's professional services. The midwife examined the patient's cervix and encountered the legs of a small fetus, which was subsequently delivered, deceased, via artificial premature birth. Though midwives were banned from surgical operations by this time, apparently they could, and did, still oversee artificial premature birth in the privacy of a patient's home. Perhaps it mattered that the product of conception was already dead, making it unlikely that the surgery would have been criminally prosecuted as an abortion. Señora G, for her part, almost died of an infection;

although she recovered, she did not bear more children.[93] Though Señora G and her family had the connections and financial resources to pay a private doctor and a midwife for in-home care, the doctor's arguably overzealous interventionism was therapeutically detrimental. At the same time, however, Señora G was not targeted for experimental care in the same way as the woman detained and imprisoned by the Sanitary Police. Señora G's class privilege positioned her to benefit from her family's protection and advocacy; most notably, her husband was able to discontinue the physician's care regime and contract a midwife instead.

Notwithstanding the particularities of individual circumstances, for Zárraga these situations indicated a larger problem relating to patients' agency and voice. When inexperienced doctors and medical students sought surgical practice in order to perfect their operational techniques, they would often "deceive the patient, falsely representing their condition and encouraging them to undergo a surgery that is sure to become tragedy."[94] "We should not operate in this way," Zárraga insisted, "we must only operate when it is perfectly justified, and we must warn the family when the surgery is likely to endanger or kill the patient."[95] His critique was not unique to Mexico: as mentioned in the introduction, British doctor James Blundell was intensely critical of the interventionist approach to obstetrics, and especially the indiscriminate and sometimes indelicate use of forceps.[96] Conflict about obstetric surgery increased in late nineteenth century Mexico, as doctors' access to antiseptic surgery and public patients increased as well.

Zárraga believed that some structural and epistemological changes would address these issues. First, he recommended an emphasis on diagnostic criteria: "We will only be able to avoid the vast majority of our surgical tragedies if we avoid making erroneous diagnoses." Second, physicians needed to "cease performing surgery except for when it is indicated and perfectly justified." Third, doctors must be honest with their prognoses and refrain from lying to patients about their conditions. Fourth, the young doctor implored his colleagues to be "serious about the risks of chloroform and consider its counter-indications." Finally, he insisted that they must not "undertake grand operations for which we have no training or prior knowledge; [even with proper training], we must focus our attention during surgery to avoid manual errors."[97]

Gendered notions about stoic and heroic surgeons also came into play. Zárraga emphasized the moral value of masculine surgeons who would "remain stone-faced instead of panicking and forgetting everything we know about anatomy. Then, and only then, will we be able to avoid the vast majority of our surgical tragedies."[98] Otherwise, he feared, the national scientific enterprise would be delegitimized in the eyes of the public and international onlookers. The young student was alarmed by professors who reportedly began to analyze extracted organs before stitching the patient's surgical wounds. After seeing these scenes, Zárraga felt that the autopsies had begun before patients were officially dead. By these accounts, late nineteenth-century reproductive surgery depended on experimental and racialized surgery that was not always therapeutically indicated. The pursuit of a moralized and masculinized brand of knowledge was at stake, similarly to when women's corporal lives had been devalued in the century prior in favor of the spiritual value of a fetal soul that demanded fetal baptism at almost any cost.

Zárraga's manifesto seemed to provoke written responses from his colleagues and professors. In particular, Ricardo Fuertes's 1886 book defended the therapeutic and scientific legitimacy of reproductive surgery, and especially ovariotomy. Fuertes had become a professor at the medical school after he received his medical degree at the University of Berlin.[99] His book seemed particularly influential and likely was used as a textbook. The goal of his study was to "rehabilitate obstetrical operations in Mexico."[100] Fuertes attributed the "decline in surgical prestige" to the "generally poor results" of nineteenth-century surgery as a whole, and not just in Mexico. In other words, it was important that his students not think this was a national problem. He moralized patient hesitancy, decrying that it was "irrational," "baseless," and "foul," and ultimately based on the outdated notion that surgery was useless and futile. Such attitudes had resulted in "an incomprehensible spirit of self-preservation" that led to an avoidance of the hospital and the operating room. Patients, Fuertes insisted, should not be afraid of "the only rational means of salvation that may help them." As a remedy, doctors needed to embrace the idea of "operating on a daily basis." Only then would they "become capable of defeating the obstacles presented."[101]

Fuertes's argument rested on the unspoken necessity of a readily available population of public, imprisoned patients, whose circumstances were previously detailed.[102] "To achieve this step forward in our national surgical tradition, we must combat antiquated ideas," Fuertes concluded. "But we will always be victorious in this fight, because progress asserts itself automatically."[103] This was a nod to the positivist and Lamarckian notion that all beings and societies are imbued with a vital force that automatically propels progress. There was a salvationism to this surgery—"the only rational means of salvation"—capable of rescuing the nation from an array of biological and professional degeneration.

Medicine and the Law, in Medical Students' Words

By 1887, the question of surgical ethics elicited legal debate, as was evidenced in the work of Alfonzo Ruíz Erdozain, who published a book on medical responsibility from a legal perspective, as part of his application for a professorial post in legal medicine in the Escuela Nacional Preparatoria (ENP).[104] Prior to the mid-century laws of reform, a doctor could suffer five years of disbarment for "practicing an operation in such an unwise manner that the patient died." Under the same regulations, if a surgeon intentionally used surgery to cause a patient's death—or when they should have known that the surgery would cause death—they were vulnerable to the permanent loss of their license.[105] "With the publication of the most recent legal code in Mexico," Ruíz Erdozain explained, "this law disappeared." He continued, "As there is no article that mentions surgical crimes, we can naturally assume that our current law does not recognize this concept."[106] "In fact," he stated, "it would only be accurate to state that the law eases the path for surgeons, by facilitating free rein in medical practice."[107] In any case, the medical student viewed it as outwardly impossible to predict how a surgical procedure would affect an individual because some people had a weaker organization than others.

One of Ruíz Erdozain's legal recommendations seemed to reference sexual intimacy, although in a pun-like manner. "Two doctors," he wrote, "attempted to terminate a woman's pregnancy by means of forceps and manual extraction. Unfortunately, they ended up rupturing her uterus instead." This example once again underscores the frequency with which women sought pregnancy termination. Yet, it is unclear whether the fetus was intended to survive the termination, and likewise, whether doctors wished to terminate the woman's pregnancy prematurely or at the end of gestation. The doctors became "fearful" after the uterine rupture and sent the woman to la Casa de Maternidad, where Dr. Juan María Rodríguez was unable to save her life. Although it was not Rodríguez's error that led to her death, the woman's family expressed its outrage to him. "From that day," Ruíz Erdozain wrote, "Professor Rodríguez and I have echoed the same recommendation: never put your hand where other men have already been."[108] Medical students rarely wrote about banter and the other forms of professional socialization they experienced during their training. Yet, Ruíz Erdozain normalized the circumstance by joking about a sexual double standard while comparing doctors to sexual suitors who expected virgin territory. He even attributed the joke to the clinic director, Rodríguez, and bragged about his inside joke with the powerful profession. Instead of commenting on the therapeutic and clinical aspects of this case, Ruíz Erdozain offered legal advice and diffused the fraught emotional scenario by invoking body-gore humor.

Ruíz Erdozain turned to religion for his last argument. God, he asserted, should be the only arbiter of surgical ethics.[109] In his view, there were two sources of interference with this natural law: professional debate about scientific knowledge on the one hand, and the regulatory state on the other. "If there were not so many schools of medical thought, theories, and systems," Ruíz Erdozain explained, "and if clinical practice could reflect *one* doctrine, followed by all—just like a religion—there would not be so many difficulties, or so much dissidence."[110] In his view, the state should not have any power to regulate surgical practice because society owes to doctors its most prized possessions: "enlightenment, prudence, and truth."

This was a strong argument for a biopower-type government by autonomous scientists and physicians, whose practices and ideologies coalesced around a uniting philosophy. Under this kind of state, scientists would be able to work quickly toward a common goal, free of legal restraints.[111] This may well have occurred at the height of the Porfirian dictatorship in Mexico, if judging by the absence of Zárraga's "surgical disgraces"-type dissent from medical students throughout the 1890s.

Ruíz Erdozain's writing further referenced religion in two ways: science as religion, and God as a benevolent supporter of science due to doctors' inherent worthiness as agents of social change. Somewhat ironically, Ruíz Erdozain insisted that a lack of surgical ethics would only be punishable in the afterlife—that is, he maintained that scientific pursuit should enjoy complete liberty and autonomy, and that the only consequences for error or misjudgment would be metaphysical and otherworldly. This invocation of religion is especially interesting in light of other Porfirian doctors' comments on the backward influence of the Catholic Church, and against the backdrop of the reforma era (and ongoing) secularization of medical practice. But perhaps it is no surprise that religion remained an important issue, given that the Porfirian government sought a reconciliation with the Catholic Church. Meanwhile, Catholic priests continued to practice cesarean operations into the 1890s, thereby continuing to exert metaphysical claims over unborn fetuses, which gave way to debates about the ethics of surgery.[112]

Another provocative argument about religion and surgery was published five years before Ruíz Erdozain's legal argument. This was a treatise by medical student Joaquin Ibáñez, who discussed the comparative ethical and religious aspects of surgical procedures, including abortion and caesarean operation.[113] Ibañez proposed a framework that he called "positive morality," and he insisted that it should guide the trajectory of these topics.

Ibañez used the concept of positive morality to argue that to sacrifice the life of the fetus in favor of the mother was an ethical wrong. Yet at the same time, he advocated for the artificial premature termination of late-term pregnancies of those women whose pelvises were seen as deficient. There were, in his view, two preferable options: to provoke abortion in early pregnancy, or to perform cesarean surgery during late pregnancy. He defended abortion in these cases by explaining that "a small fetus is far from viable, and many things could happen before viability: first of all, the narrowness of the pelvis could prevent the development of the uterus, which could provoke miscarriage, or otherwise create unnatural conditions for fetal survival."[114] Meanwhile, the termination of pregnancy via artificial labor or abortion had, for him, "a powerful and logical rationale, under positive morality."[115] As more doctors turned to the caesarean operation as a logical intervention in the face of alleged pelvic deficiencies, it is plausible that they did so because it was seen by authorities as a more acceptable intervention than abortion. This was certainly Ibáñez's opinion. He wrote, "Positive morality should prove that feticide is illicit, and as such, the caesarean operation is the safest, and most moral of all options—in the religious sense, at least."

Ibáñez framed this argument not just in terms of positive morality but also with the language of liberal rights. Ibáñez viewed the "right to life" as a "fundamental right, and that which underpins all the other rights." "Without life," he wrote, "there are no rights, and so we must view rights as that which begins when the first seed is deposited within the mother." Ibáñez insisted that women themselves did not have the right to terminate a pregnancy, even if that pregnancy threatened their life. On the contrary, women exhibiting a "faulty organization" should take it upon themselves to avoid bearing children, given that those pregnancies ran a higher risk of failure. Women in this situation were guilty of "voluntarily seeking conflict with their own fetus."[116]

This constituted a shift in medical thought. A mere ten years before, as demonstrated in chapter 4, the medico-legal argument took the opposite position—namely, that fetuses endangered some women's emotional and sociocultural lives. During the Porfiriato, the rhetoric became racialized and biologically deterministic, with an emphasis on "defective organization." Now for the first time in postcolonial Mexican medicine, obstetricians wrote about the mother as an enemy of the fetus. Though cast in liberal and scientific terms, this was a callback to eighteenth-century ideas about surgeons' responsibility to prioritize fetal over maternal life. These were salvational surgical arguments indeed. With the right argumentation, men could be saved from women's irrational reproduction, and elites could be saved from the socioeconomically oppressed classes' faulty biological organization. At this time in the United States, the American Medical Association was consolidating its position against women's access to contraception and abortion, inspired by rabid anti-sex activist Anthony Comstock. In Mexico, on the other hand, medical arguments vacillated between decrying abortion and supporting it, depending on how the topic could be reconciled, or not, with the biologically essentialist or interventionist prerogatives at hand. Mexican postcolonial doctors, as a whole, did not seem as committed as American doctors to preventing women from accessing contraception and abortion. Nonetheless, they shared the paternalistic belief that male scientific authorities should influence reproduction while exerting social control over women's lives.

Ultimately, Ibañez equivocated on abortion and clinical experimentation in the same breath, stating simply his belief that a loss of life was unavoidable in reproductive medicine: "There are inevitable life and death conflicts among finite beings, and these often become tragedies; these should be handled by moral men, whenever possible, lest they become criminal acts."[117] Porfirian doctors saw some surgeries as tragedies, but they were the moralistic, even priestly, facilitators of human tragedy. Thus the origins of the "right to life" legal discourse in the Americas was undergirded by structurally and epistemologically ingrained obstetric racism and violence.

As the Porfiriato progressed, scientific politics effectively reshaped higher education and led doctors to treat some of Mexico City's lower-class women as they had treated the girl of Devil's Alley. This chapter has demonstrated how elite preconceptions of race, class, and gender influenced medical practices in public hospitals, and how positivist thought impacted state relations with marginalized groups by embedding racial and social prejudices in purportedly neutral bodies of scientific knowledge.[118] Indeed, the Porfiriato witnessed a great deal of elite insecurity about the racial standing of the nation and its progress toward modernity. The Porfirian liberal establishment was heavily influenced by *los científicos,* who sought to apply science to politics in the hopes of social regeneration for Mexico. The heart of their philosophy was "the search for an ever-diminishing number of laws or 'general facts' of which all observable phenomena are observable cases."[119] According to positivists, communities and nations functioned like a set of organs, so the whole was only as strong as the weakest part. Some Mexican doctors came to view natural selection as either ineffective among such a physiologically disadvantaged population or believed that it was working too slowly for the nation to effectively modernize and industrialize. The solution was to further scientific research through anthropometric research and clinical innovation.

The obstetric writings examined in this chapter were a core part of this quest for regenerative scientific laws. Meanwhile, some experimental approaches to surgery endangered public patients' reproductive health and may have compelled them to seek further experimental care in the future. While elite women were seen as more delicate and therefore in need of pain control, doctors simultaneously believed that they were inappropriate subjects of some kinds of therapeutic intervention. At times, elite women's class and racial privilege afforded them more agency in choosing a health care provider and pursuing alternate treatments. This was not the case for the majority of reproductive-age women in Mexico City, and certainly not for the thousands of women detained and imprisoned by the sanitary police. Racist ideologies manifested in tangible ways in public clinics, where interventions became embedded in a moral rhetoric about scientific progress and sociobiological evolution.

Part IV
Surgery and Revolutionary Salvation

CHAPTER SEVEN

A True Professional Sacrament

Tubal Ligation and Eugenic Sterilization, 1920s–30s

By the early 1930s, thousands of pregnant women per year approached the steely gates of the General Hospital in search of resources like food, medicine, and health care services during the vulnerable and painful time of labor and childbirth. The administrators of the General Hospital did not wish to leave them in need. The General Hospital had been at the center of health care in the city since 1905, when President Porfirio Díaz inaugurated the massive institution. He did so in response to Eduardo Licéaga's pleas for a "project that would unite all of the offices and functions of the Office of Public Health and Welfare under one administration, with the goal of improving the lives of the people who go there in search of shelter and care."[1] Hospital Morelos and the Casa de Maternidad, institutions that figured prominently in previous chapters, were no longer the primary spaces where women received reproductive treatments and surgeries.[2] Chapters seven, eight, and nine focus primarily on the General Hospital, where struggles over reproductive surgery grew in both size and scope while inflecting social-salvational debates about eugenics, feminism, fertility control, and the Mexican Revolution.

Beginning in 1910, the Mexican Revolution became internationally significant as the first grassroots social revolution of the twentieth century. The movement enveloped a massive uprising of Mexicans from all parts of the country who were exhausted for having been exploited by Díaz's extractive regime and by foreign investors who owned most of Mexico's wealth, land, and resources. Demanding "land and liberty," communities rose up in revolt, burning the estates of wealthy landowners and taking over their properties, factories, and haciendas.

After almost a decade of civil war, 1917 brought agreement on a constitution enshrining many socially progressive rights and benefits. Significantly, for example, the constitution made Mexico the first nation in the world to guarantee health care as a right to all Mexicans. Sadly 1917 did not mark the end of revolutionary warfare, and substantial strife and civil warfare persisted throughout the 1920s. In particular, the Catholic Church declared a revolt in 1927 when they felt that their privileges were being limited by radical anticlericalist politicians. The religious question loomed large, as politicians, expelled priests, shuttered churches, and assassinated Catholic militants while blaming the Church for stymying political, social, and economic progress. Many Mexicans, for their part, insisted on the importance of religion in their day-to-day lives.

Many other factors exacerbated the nation's challenges. Among these were material shortages resulting from World War I, the Revolution, and reconstruction, and depopulation from over 1 million deaths from revolutionary warfare. An additional half a million deaths from the 1917–18 influenza pandemic worried state-builders, who fretted about whether Mexico had the human capital for reconstruction and economic revitalization. It did not help that the depression of 1931–33 sent impoverished Mexicans from across the country to the capital city in search of government aid and welfare. Another social problem stemmed from the repatriation of at least 350,000 Mexicans who had been living in the United States and were deported to Mexico City. There they lacked resources and social networks and reportedly overwhelmed the welfare system.[3]

By the early 1930s, Mexico was in a strongly progressivist phase with a leftist and uniting president, Lázaro Cárdenas, who had helped pull the country from the religious *Cristero* war of the 1920s, in which some 90,000 people died. Cárdenas's proposals for land reform and state-sponsored health care, schooling, and industrialization gained support from the populace, and it seemed that the promises of the Mexican Revolution might finally be fulfilled. Mexican women helped lead the Revolution, and many were deeply invested in and inspired by revolutionary politics. Mexican feminists and others mounted vibrant campaigns for a multitude of rights, including voting, divorce, entrance into the workforce, and access to fertility control. Sexual mores were in flux in the 1920s and 1930s, in part due to cultural changes brought by film and radio, the faster circulation of feminist ideas through media and print, and the roiling transnational suffrage and fertility-control movements.[4]

Racial politics were shifting as well, though like gender politics they saw considerable continuity as well as change. Starting in the 1920s, the nation turned to what Andrés Molina Enríquez, Manuel Gamio, José Vasconcelos, and others called the "Indian problem."[5] State leaders obsessed over how state projects could incorporate long-marginalized communities into the national fabric. Public health authorities in Mexico City promoted medical and hygiene campaigns, targeting poor urban women and Indigenous internal migrants whom they saw as culturally backward but potentially redeemable. As in the United States, progressive-era officials addressed a range of public health issues like alcoholism, syphilis, tuberculosis, and hereditary ailments, which they believed posed a grave danger to the national "race."

By focusing on racialized obstetric surgeries, this chapter addresses the largely unknown history of eugenic sterilizations in 1930s Mexico. On an international scale, sterilizing surgeries were extremely common at the time. Indiana became the first US state to legalize sterilization in 1907, a development that several Mexican eugenicists emphasized in their contemporaneous writings.[6] The majority of US states soon followed suit, and hundreds of thousands of women lost their procreative capacities as a result of state and scientific class, racial, and disability-based prejudices. Some governors in the United States are beginning to grapple with this legacy and offer apologies and redress.[7]

Although many have explored the politics of eugenic sterilization in the United States and western Europe, the topic has received much less scholarly attention in Mexico and Latin America. Historians of science and medicine have tended to view Latin eugenics as less interventionist, more opposed to permanent sterilization, and generally "softer" and environmentally focused, in contradistinction to the "harder," more hereditarian, US and western European traditions. The idea of a comparatively mild eugenics in Latin America stemmed from many factors, including a strong tradition of progressive social medicine in the region. It was also rare for Latin American countries to implement nonconsensual sterilization laws. The only exception appears to be the Mexican state of Veracruz, which legalized state-mandated sterilization in 1932. Historians' understanding of Latin eugenics has become much more nuanced in recent decades, as scholars like Alexandra Minna Stern and Marius Turda have explored the situated and interconnected questions of racism, nationalism, religion, economics, politics, and culture throughout the "Latin" world and its borderlands.[8]

Decades of historians and other scholars of Latin America and the Caribbean have explored how racism manifested in colonizing nations as compared to colonized and formerly colonized regions. Scientific racism was unique, but still pervasive, in the racially mixed, politically progressive, and so-called racial paradises and mestizo nations of Latin America. On the one hand, and as Nancy Stepan compelling analyzed in the 1990s, eugenicists throughout Latin America lent considerable credence to neo-Lamarckian theories of genetic inheritance and did so well into the twentieth century. But on the other hand, eugenicists in Latin America did not ignore hereditarian questions, eschew Mendelian-inspired eugenics, or remain immune to sociopolitical debates about the germ plasm. As seen in previous chapters, they also embraced Spencerian and Malthusian thought, though their discussions of such ideologies were almost always underpinned by Comtean positivism. Nor was Latin America a mirror image of US racial ideologies. Like in the United States and other nations, Mexican scientists and authorities racialized groups on the basis of myriad factors, including economic status, cultural difference, language, diet, lifestyle, and behavior. As historian Karin Rosemblatt has recently shown, not only was race a "scientific category that enabled cross-border discussions," but Mexican eugenic ideas were as influenced by racial scientists to the North as by Latin eugenicists in Spanish, Portuguese, Italian, and French nations and colonies.[9]

Laura Suárez joins other historians in refuting the notion that Mexican eugenicists were less wedded to racialized and hereditarian prejudices than their Western European and American counterparts.[10] Through an examination of the Mexican Eugenics Society (established in 1928), Suárez shows that eugenic thought strongly influenced Mexican governance, and that it continued to do so until the 1970s. More recently, historian Sarah Walsh has added significant nuance to the idea that Latin eugenicists were broadly opposed to surgical sterilization. Focusing on Chile, Walsh argues that "there was no uniquely Latin objection to the practice initially," and "it was not until the implementation of the 1933 German racial purity laws" that Chileans "began to define their objections to the practice as explicitly Latin."[11] Latin eugenics was not some foregone, culturally rooted phenomenon: it was, at least in part, a rejection of genocidal eugenics as they played out in Germany.

Because the historiography on Mexican eugenics is relatively new, sterilization has almost always been studied through state and legislative sources—as a matter of law, and not clinical practice. Historians have also drawn on conference proceedings and medical journals, but these were mediated and public-facing venues in which students were less likely to discuss federally banned surgeries. Through an examination of student writings, General Hospital records, and reports from the secretary of health, this chapter joins others in correcting the long-standing assumption that Mexican women were not targeted for coercive eugenic sterilization. It reveals that surgeons, professors of medicine, and medical students regularly subverted federal laws prohibiting sterilization in order to perform a range of surgical interventions to alter women's reproductive capacities. Many doctors sterilized women in the service of eugenic ideology, but compelling evidence also shows that they were aware of, and reacted to, women's own demands for fertility control. Although nation-states are almost always viewed as the main drivers of eugenic ideology, this chapter highlights spaces in which medical doctors—who were at that time state employees—subverted state policies, pursuing the operations frequently, clandestinely, and as a kind of open secret.

Racial Discourse and Sterilizing Surgeries in 1930s Mexico

Let us return to the women who sought reproductive health care in the General Hospital. The massive compound, which consisted of small, contiguous buildings, occupied more than 170,000 square meters in the heart of Mexico City. Nestled near the Rio de la Piedad, the complex had 55,000 meters dedicated to gardens and open space, which must have provided pleasant scenery for patients, students, and employees alike. When the sick, injured, homeless, and hungry entered the complex, they traversed a complex network of wide, clean corridors that ran between the small buildings. The institution was widely celebrated as the embodiment of modernity and as a symbol of Mexico's dedication to care for its citizens' health.

In the largest building lived the director of the hospital with his family, near the intake and administrative offices; thus, when a person approached the hospital in search of care, they stepped into the home of the institution's most powerful and influential figure. Other buildings contained wards for patients with leprosy, tuberculosis, and venereal diseases, as well as those for surgery and reserved for "distinguished patients," who presumably paid top dollar for their stay. A large kitchen provided a place to prepare food for the thousands of patients and workers of the hospital; it was also where dozens of children toiled and played, given that the offspring of the nurses, laundresses, cooks, and patients were part of the hospital community. When a pregnant patient received obstetric care at the General Hospital, she became part of a larger community, for a short time at least. The community comprised the public health officials who squabbled over the distribution of resources, the laborers whose daily toil of laundering, cooking, and scrubbing made the institution work, and a host of patients whose patronage, requests, and complaints reflected their expectations for health care as well as their demands on the state.

The hospital community was profoundly influenced by those who exerted the most power over other people's bodies: the professors of medicine whose instruction was based there, and the medical students who shadowed those professors while practicing in the wards and while observing and performing surgeries. Their practices, their writings, and their ideologies were a product of Porfirian epistemological legacies, progressive revolutionary politics, and the international dialogues in which they participated.

Obstetrics after the Revolution showed strong clinical continuity from the late nineteenth century, in which doctors pursued interventionist surgeries on racially marginalized women as part of a larger national project that pathologized Mexican women and disparaged their biological capacities. This much was clear to medical student Genaro Ramírez Elliot, who wrote in 1932, "In Mexico, surgical sterilization was born with the desire to prevent women with small pelvic measurements from giving birth. For many years, that was the only scientifically acceptable rationale for sterilization. Sterilization has expanded in subsequent years. But even today, Mexican doctors always experiment with sterilization techniques on women with small pelvises first. Following these preliminary experimentations, we then begin to use new surgical techniques on other women, as well."[12] Ramírez Elliot's blunt comments demonstrate the perpetuation of racial prejudice in Mexican obstetrics. He evoked nineteenth-century rhetoric concerning anatomical deficiency to claim that some patients could not successfully birth without scientific intervention; this provided the therapeutic and clinical pretext for eugenic sterilization.

Despite the egalitarian aims of Mexico's social revolution, postrevolutionary hospitals continued to be spaces of social and national exclusion and race-making, specifically through the state's efforts to cultivate culturally reformed, and even revolutionized, subjects through the application of eugenic medicine.

Although women from all social groups and statuses frequented Mexico City's reproductive health care services in the 1920s and 1930s, parsing patients' racial and ethnic identities is a complex task. In a sample of eighty medical theses from the 1930s, doctors described 114 women as *mujer india* ("Indian woman") and another thirty-eight as *indigena* ("Indigenous"). They referred to seven patients as speaking a dialect, which presumably referred to an Indigenous language. Doctors used the word *morena* (dark-skinned or Black) to refer to fifteen women, and *mestiza* ("mixed") for eleven. Nine women were marked *sajón,* as in Anglo-Saxon. Physicians noted their patients' class status 604 times but referred to *clase campesina* (peasant class) only ten times. Patients were categorized as *clase analfabética,* or "illiterate class," on nineteen occasions, and as *clase humilde,* or "of a humble class" in 114 references. Finally, doctors mentioned the "culture" of their patients 216 times, using describers such as "none," "rudimentary," "medium," or "elevated."

Doctors were invested in making categorical distinctions among their patients, even if those were inconsistent and highly variable. They commented on a range of characteristics, from phenotype, to occupation, to literacy. As

Karin Rosemblatt has noted, racial categories were always intricately intertwined with, among other criteria, "ideas about religion; soils and climates; urban and rural landscapes; genotypes; phenotypes; natural and social environments; gender; upbringing; inheritance; diets; exercise; and culture."[13] These are all racialized constructs, as race itself is a biosocial construct like culture.

Although eugenics was a classificatory project, doctors made inconsistent notes on patients' social status. Sometimes medics included detailed information about "race," "class," "culture," and "education," which are, of course, contested and contingent categories. Though racial discourse permeated the doctors' writings, racial categories remained slippery, malleable, and fleeting. Physicians sometimes casually mentioned "Indian" patients, as though it was obvious that they were of Indigenous descent. For example, in 1932 when one inspector made a complaint about a doctor in Ixtacalco, he casually mentioned that the doctor had been treating "some Indians" for various ailments.[14]

More evidence for the widespread nature of racial discourses appears in the writings of Dr. Rafael Carrillo, who was the president of Mexico's Puericulture Society in the early 1930s. In an article he described as a "defense of eugenic ideas for racial betterment," Carrillo especially "sought to defend the hereditary ideas of Galton and Mendel" against neo-Lamarckian trends. Like the clinicians cited in previous chapters, Carrillo emphasized the importance of anthropometric studies; because Mexico had a "mosaic of races," he believed anthropometry was one of the most important ways to "distinguish races." Classifying "ethnological typologies" would allow scientists to understand a litany of biologized and behavioral factors, including "biological functions, mentality, attitudes toward various activities, resistance to work, and degree of initiative and moral values, as well as the somatic, psychiatric, and moral functions and the rules that guide those functions."[15] If Mendelian genetics could become experimental, he posited, anthropometry offered a mathematical solution that could usher in solutions to "complex problems."[16] At the same time, like many puericulturalists, he emphasized that eugenicists' goal should always be to create environmentally optimal conditions for racial regeneration. One of Mexico's most important public health doctors, Carrillo was not shy about his racist opinion: that Mexico needed eugenics in order to "elicit something clean from something dirty."[17]

Mestizaje, or racial and cultural mixture, was of particular interest to Carrillo. He believed that about 50 percent of the Mexican population was already mestizo, and that only 30 percent was Indigenous. Spaniards allegedly comprised 15 percent of the nation, though he did not clarify whether he referred to Spanish nationality or heredity. Carrillo believed that 1 percent of Mexico's population was Black, and that the rest, or 4 percent of the country, were of Asian and other descent.[18] On the one hand, this doctor seemed influenced by Vasconcelos's idea that the "mestizo race" would gradually become biologically and culturally stronger via increased admixture with other groups, under the principle that the stronger races "win out" against the "weaker ones."[19] He believed that miscegenation would slowly dilute undesirable physiological characteristics. On the other hand, Carrillo referred to Indigenous groups as separate races and proposed that it would be advantageous to prohibit sexual unions between the "lower races" and those that showed a higher degree of civilization in their ancient societies, like the Nahua, which he called "ancient Mexicans," as well as the Mixtec, Zapotec, and Maya. Other groups, he proposed, could be treated like the Indigenous peoples of the United States and placed on reservations in mountainous areas.[20]

As postrevolutionary doctors expanded debate on the social and biological circumstances surrounding eugenics and sterilization, the alteration or removal of reproductive organs increased in frequency from earlier times. Between 1911 and 1936, 415 students in the national medical school designed and conducted studies on obstetrics, gynecology, or reproduction. These studies generally referenced between thirty to fifty patients, although sometimes they included demographic and clinical data from as many as 800 women. One report from the Hospital Juárez in 1926 illuminates the widespread performance of obstetric and gynecological surgery. Of 1,946 operations reported that year, 503 were hysterectomies. Another 201 surgeries were laparotomies, in which the abdomen was opened, allowing doctors to tie the patients' fallopian tubes or perform other major surgeries. Eighty-four of the surgeries were designated as "resulting from childbirth," without additional information, and another twenty were cesarean operations. The remaining 707 surgeries were nondescript.[21]

A detailed enumeration of interventions in one Mexico City clinic can be found in Francisco Ortega Fuentes's quantitative study, which was published in 1917 despite the lack of theses produced during the Revolution.[22] Fuentes's study, which was entitled "Sixteen months of observations in a gynecological clinic," reveals that between January 1916 and March 1917, 309 patients were admitted to the clinic where he worked, of which 207 of the 309 underwent surgery during their stay. Of the 207 operations performed, 105 involved some form of hysterectomy (removal of the uterus). At least six other women received a salpingectomy (elimination of the fallopian tubes), and three underwent oophorectomy (extraction of the ovaries). Furthermore, nine experienced annexations of the uterus (a form of partial hysterectomy). The unit admitted patients for a variety of reasons, including general health problems such as appendicitis. The most common conditions that Fuentes recorded were genital warts, kidney pain, and vulvitis or inflammation caused by allergens or other irritants such as bacteria or yeast. Fuentes additionally listed patients who reported no health problems and left the hospital without treatment. In other words, the evidence strongly suggests that Fuentes based his observations on an ordinary group of patients.

In the clinic where Fuentes worked, the primary rationale for surgical intervention was diagnosis of a "backward-slanted uterus." Fuentes reported that 156 of the 309 women in his study were affected. The young medical student proposed that hysterectomy should be performed "as soon as a uterine tilt was diagnosed." At the same time, however, he mentioned that the condition was not painful, and that there was no medical consensus concerning its proper treatment. Fuentes worried that a tilted uterus might provoke hysteria as well as inhibit the elimination of menstrual fluid, which he believed would cause "self-poisoning, given that menstrual fluid is toxic." Echoing these ideas, one of Fuentes's classmates recommended that uterine tilts justified extremely high levels of surgical intervention. Writing in 1929, he diagnosed a primary or secondary tilt in 600 of 1,000 patients he examined in wing fourteen of the General Hospital. "The only proven cure for backward tilts," he insisted, "is surgery. Of every three women with the condition, at least two should be 'operable.'"[23]

Apart from reifying and contributing to commonplace notions about female pathology, Fuentes's writings indicated the degree to which the diagnosis and treatment of uterine tilts became racialized in Mexico. First, the student equated one variety of problematic uterine placement as a "primitive state," and reported that a common type of uterine tilt was a "primitive backward slant." Of the 105 hysterectomies that he reported, thirty-one were performed on women with a "primitively located uterus." Second, he placed a familiar emphasis on pelvic deficiency when discussing the origins of the "primitively placed uterus." The foremost "debilitating influence on uterine suspension" was, according to Fuentes, "subnormal pelvic amplitude."

Fuentes's reference to backward-slant was noticeable for its continuation of nineteenth-century scientific racism. Another doctor exemplifying this trend was Juan Duque de Estrada, who worked as a professor of obstetrics from the late Porfiriato through the 1920s. In many ways Duque de Estrada pioneered the science of pelvimetry in Mexico: between 1897 and 1919, the obstetrician published at least nine studies (totaling over 300 pages) on the prevalence of the "infantile-type" pelvis in Mexico, which bore great resemblance to the "faulty" pelvis that Francisco de Asís Flores y Troncoso described in 1888.[24] Upon observing women with "infantile pelvises" and "retarded pelvic development," Duque de Estrada began to perform autopsies to further national pelviology. His findings eventually formed a main part of the medical school's curriculum, and as a result he became the head professor of the obstetric clinic and oversaw student training there for thirty years.

In 1917, Duque de Estrada published an article entitled "Mexican Pelvimetry: Description of an Infantile-Type Pelvis. Summary of a Lecture I Gave in the Obstetrical Clinic Regarding Sara Rodríguez."[25] "Sara Rodríguez," wrote the doctor, "was a tiny woman, who was infantile, and of incomplete development." Although Sara visited the General Hospital for her first two pregnancies, in 1916 she became a patient at the maternity clinic, where Duque de Estrada elected to perform a cesarean section to extract the child. Sara died during the procedure along with her third child, and Duque de Estrada conducted an autopsy to study her pelvis. Upon investigation, the surgeon found that Sara's "pelvic cavity was inclined downward," and that she had a "backward slanting spine." Duque de Estrada concluded that Sara's skeletal structure was not only developmentally retarded but also slanted in a downward and backward manner. He asserted that Sara's physique was pathologically small and classically infantile, and he pointed to her "underdeveloped vagina and vulva" as evidence.

Sara's figure, according to Duque de Estrada, was underdeveloped and weak, and even her spine pointed in a rearward direction. In short, her biological inheritance rebelled against progress and symbolized a stumbling block in the nation's halting march toward modernity. Duque de Estrada insisted that cesarean sections should be performed on women who displayed signs of pelvic deficiency, despite the fact that the procedure still usually resulted in maternal death during his time as a professor of obstetrics.

Similar rhetoric surrounded procedures like the hysterectomy, as discussed in student Guillermo Souza Vásquez's thesis. His 1932 study featured thirty-nine case-studies of an experimental hysterectomy technique, in which the uterus is extracted through the vagina, thus eliminating the need for abdominal incision. Vásquez recognized that this "operation mutilates women in their childbearing years" and that it "has a very high mortality rate." At the same time, however, he insisted "we must attempt to practice this surgery whenever possible. It is better to sin by means of excess than to fail by neglecting to perfect our technique."[26] Vásquez mentioned the Church's concerns about "mutilating" operations and also "sins" and "perfection" in relation to surgery, thereby positioning surgical progress as the cure for religious preoccupations.

Vásquez's colleagues discussed many different kinds of sterilizing surgeries. Doctors cited the most common of these as ligation of the fallopian tubes, hysterectomy, removal of the ovaries, and electrocution of the ovaries. Previous chapters examined the roots of oophorectomy in the 1870s, and electrocution of the ovaries in the 1890s, during which time doctors insisted that the electrocution was for the purpose of "vital regeneration," generally without discussing its abortive or contraceptive effects. By the twentieth century, other common sterilization methods included incising part of the fallopian tube or creating scar tissue on the inside to interrupt normal gestation.

By the late 1920s doctors sometimes radiographed the ovaries and uterus to achieve sterilization, usually citing contemporaneous German experiments with the same. This, however, was an inconsistent and unreliable approach. The correct dosage for sterilizing effects was unknown, and although the women so treated generally ceased to menstruate, some still became pregnant again. Doctors rightly feared that radiated eggs produced damaged or inferior fetuses. Hence, one medical student suggested that any pregnancy following a radiograph should be terminated by means of abortion.[27]

Obstetric training and practice had fully recovered from its revolutionary-decade lull by the 1930s. Clinical records from that decade show that pelvimetric science was fully institutionalized as part of the intake process in public hospitals. In the General Hospital, for example, doctors took nine pelvimetric measurements when they admitted new patients.[28] Yet pelviological theory and pelvimetric methods were still hotly contested. In 1935, medical student Alfonso Mejía Schroeder wrote that women with pelvic "deficiencies" were essentially "incapable of healthy reproduction,"[29] and, using the language of social Darwinism, he referred to "pelvic deficiency" as symptomatic of "recapitulation" and "infantilism."[30] These ideologies affected large swaths of women: in 1934, José Figueroa Ortíz presented data for sixty-two women whom he had studied for signs of pelvic deficiency. Figueroa Ortíz's study took place in the Casa de Maternidad, where all patients were there to receive pregnancy-related care; 57.5 percent of the women in Figueroa Ortíz's study underwent cesarean surgery.[31]

In 1936, Rufino García Rodríguez published another influential work on the pelvis, entitled *Diagnosing a Narrow Pelvis and the Classic Cesarean Operation.*[32] In it, Rodríguez acknowledged that the diagnostic criteria for pelvic narrowness revealed several inconsistencies. More specifically, he stated that there were large discrepancies in the data because "neither the position of the patient, nor the points of reference, nor, in many cases, the instrument employed" were "exactly the same."[33] Notwithstanding, Rodríguez insisted that it was "fitting to assume that all 42 percent of Mexican women with small pelvic measurements would experience difficulty during birth."[34] Thus, according to him, "surely one of the most precise criteria for cesarean sections is pelvic narrowness of any kind."[35]

Yet Rodríguez placed a caveat on his own claim when he wrote, "nonetheless, all of the data in respect to the diameters I just indicated are, necessarily, very theoretical." "In reality" he explained, "it is a theoretical axis we measure."[36] Yet, Rodríguez eagerly mapped the "theoretical" axis onto other forms of alterity. In a clear indication of somatic and socioeconomic prejudice, he proposed that a "square body type" and "bad teeth" were indicators of a deficient pelvis. Juan Antonio Torres Septién, writing in 1934, specified "short stature," a "poor moral attitude," and "poor integrity of bodily movements" as symptoms of the same.[37]

Underlying these works were social Darwinist notions concerning biological worth and the hierarchical classifications of human groups or "races." Medical student Gustavo Trangay, for his part, referred to some Mexicans as being "incapable of the struggle for life," and he listed a number of circumstantial, behavioral, and physical characteristics that supposedly identified such a person. Pelvis size topped the list in his mind, at least. He asserted, "The doctor's actions should always combat or prevent social ills or ailments that have no other humane solution: for example, sterilization for undisputable pelvic narrowness."[38]

Like other social Darwinists, Trangay presented a culturalized take on Darwin's thesis about the survival of those most able to adapt to their environment. He wrote, "A responsible mother has the number of children that are proportional to her ability to take care of them; and, first, to care for them, she seeks out men who are capable of providing to them food, clothing, culture, and education. Second, responsible maternity shall consist of the judicious election of a partner who will father healthy and robust children. These will have the highest chances of survival."[39] The student also asserted, à la Spencer, that humans were worse than animals when it came to survival of the fittest due to their tendency to disregard economics, and à la Darwin, that they similarly ignored biological strength.[40] He included direct references to Malthusianism as well as Mendelian genetics. Accordingly, he insisted that the limitation of reproduction—permanent sterilization and medically supervised birth control—should be the domain of the clinic because a doctor's task is never limited to the protection of individual health. A doctor's task, Trangay insisted, was to regenerate the entire populace through eugenic principles. Thus it followed that doctors were more well-equipped than state officials for this aspect of national planning.

Nevertheless, Trangay believed an outright eugenic sterilization campaign should only be implemented in Mexico on a conditional basis. He proposed that if eugenics resulted in a collective improvement, the program should be continued; if it somehow produced the opposite outcome, it should be condemned. His proposal rested heavily on eugenic theories of racial regeneration, even if he himself avoided strictly racialized categories like those described by Rafael Carrillo. Perhaps medical students were more inclined than public health officials to see the gray zones of racial and ethnic groups, having done autopsies on people of all phenotypes, during which they must have observed that physiological classification defied all rules. In addition, whereas nineteenth-century obstetricians believed that small pelvises were identifying criteria for Indigenous women, postrevolutionary eugenicists were likely ambiguous because they wished to extend the label of "unfit" to many mixed-ethnicity, "culturally degenerate" Mexicans in addition to Indigenous people.

Nonetheless, many medical students, like Gustavo Trangay, certainly shared nineteenth-century concerns about miscegenation. On this topic, the obstetrician-in-training wrote, "Not long ago there lived a strong and pure race in Mexico," which, he reported, had "declined due to environmental factors, inadequate parenting, and racial mixture."[41] In his words, the health of the nation depended on "homes with children who were numerically, biologically, and culturally controlled."[42] This conflation of biology and culture was significant because he assumed that "cultural pathologies" were predetermined and shared within social groups, much like biological traits inherited. Yet, unlike cultural theorists and state-builders Manuel Gamio and José Vasconcelos, who dreamed of creating a superior mestizo race via gradual whitening and acculturation, Trangay was pessimistic. "From the eugenic point of view," he wrote, "it appears that we have weak prospects for elevating our race."[43]

Trangay seemed to be writing for an audience of state-builders when he stressed his belief that science—and especially the "hard laws of heredity"—should constitute a moral authority above the state, the Church, and individual autonomy. His thesis included a quote from UNAM professor

Mario Fuentes, who linked Mendelian heredity and Lombrosian positivism to racial fitness during a classroom lecture. He reportedly stated, "I believe that racial evolution should be our first priority in discussions about fertility control"; and "our country is already saturated. Furthermore, many of our people are so lowly evolved that their conduct is limited to poorly controlled reactions, which stem from the frontal lobe."[44] This attitude turned away from Lamarckian and neo-Lamarckian theories regarding moral and behavioral characteristics, representing a much more fixed, hereditarian, and brain-based view of hereditary behavioralism. In the same way, twentieth century doctors like Fuentes, Rodríguez, and Trangay placed less emphasis on the intergenerational alteration of hereditary traits and more emphasis on the experimental abolition of some traits through sterilization.

Paternalism in Obstetrics and in Medical Student Writings

An ethos of patriarchal control over women's fertility and reproduction underpinned much eugenic pontification in the twentieth century. Drawing further on Trangay's work, "Responsible Maternity and the Clinic," this section contextualizes eugenic and post-revolutionary notions about cultural maternal norms. Emphasizing that the state could, and should, influence individual behavior, the medical student pontificated about women's duties to the nation: "A responsible mother solicits the assistance of a doctor for the purpose of controlling her disorderly childbearing habits; a responsible mother harmonizes the demands of nature with the social and economic demands of the society within which she lives."[45] Gender, then, formed a main focus of the treatise, along with virtuous citizenship—in fact, the doctor focused explicitly on women, and he wished for scientific control over maternity but not paternity or a combination of the two. Targeting the population and imagined values of small and marginalized Indigenous and Afro-Mexican communities, the student opined that "rural Mexican women birthed like beasts" and explained that, in response, his "cohort presented a plan for female sterilization."[46] Because he explicitly rejected the idea of male sterilization, this proposal construed the female body as the most important venue for the enactment of scientific solutions for social problems.[47]

Such were the ideologies shaping the clinical treatment for a woman whose name historians do not know, but whose experience shines light on the gendered dynamics of 1930s eugenic thought. Heavily pregnant, this patient approached the enormous courtyard of the General Hospital in Mexico

City in the latter months of 1930. Unaccompanied, dressed in humble clothing, and lacking resources, she likely felt some trepidation regarding the impending birth of her child. Following the intake examination, Trangay and his colleagues decided to pursue sterilization due to class-based prejudice regarding her humble conditions, and due to racist ideas about her pelvic size:

> After successfully performing the [cesarean] operation—and before closing her uterus—in the most natural of manners, and with the understanding that the other doctors present were to remain silent, we proceeded to tie her tubes. It was a true professional sacrament, as plenty could be said about why Mother Nature permitted a vital organ to such a miserable life. We believe that neither moralists, nor prudes, nor demanding sociologists can deny that to have done anything else in this case would have been to tacitly accept abortion, or to expose the woman in question to the risks of another cesarean. In other words, to do anything else would have been absolute medical negligence. And what we have explained about this concrete case is completely applicable to the one before it and all similar cases. In every single case, sterilization is necessary.[48]

It is telling that Trangay referred to this illegal and clandestine sterilization as a "professional sacrament": his insistence on social control through eugenic sterilization converted surgery, once again, into a source of redemption and salvation, but now with revolutionary inflections. Many students agreed with Trangay, and at least fifteen others in the 1920s and 1930s dedicated large portions of their work to praising the potentially redemptive aspects of eugenics.[49]

Archival records are silent about other details of the aforementioned patient's interactions with the doctors who would decide her reproductive fate. We only know what we can glean from the student's indication: namely, that the surgery was not consented ("we decided that abdominal cesarean was the only consideration"). He reasoned that "she could not possibly attempt a spontaneous birth" due to her "excessively small pelvic measurements."[50] Did the medical students or professors likely have a conversation with this patient about the cesarean surgery? Or did they simply place a chloroform mask over her face, as they had done for young woman of Devil's Alley? Some protocols must have shifted since the 1880s, despite the persistence of racial and economic criteria that typologized women as ideal candidates for sociopolitically influenced surgeries. Trangay focused on the woman's "humble class," and her "pathologically deplorable conditions." One wonders if the team of doctors and medical students said anything to make her feel ashamed of her humble circumstances, or if their contempt was conveyed primarily through judgmental gazes during pre-and-post operative procedures.

Notably, this patient's tubal ligation occurred "with the understanding that the other doctors present were to remain silent." The surgeons needed to remain silent to avoid legal sanctions for their actions; at the time, sterilization was illegal in Mexico City unless performed on convicted criminals. Articles 949 and 955 of the federal Penal Code prohibited doctors from performing "sterilization aimed to limit childbearing," and deemed that this was punishable by up to "twelve years in prison and a fine for the first offense."[51]

Trangay interpreted these codes as evidence of biopolitical negligence by the state. Decrying that the state should be more attentive to the birth of "deformed individuals," "sick individuals," and "inept [family] units," he lamented that Mexico's antisterilization laws sought to prevent doctors from surgical decision-making.[52] Claiming that allowing natural birth would have been "absolute medical negligence," he emphasized the importance of sterilization "in every case."[53] Although state prerogatives often drive historical narratives about eugenic sterilization, in Mexico City individual surgeons took the question of sterilization into their own hands, deciding which women to sterilize and under what rubrics. While some students—like Trangay's classmate and fellow eugenicist José Vilchis Vilchis—emphasized biological and medical reasons for sterilization and particularly emphasized pelvic width and tuberculosis, others insisted on the importance of social criteria for tubal ligation and hysterectomy.[54]

For his part, Trangay sought a legislative loophole that could help sterilizing doctors evade the law. "The article that banned sterilization," he explained, "speaks of an operation that is 'completely unnecessary': unnecessary for the individual's health, for their well-being, or what exactly?" He continued, exploring the semantics of necessity in its social, political, and biological nuances: "a doctor who sterilized a woman suffering from an ailment incompatible with reproductive functions would perform a necessary operation for that woman. A doctor who sterilized a woman who already had the number of children she could support and educate would perform a necessary and beneficial operation for the economic well-being of that woman."[55] In cases such as these, he explained, "we believe that sterilization would be the only effective route" and for that reason "necessary sterilization, which is how we baptize it from the juridical viewpoint . . . remains plainly justified."[56]

Trangay's reference to "baptizing" a surgery reflected another socio-cultural interpolation of surgery with revitalizing aims. Evoking a wide range of ailments—tumors, tuberculosis, mental health disturbances, and poverty—the student listed a litany of examples in which doctors should be exempt from punishment for sterilizing a patient "for their own good." Therapeutic, medical, racist, and cultural forms of salvation all intersected to endow sterilizing operations with a salvific veneer. In sum, then, the obstetrician-in-training claimed that ambiguities and loopholes in the penal code actually freed doctors of potential punishment for effectuating sterilizing surgeries, and for doing so without patient's consent. In his words, "no Penal Code insists on the value of surgical consent."[57]

Though Trangay's voice is particularly prominent in this chapter, he seemed to speak for an important cadre of fellow students and professors. He wrote with the collective "we" (*nosotros*), and arguably did so to a greater degree than most students. He also referred to his "cohort," who reportedly "had to resort to clandestine sterilizations due to state inaction."[58] This circumstance made his ideas seem more, not less, typical. Given that Trangay was a medical student at the time of writing, he must have acted under the supervision of professors, practitioners, or both. Although he clearly assumed the stance that doctors should mandate forced sterilization, it is unlikely that he was the agent pressuring his supervisors into allowing or performing the surgeries. On the contrary, he probably always acted under their direction, and the references to his professors' lectures confirmed eugenics as a significant topic of discussion in classrooms and clinics during his time as a medical student.

Historians might see Trangay's tract as emblematic of the Mexican state's revolutionary take on fertility control—a take that seemed to set the terms of debate for the rest of the twentieth century. In the 1930s, deliberations about the unborn acquired a primarily cultural tone, as authorities became less focused on adjudicating the spiritual, legal, and biological parameters of incipient human life. Whereas Porfirian scientists advanced biological arguments against religion and legalistic arguments against women's freedom to end their pregnancies, revolutionary physicians took this argument and overlaid it with a cultural analysis.

Because they believed that some individuals presented economic, cultural, or biological threats to the nation, eugenicists emphasized that the medical establishment was the ideal institution to protect state interests, and that states were antihuman if they stood in the way of eugenicists' work. In general, medical students' eugenic treatises shared five relevant themes: the desirability of scientific control over women's sexual behavior; knowledge of a secular morality that could correct rural backwardness; a conviction that irresponsible reproduction posed a threat to economic productivity; the belief that Mexico needed racial regeneration; and finally the opposition of the medical establishment to federal legislation that disallowed forced sterilization.[59] Faced with what they saw as a weak and inept state eugenics apparatus, prominent surgeons seemed to view it as their moral responsibility to develop and implement a program for eugenic sterilization themselves.

Trangay, for example, insisted that eugenic sterilization would provide economic benefit to the nation and its citizens. This argument moralized socio-economic stability, therein making fertility control into an ethical mandate.[60] "The state," he wrote, "could not possibly provide adequate support for the poor women in this country [because they] become pregnant again at delivery." Apparently Trangay's professor had made this joke in class, and it was a topic of frequent conversation. Yet, the joke overlaid the construction of irrational reproduction as a threat, or even as a quasi-sin. For the young obstetrician, the expectation of a "professional morality"—presumably, obedience of the anti-sterilization laws—"condemned the realization of a moral end: to exterminate misery and limit the number of beggars and thieves in incubation."[61] A truly moral medic would serve a higher behavioral prerogative instead of a capricious state. Though Trangay's rhetoric may have been altruistic and papered with concern for the poor, it was racist just below the surface, if not on it. For example, the doctor's reference to the "incubation" of lower-class criminals suggested that criminality and poverty were innate character traits, not learned behaviors. It was also slippery, even by his own parameters: although socioeconomics composed a central theme of his argument, he extended the definition of an "irresponsible mother" not only to "our lower-class women," but likewise to "many of our middle-class ones."[62]

Trangay believed that Mexico's institutions failed to support women in the challenges of raising a family. Insisting that orphanages and maternity hospitals often served an antisocial purpose, he noted, "Maternity hospitals do not offer a true form of protection for women while those women produce the long-awaited fruit. Doctors kidnap the product of their wombs after birth, and the infant mortality rate is higher in the maternity hospitals than it would be if the mothers raised the children themselves, despite their economically precarious situation."[63] This was a radical critique of the Porfirian legacies of the maternal health care system, in which so-called fallen women who gave birth anonymously in la Casa de Maternidad were sometimes coerced into surrendering their infants to an orphanage.[64] It is unclear whether the post-revolutionary state continued this practice, but the accusations are suggestive at least.

Per Trangay, for example, a "truly socialist government" would recognize that a fit and healthy citizenry would benefit the collective whole. This necessitated the elimination of poverty and hunger, a point that he emphasized repeatedly. In his view, the fascist government of Italy epitomized the antithesis of a scientific utopia, because it had since 1927 proposed severe penalties for those who attempted to limit natality. This was a kind of "Catholic fascism," the medical student wrote, and it was opposite the forward-thinking government that Mexico needed.[65] "I refer to a real protection for the poor," he explained. "A monthly subsidy for women with more than three children, for example."[66] Yet because this was not possible in Mexico, limiting maternity was the only immediate solution that he could endorse.

Through an investigation of eugenic discourse and reproductive surgery, this chapter has highlighted how the postrevolutionary medical establishment adopted late nineteenth-century articulations of biological worth, and how doctors adapted these ideas into a brand of revolutionary clinical medicine with which they could assert control over women's reproduction. This was ostensibly done in the interests of secular morality, economic productivity, and racial regeneration. Bolstered by international eugenic reforms, postrevolutionary scientists took Porfirian prejudices to their extreme conclusions, sometimes removing the organs that nineteenth-century scientists had previously sought to reform or regenerate. In the next chapter we will see that they altered reproductive organs in radical or "revolutionary" ways by means of vaginal bifurcation. Meanwhile, doctors wanted the state to exalt them as a paternalistic and morally righteous class, perhaps even poised to replace the clerics recently ousted by General Plutarco Elías Calles—so long as authorities did not try to regulate them excessively.

Discourses of biology and culture meshed in new ways after the Mexican Revolution. On the one hand, doctors were influenced by the Mendelian, Galtonian, and anthropometric discourses, as promoted for example by Rafael Carrillo, president of Mexico's Puericulture Society. On the other hand, their practices were now couched in a political rhetoric that sought to wield clinical medicine in salvational manners that were compatible with the cultural politics of postrevolutionary state consolidation. Whereas Porfirian doctors very rarely commented on women's personal or structural conditions, postrevolutionary surgeons believed that women's social lives were in need of reform. They viewed medicine as the best form of salvation, akin to the liberal reforma-era doctors who wrote about therapeutic abortion in the 1870s. Twentieth-century surgeons thus combined a positivist and racialized obstetric tradition with a new nationalist optimism about the benefits of eugenic sterilization. Thus arose a revolutionary salvation through surgery: inseparable from eugenics on the one hand, and the nation's relationship with the Catholic Church on the other.

This new nationalist optimism ushered in emergence of a "right to health" discourse, likely bolstered by the 1917 constitution.[67] The medical students who embraced this worldview tended to focus on the potentiality of fetal life, as opposed to its so-called actuality. Instead of deliberating the spiritual or legal standing of the unborn, as before, post-revolutionary obstetricians tended to phrase all concerns about reproduction under the umbrella of revolutionizing society by controlling women's reproduction. If the fetus was a religious subject in the eighteenth century and a biological object in the nineteenth, by the twentieth century it became a potential, realizable citizen of the state. By the early 1930s, eugenicist students built on more than a century of interventionist discourse to insist that maternity should be dictated by the state's interests and not by individual will. At the same time, they were influenced by the right to health discourse, and believed that an ideal scientific state would meet the basic needs of its populace.

Reproduction is thus key to understanding how racism functioned to stratify Mexico even after the nation's egalitarian and justice-oriented social revolution. Lamarckian genetics gave the impression of a "softer" scientific racism in Latin American nations, and some prominent Latin American thinkers proposed that Indigenous people could be identified based on cultural—and not somatic—criteria. However, when it came to medical practice, biologized discourses about race and the body underscore the tenacity of twentieth century racial prejudice, which was part of a sociopolitical effort to create mestizos through cultural assimilation and the biologically essentialist devaluation of Mexican people of Indigenous and African descent. While many non-physician state-builders sought to whiten the population through racial mixture and cultural adaptation, medical students' writings point to widespread surgical sterilization practices. Medical students apparently practiced racialized sterilizing operations on a frequent basis, referring to the operations as "clandestine" and "open secrets." State-building authorities worried about depopulation; many high-level eugenicists were pro-natalists too, arguing that the nation's economic strength depended on population increase. Clinical doctors, on the other hand, saw patients on a more intimate level, and believed that many should not contribute to the country's hereditary stock.

Multiple factors apparently enabled doctors to perform sterilizations without legal repercussions during the *Maximato*—the formal and informal presidencies of Plutarco Elías Calles (1928–34). At first, little oversight over the national university gave scientists and doctors wide breadth to pursue their own treatments. Heads of institutions and politicians seemed to turn a blind eye to sterilizations, which were simultaneously seen as part of a postrevolutionary project to create a utopian scientific authority for Mexican society and as part of the regime's anticlerical campaigns against the Catholic Church.

Because sterilizations were not sanctioned by law and bureaucracy in Mexico the same way as in other countries, notably western Europe and the United States, it will likely be impossible to know how many occurred. Nonetheless, medical commentary on rubrics for sterilization provides valuable insights into logics of racialization, gendered mores around sexuality, and notions of physical and mental debility. Thus, obstetric surgery exemplifies one sector in which doctors drew on international eugenic ideology to pursue their own programs of social regeneration and reform via sterilization in the decades before the rise of mid-twentieth-century biotypology.[68]

Although these discourses arose dialogically from Mexico's relationship with Indigeneity and urban modernization, their transnational lives were undeniable. For example, when two obstetricians at Johns Hopkins University in Baltimore wrote about pelvimetry in 1922 and 1932, they both cited international research on the topic. Racial prejudices sadly affected their conclusions as well, though in distinct ways: specifically, the doctors concluded that African American girls' pelvises were pathologically narrow, even though the median age of that group of patients was thirteen compared with the median age of the white patients in their study, which was sixteen.[69] Like many of the studies cited in this chapter, the Johns Hopkins researchers' work suffered from poor survey and statistical methods, reification, and false quantification. In both nations, racialized research prerogatives shaped childbearing people's experiences with health care.

CHAPTER EIGHT

Temporary Sterilization Could Be Our Daily Bread

Vaginal Bifurcation, 1930s

In 1932, a twenty-eight-year-old woman by the last name of Ríos traveled several hours from her home in the state of Mexico, which surrounds Mexico City, to arrive at the grand General Hospital. Ríos's painful cough had been worsening for months, and she worried about the blood that she had begun to produce from her lungs. Breathing became a laborious task that felt more like drowning. Mexico City had undertaken an extensive informational campaign about tuberculosis; as a result, Ríos may have connected her symptoms to the disease's etiology. Perhaps she dragged herself to the hospital hoping someone would provide medicine and alleviate her pain. Naturally, no one knew that another twenty years would pass before tuberculosis-curing antibiotics were developed.[1] A medical student greeted Ríos near the entrance of the hospital and asked her to wait in the pleasant, grassy corridor near the obstetrics wing. She likely watched as pregnant women entered, some crying out with labor pains, and as others left—some alone, and some with bundled babies.

Genaro Ramírez Elliot was the medical student who greeted Ríos and spoke with her to learn about her medical history and ailments. A contemporary of Trangay's, Ramírez Elliot shared his classmate's enthusiasm for surgery as well as eugenics. After thoroughly examining his compliant patient and confirming that her lungs were diseased, Ramírez Elliot told her that he hoped to make space for her in the tuberculosis wing. Ríos, for her part, may have been worried about the idea of hospitalization because she had several children and did not have anyone with whom to leave them. Or perhaps she wanted a break from the daily toil of feeding and providing for all her young ones. It seems that her sickness made her feel incapable of carrying another pregnancy to term and caring for another baby.

Straining under the dual burden of reproductive labor and illness, Ríos broached the topic of fertility control in conversation with the medical student. She had likely heard from friends and family that doctors could help prevent pregnancies; they could tell her where to buy a diaphragm or spermicide, but those were expensive options, and their use required the consent and cooperation of a partner. Many women knew that the General Hospital's physicians could perform permanently sterilizing surgeries. Surgery outcomes had improved due to the spinal and intravenous anesthesia that replaced noxious gases like chloroform and ether. Nevertheless, major abdominal surgery remained a risky undertaking prior to the discovery of penicillin antibiotics, due to the risk of serious post-operative infection.

Ramírez Elliot shared in his colleagues' eugenic ideas about scientifically improving the so-called national race, and this concern seemed to be pressing while he listened to Ríos's fears about becoming pregnant again. His assessment of Ríos's womb and pelvis found that her pelvic capacity was ample. She did not have syphilis, the disease that he and his colleagues viewed as a degenerating racial poison, and her uterus had only a slight backward tilt. Though she was temporarily too sick and weak to reproduce, he hoped that in the future she could bear healthy children. The young doctor was extremely interested in questions of futurity, and his approach to eugenics and sterilization reflected these interests.

Ramírez Elliot unmistakably viewed this patient through a racializing lens, describing her as "light-skinned" in his notes. Because she had some markers of "racial fitness," Ramírez Elliot believed that Ríos was an excellent candidate for an experimental surgery that excited him immensely. The procedure had been developed by Don Carlos Colín, his professor of obstetrics and gynecology, and he was proud that it represented an innovation from Mexican medics to international surgeons.[2] Although it is unclear if vaginal bifurcation was original to the Mexican context, it is worth noting that there is no evidence of the procedure having been performed elsewhere. Ramírez Elliot called the surgery "temporary sterilization without mutilation." Historians might describe it as "temporary sterilization via vaginal bifurcation" or, in cruder terms, "the creation of a double vagina."

When Ramírez Elliot explained the idea behind the surgery to his patient, he emphasized that it was a "a revolutionary one that creates two vaginas: one that could become pregnant, and one that could not."[3] Ríos may have felt trepidation when she heard this inexperienced surgeon so enthusiastically describing the strange operation, which bifurcated the vagina so that the top section was closed off to the cervix via flaps of tissue united with a line of sutures. When the tissue and sutures healed, they left a stretch of scarring that ran from a half-inch below the cervix down the length of the birth canal. This created a canal in the upper part of the vagina that could be used for sexual intercourse. Because scar tissue occluded the cervix, ejaculation into this upper vessel would not result in pregnancy. The smaller bottom channel allowed fluids to drain from the uterus as they normally would. The resulting bifurcation created one orifice for male use and the other for female use, if viewed in the light of the problematic social ideologies that made these categories possible.

Presumably Ramírez Elliot even explained the surgery to Ríos analogously, emphasizing that one orifice would remain useful for menstruation and future pregnancy, while another could receive semen without making her pregnant. Vaginal bifurcation underscores the extent of eugenic sterilization in 1930s Mexico, which appeared to be so common that it gave way to novel surgical forms of contraception. It also highlights Mexico's role in the production of knowledge about experimental surgeries, a topic that is more closely associated with Germany in the early 1930s; indeed, many Mexican surgeons were primarily citing German research by the 1930s, representing a shift from predominantly French citations through the 1870s and U.S. citations between 1880 and 1920.

A special appeal of temporary sterilization was the reversible nature of the procedure, even if there is no evidence that it was ever reversed. The women featured here appear to have lived their whole lives with a "double vagina." For their part, doctors likely saw vaginal bifurcation as a satisfactory manner of addressing religious concerns about the eugenic mutilation of human reproductive functions. In Ramírez Elliot's words, "the advantage of temporary sterilization is that it has no mutilating effect, in that it does not alter the anatomy or function of the feminine organ."[4] When legislation addressed sterilization, it heeded this concern by stipulating that operations should never have a disfiguring effect; though they had been sterilized, the patients should retain the ability to engage in sexual intercourse, which partially explains the political reluctance behind male castration. Ironically, of course, bifurcation mutilated a woman's birth canal invasively. From this perspective, the medical construction of two vaginas would seem to be the least natural surgical pursuit of sterilization thus far, even if it was the most revolutionary.

By defining mutilation as that which results from permanent surgery, instead of that which related to disfigurement, Ramírez challenged what could be considered "mutilation" from the surgeon's standpoint. Thus the student's use of the phrase "without mutilation" must have been a dog whistle for papal politics. Although mutilation was a serious concern when male eugenicists wrote about male bodies, most were not similarly concerned for women's bodily integrity. Because women's bodies and behavior had long been sites of medico-moral intervention and inquiry, surgeons invisibilized mutilation-based ethical concerns when occurring on feminized organs. Simply put, and as Nancy Stepan has argued, eugenic discourses took women's reproductive bodies as primary sites of intervention while naturalizing categories of masculinity and femininity.[5]

Vaginal bifurcation was particularly notable for how it reconciled eugenic sterilization with Catholic prohibitions on the same, thereby allowing physicians to pursue revolutionary eugenics with surprising Catholic inflections. As another kind of salvational surgery, temporary sterilization sought to save Mexico from racial and cultural degeneration while protecting eugenicists from accusations of violating religious and legal prohibitions. I refer to this as a co-production because it represented a reconciliation of Catholic gender mores with a scientized approach to exerting paternalistic influence over childbearing.

This chapter explores these politics by juxtaposing religious and medical views on sterilization, with attention to Catholic eugenics, on the one hand, and what Karin Rosemblatt has described as the modernization of patriarchal values under radical regimes, on the other.[6] In the end, both Church and state policies marginalized women's agency, viewing them as corporeal pawns in political platforms. Meanwhile, reproductive people and surgeons acted within the interstitial spaces of Church and state ideologies, advocating for their own interests and pursuing their own solutions to fertility control.

AS MENTIONED IN THE previous chapter, the postrevolutionary and progressive era witnessed a surge of popular pleas for birth control among women whose demands were reflected in medical literature. Surgical records offer new historical insight into this matter inasmuch as they show that women sought services to prevent future pregnancies and terminate actual ones. In this decade ordinary women undertook violent efforts to control their own reproduction, for example, by puncturing their wombs with sharp objects and then presenting to the General Hospital hoping to receive a hysterectomy.[7] These measures represented a shift from previous eras, in which women had predominantly solicited the assistance of midwives and doctors for fertility control and pregnancy interruption, including herbal abortifacients, uterine flushing, and bloodletting to induce miscarriage. Before the 1930s, women generally recurred to physicians when compelled by their own family or when coerced by state officials.

By the 1930s, reproductive surgery was such an important part of Mexico City's landscape that even popular approaches to the termination of pregnancy became surgicalized, and more women of all classes voluntarily sought reproductive health care in hospitals. While evidence in the previous chapter demonstrated that many sterilizations in Mexico City were unconsented, this chapter suggests that others were likely done at the patient's request. This trend mirrors the concurrent history of abortion, which was criminalized at the time (and remained so until the supreme court ruled in 2021 that it is unconstitutional to punish abortion as a crime). Although evidence makes clear that some women sought abortion care in hospitals, it is also obvious that many doctors paternalistically assumed control over women's decisions about surgical abortion, deciding which patients fit their criteria for the procedure and which would be subject to sterilization or forced childbearing instead.

Medical student Ramírez Elliot fit this trend. One the one hand, he emphasized that a mother should be "self-sacrificing" for her family; on the other hand, in the opening pages of his book he lamented that women "still did not have the rights they deserved."[8] The student did not specify to which rights he referred. Echoing a standard eugenicist line, he insisted that fertility control technologies, such as diaphragms, condoms, and spermicides, were not suitable for fertility regulation. Even though these were "easy to use and cheap," they were "of no use—because women would have to use it without medical supervision, and so they will forego it easily whenever they have the incentive to do so."[9]

The medical student was more compelled by technologically innovative and difficult-to-access contraception. He was keenly attuned to updates on experimental hormonal methods: consuming small pieces of placenta seemed to prevent pregnancy, as did swallowing ovary tissue from pregnant animals. Another form of contraception under trial included the intravenous injection of sperm, which doctors hoped would provoke women's bodies to produce a natural spermotoxin that would prevent fertilization. Ramírez Elliot showcased racist beliefs when he pondered whether a given person's natural spermotoxin would be similarly effective against all "races" of sperm.[10]

In the same line that the medical student recognized the "vast" prevalence of sterilizing surgeries like ovariotomy and tubal sectioning, he insisted that a surgeons must not "cave to a woman's capricious insistence on limiting family growth."[11] Like many of his classmates, Ramírez Elliot did not intend reproductive surgery to have emancipatory consequences but rather to further patriarchal influence over women's reproductive capacities in light of their widespread demands for fertility control. Women's irresponsibility and untrustworthiness emphasized the utility of medically guided fertility control. Much as religious discourses were appropriated, physicians co-opted aspects of the feminists' contraceptive demands. Yet instead of advocating for an liberatory approach to fertility control, eugenicists argued that they were dealing with a culturally sick nation. Sterilization, temporary or not, seemed to be an important cure.

Obstetricians worried that women were rejecting the nuclear family, given that almost 30 percent of Mexico City's mothers were unmarried in the 1930s. Authorities wondered how they would rebuild a nation in the absence of patriarchal family structures. Furthermore, between 1922 and 1930, 45 to 60 percent of infants born in the city were deemed "illegitimate," a classification that referred to their parents' unmarried status. Public health authorities and physicians moved swiftly to affirm their clout in this era of rapid cultural and political national change. They did so by asserting a modernized and patriarchal brand of authority, one that was based on scientific morality and respect for masculine expertise. Throughout, they appealed to the goals of the bureaucratizing twentieth-century welfare state.[12] In the last line of his thesis, for example, Ramírez Elliot underscored that temporary sterilization was valuable as "some degree" of a social safety net for women who were sick and suffering.

One of Ramírez Elliot's cohort mates, Alfredo Islas Hernández, expressed similarly paternalistic views in his pronatalist stance. He wrote, "Any woman who does not wish to contribute to building the population should not have any faith in the nation" and, what was more, "any woman who consents to intercourse enters into a tacit pact with the State, in which she agrees to birth its children."[13] This was ironically a proto-Catholic view, as some church authorities believed that any woman who consented to intercourse also consented to bear children. The difference was that Hernández insisted that a woman was bound to bear children for the state, not for God or her family. In this view of twentieth-century citizenship, a woman's inclusion in the polity depended on her willingness to provide it with future citizens. Hernández clearly took these gendered ideals of citizenship to the extreme when he suggested that women should not enjoy sexual relations without a willingness to bear children.

Nonetheless, it is important to note that women's popular demands for reproductive health care altered the landscape of fertility control services in the nation. Those thousands of women who approached the steely gates of the General Hospital came with their own prerogatives. Their doctors responded imperfectly, but there is no doubt that medic's responses were shaped by women patients and their families. Physicians, for their part, were sometimes selectively attentive to women's concerns about the structural factors that constrained their reproductive choices, though they still emphasized the value of state and medical control over reproduction in which male authorities decided which women should have access to fertility control and in which contexts.

The postpartum interval became the ideal time for temporary sterilization, especially as surgical outcomes continued to improve over time. An operation while women were recovering from childbirth seemed particularly convenient because the women were already in the hospital and receiving antiseptic washes. They were confined and in pain, circumstances that made them uniquely vulnerable to intervention. Again, these examples underscore that a simplistic liberal notion of individual consent is inadequate for understanding vaginal bifurcation within its context: many conditions drove women to seek reproductive health care, and many factors, including class and racial status, shaped their interactions with physicians and inveigled the interventions doctors chose on their behalf. Although women in 1930s Mexico City may have requested surgical forms of fertility control, they are unlikely to have desired such a probationary procedure.

ONE OF THE MOST striking aspects of temporary sterilization is that it seems to have been conceived for lighter-skinned women who were sick or impoverished but who would, according to eugenicists, subsequently birth biologically fit children. Although historians no longer refer to positive and negative eugenics, here is a particular interventionist example of doctors encouraging the reproduction of some Mexicans—a phenomenon that would have previously been called positive eugenics.

The experience of A. Rios, the woman whose story opens this chapter, echoed those of ten other patients who underwent vaginal bifurcation in the General Hospital in the space of a month. All were overworked, thin, hungry, and sick, and suffered from cough or tuberculosis. Apart from those conditions, their health showed hope for improvement, prompting Ramírez Elliot to describe them as good candidates for the operation. The patients were from San Luis Potosí, Guerrero, Guadalajara Jalisco, Pachuca Hidalgo, the state of Mexico, and Mexico City. Three were caring for children at home, one worked as a seamstress, one was a cook, and the others' professions were not specified.

Ramírez Elliot made no mention of these patients' "rudimentary culture" or "illiterate class," as was so common in the previous chapters' examples of forthrightly racist tubal ligations and hysterectomies. While Indigenous and

Afro-Mexican women were much more likely to be permanently sterilized, lighter-skinned women were supposed to reproduce the nation and therefore became the subjects of this attempt to pioneer a kind of temporary sterilization firmly under medical authority. By targeting lighter-skinned women, vaginal bifurcation too acquired and reified distinct racial meanings in the context of eugenics and the birth control movement. The medical student cast a wide net regarding which conditions made women perfect candidates for the surgery. Apart from tuberculosis, indications included anemia, disturbances of the nervous system, heart problems, ulcers or other chronic stomach problems, kidney disease, and depression.

After several weeks of rest and recovery, Ríos left the General Hospital "with a double vagina." Ramírez Elliot must have written with tongue-in-cheek when he declared that she was "released in better condition than when she arrived."[14] Unfortunately, the other bifurcation patients did not fare so well. One woman died from heart failure during the surgery. Others seem to have survived, although only one, Ríos, was free of postoperative complications. The remaining patients developed infection, fever, and incomplete wound recovery. Post-operative coital pain seemed to preoccupy some of the student's interlocutors. He recognized that the vaginal canal swells during the more "sensuous acts" of intercourse, and that this could complicate the intended use of the pocket of flesh designed for sex. His recommendation was that couples reduce foreplay to avoid this swelling. He reassured readers, and presumably patients, that sex, and even fertilization, were possible without high levels of stimulation and excitement. For proof he invoked the disconcerting "common knowledge" that women are able to receive penetration and become pregnant while under the influence of both chloroform and alcohol, and that there is relatively less swelling and "voluptuosity of movement" during incapacitated copulation.[15] If lack of unconsciousness provided the physiological baseline, it would appear that post-operative care required some delicacy to say the least.

Notwithstanding the complications, Ramírez Elliot underscored the social value of the surgery by insisting that temporary sterilization was an ideal solution for women who were exhausted from reproductive labor and who could not pay for others to care for their children. Making references to the potential of science to improve humanity, the medical student wistfully adjured, "Temporary sterilization could be our daily bread; it could revolutionize and transform this wrecked human race." His plaintive appeal to "daily bread" strongly invoked religious imagery because bread symbolizes the body of Christ in Catholicism, and because many pastoral figures refer to daily spiritual care as "daily bread." Ramírez Elliot sought a therapeutic salve for the nation, for its families, and for its health care landscape, and he insisted that surgery was a recourse for this salvation.

Another medical student, Guillermo Souza Vásquez, voiced concern about the mutilating nature of sterilizing surgeries. Vásquez's thesis chronicled thirty-nine surgeries he practiced, which he called "experimental vaginal hysterectomies." This rarely implemented procedure extracted the uterus through the vagina, thus eliminating the need for abdominal incision. Vásquez recognized that this "operation mutilates women in their childbearing years," and that it "has a very high mortality rate." At the same time, however, he insisted, "we must attempt to practice this surgery whenever possible. It is better to sin by means of excess than to fail by neglecting to perfect our technique." Vásquez nodded to the Church's concerns about "mutilating" operations, at the same time that he invoked the language of "sins" and "perfection" in relation to surgery. At least rhetorically, Vásquez too reconciled surgical progress (or perfection) with religious concerns about bodily integrity.[16]

Notions of responsible maternity inflected strongly on surgical approaches to sterilization, just as they formed the basis for the permanent sterilization discourses highlighted in chapter 7. Most women, Ramírez Elliot insisted, were generally capable of becoming the kind of mothers and wives who attended to their responsibilities while enjoying life enough to offer their husbands pleasant company in the home. Thus, vaginal bifurcation promised to be a transitional and regenerative surgery that would lead women to a superior reproductive and maternal state. Not only did it encourage women's productivity, but it would also make them less stressed, less overburdened, and more keen to serve their families cheerily.

Temporary sterilization may have been a radical and perhaps unprecedented procedure, but it was underpinned by antiquated patriarchal ideals that emphasized women's sexual usefulness and labor-servitude to those around them. Apparently, women "knew that men would cheat on them if they declined to have sex"; therefore, according to the young medical student, "any humane doctor knows that it is less cruel to temporarily sterilize a woman than to risk the loss of conjugal peace."[17] Responsible maternity demanded many kinds of corporeal sacrifice, balancing a woman's sexual services to her husband; her domestic service as a caretaker of existent children; the hygienic and eugenic responsibility to not bear children while ill with a disease; and pro-natal State and Catholic expectations to bear children for God and country.

The View from Rome: The "Spiritual Campaign for Mexico's Children"

As emphasized, the reversibility of temporary sterilization excited some eugenicist physicians. Perhaps some women also saw this as an advantage, though if this was the case, it went unrecorded. The framing of the operation seemed to address concerns in Pope Pius XI's *Casti Connubii* of 1930, which condemned the use of fertility control and contraception, pregnancy termination, and the mutilating aspect of sterilizations. At the same time, however, *Casti Connubii* sympathized for the plight of impoverished families who were unable to support children and wanting to limit births. Overall, Pope Pius XI defended the institution of marriage against the perceived threats of divorce, abortion, contraception, and eugenics.[18]

Within all this, medical debates about the life of the unborn took a notably cultural turn in postrevolutionary Mexico. Discourses about the unborn were no longer primarily rooted in theological claims, as had been the case until the 1830s. Nor did doctors seem to be preoccupied with Hackaelian and Darwinian questions about evolution, topics that predominated between 1860 and 1900.[19] Instead, the unborn morphed into cultural icons during the twentieth century, and debates about them centered on politicized extrapolations about cultural norms (marriage, divorce, and gender relations) and state institutions, especially as related to the creation of scientific knowledge in the service of the nation.

These discourses were particularly evident in Mexico's *Gaceta Oficial del Arzobispado de México*, especially when the monthly publication reproduced the *Casti Connubii* over the course of three issues.[20] In the first of these, dated February 1931, Mexico's archbishop, Pascual Díaz, prefaced the encyclical by laying out a platform for what he called a "spiritual campaign for Mexico's children."[21] Following publication in *la Gaceta*, priests read the encyclical out at masses across the archdiocese. This meant that the views espoused by Pius XI and Pascual Díaz were consequential to the development of popular ideologies regarding maternity and childbearing.[22] The opening lines referenced the problem of the "demographic battle: or, moral, social, and religious issues" faced by nations, religious authorities, and common people. Of particular concern to Pius XI were those who expressed the desire to "limit birth rates," as well as the so-called "missionaries of eugenics and divorce." (Even allegedly irreligious platforms were expressed in evangelizing terms.) Pascual Díaz understood this problem in the context of the marriage sacrament and underscored the questions of gender and maternity at the heart of this debate:

marriage was indissoluble, he insisted, because it was a sacred sacrament and because reproduction was God's intended outcome for marriage.

Because the social duty of a Christian mother was to oversee the regeneration of her husband's and children's souls, Pascual Díaz insisted that she maintain loyalty to Christian practices and beliefs. The pope emphasized that it was "shameful and heartbreaking when married women are not dedicated in this way to their children." Perhaps, he speculated, some even saw marriage as a "convenient way to avoid social problems." Marriage was incomplete, or even a farce, if not accompanied by childbearing. It was in this vein that Pius XI underscored the spiritual and social importance of women's reproductive labor, and the idea that religion was the appropriate guiding force for that labor. In his words, "to eschew motherhood would destroy the nobility of women's calling."[23] When discussing "assaults on Fertility," Pius XI underscored this point. He emphasized that because sex and generation were "natural," childbearing was thus the most logical act within a marriage. At the same time, he deemed acceptable that a couple would take a mutual and consensual pact of abstinence. Apart from abstinence, Pius XI pulpiteered that sexual activity without reproduction was a sin of the flesh, even when this occurred with the consent of both partners. Not only was this a "poor use of marriage," but it was also allegedly criminal, indulgent, and an assault on the young.[24]

So too did Pius XI address medical pretexts for fertility control. In a section entitled "Exaggerations," the pope argued that abortion was never acceptable, even when it was intended to save a woman's life. He insisted that the medical rationales given for these procedures often justified them with "gross exaggerations," and "outright fabrications." "And this," Pius XI wrote, "is not to mention those [medical justifications] that are just plain shameful."

Pius XI's discussion was provocative for how it reasserted eighteenth-century ideas about the sacrifice of maternal life for fetal survival, especially during complicated or dangerous pregnancies. The pope modernized these ideas by insinuating that doctors rationalized the termination of pregnancy by making false claims about threats to maternal survival. "The Church," Pius wrote, "merciful mother, understands perfectly what occurs with these claims about [danger to the] mother's life." Clearly skeptical about the medical rationales for therapeutic abortion, he asked, "Who would fail to admire the extraordinary mother who submits herself to near certain death—with heroic strength—to conserve the fruit of her womb?" All might admire this sacrifice, the pope insisted. And yet, "Only one, God, immensely rich and merciful, will repay her suffering."[25] Such sentiments clearly reavowed the words of eighteenth-century theologians who insisted women die to save the spiritual lives of their unborn. Although the eighteenth-century impetus to extract and baptize the unborn had faded with the onset of scientific and state-based modernity, Catholic authorities continued to insist on prioritizing fetal life at the cost of maternal survival.[26]

Pius XI thus viewed therapeutic abortion as a grave crime, no matter if the justification were medical, social, or eugenic. Under a section heading entitled "Thou shalt not kill," Pius XI emphasized that "the right of life or death, can only be used against criminals; by the same logic, the 'right to self-defense' is also inapplicable in this circumstance, given that an innocent child can never be seen as an aggressor." Likewise, Pius XI insisted, the "so-called 'right of extreme circumstance' is not applicable." In this vein, the pope denounced forms of "chemical sterilization," and decried, in graphic detail, the idea that surgeons "open the womb and destroy the child within."[27] These were the papal battle lines drawn in the metaphysical battle over the souls of Mexico's unborn.

In a section entitled "Economic pretexts," Pius XI addressed the financial aspects of fertility control. He wrote, "It is with bitter pity that we hear the moans of those married couples who are so oppressed by harsh poverty that they find it difficult to feed their children." "But," he insisted, "those acts against [unborn] children are the worst of all: they are even more evil because they are of an intimate nature." By 'intimate,' Pius XI presumably did not refer to sexual reproduction. Intimacy, here, would likely rather be a reference to the intimate location of the unborn (within the mother), and the spiritual intimacy of a supernatural connection between the child and God. According to the pope, those too poor to reproduce should abstain from marriage; by choosing this option, they would "be pure and chaste, and they would avoid a shameful stain."[28]

On eugenics, Pius XI emphasized that it was the responsibility of the authorities and the state to protect the innocent and unborn by means of imposing laws and criminal penalties. The state, he insisted, must be the entity that establishes that it is unacceptable to commit moral wrongs, even if they might lead to desirable outcomes. Here Pius pivoted to a discussion of eugenic sterilizations for those with defective hereditary transmission. In his view, eugenicists "forget that the family is more sacred than the state, and that humans do not reproduce only according to their place in time and space, but also for the heavens and all of eternity."[29] This morphed into a metaphysical claim about the nature and aims of reproduction, and about the state's right to stake authority over those processes. Governments should protect and defend children, Pius XI emphasized, and should not "allow their laws and regulations to create situations in which children are delivered to the hands of doctors and others who murder them; the authorities should recall that God judges them, and that he will avenge innocent blood, which calls out, from earth to the heavens."[30] The pope believed that even a secular state must reflect Church teachings.

It is worth underscoring that Pius XI predominantly equated "eugenics" with abortion and not sterilization. Eugenic surgeries clearly encompassed more than abortive procedures, but abortion was the issue that Pius XI argued against most forcefully, framing it as a tragedy that doomed "children who are still trapped in their mothers' wombs."[31] This phrase also appeared in Cangiamila's 1745 work, and was even incorporated in the title of González Laguna's 1781 tome on cesarean operations. Religious defenses of the unborn no longer focused on their embryonic development, nor on the insistence that life begins at conception, which was, by this time, taken for granted by Catholic authorities. Instead, connections between the family and the state became the main point of contention.

Discourses about how sexual reproduction inflected on state formation were fundamentally connected to eugenic ideology and practice. While physicians viewed male sexual exploits as gender-appropriate, they saw "feeble-minded" and "irrational" women as moral deviants and a potential threat to national stability. Reproductive control was of particular concern because postrevolutionary women increasingly challenged repressive sexual mores, and because doctors feared that the "extremely common" practice of illicit abortions would destabilize the nation by causing women "psychic damage."[32]

Gustavo Trangay, the doctor introduced in the previous chapter, joined many revolutionaries and postrevolutionary state builders in asseverating that religion was the main barrier to scientific morality and state reformism. He viewed the Catholic Church as antireformist, prescientific, and the antithesis of progress; for Trangay and his colleagues, Catholicism had a biologically retarding effect, like a virus that zombified their society. Trangay's statements thus represented a paradox: revolutionary obstetricians accepted religious views on female chastity and female subservience, but rejected the underlying philosophy that produced these social mores. It was this logic that made sterilization into a moral issue, which he expressed with the following statement: "Even moralists, sociologists, and the religious should agree that that it is less moral—and more offensive to God—to kill innocent people with hunger than to prevent their arrival in the world."[33] The student noted that the

Church was responsible for one form of sterilization, at least: the castration of young boys, which was done until the eighteenth century to preserve their soprano voices. In all, Trangay claimed that a scientific brand of secular morality legitimized his authority, which he constructed in opposition to the Church.[34] He explained,

> Religion has always been the most powerful enemy of Science, and that which has most impeded its evolution. Now, it is perfectly understandable that the brainwashed masses would sacrifice their vitality and their well-being to honor the prejudices of a conventional morality and unfounded religious precepts. But it is inexplicable that these prejudices and precepts could be capable of impacting those who, due to their knowledge, are obligated to resolve problems that profoundly affect the vitality of the community. If doctors possess scientific knowledge, with which, like laws of inheritance, they may legitimately impede the birth of children to sick parents; if clinicians rightfully take charge and help to inhibit the birth of infants to homes that are economically unstable; if physicians were permitted to do their work well, they would help avoid the onslaught of sick individuals who are incapable of the struggle for life. Indeed, it is ultimately the healthy and capable that society must support. Those surgeons, in sum, would act in agreement with Morality, because Morality is the science of well-being.[35]

Like others before him, and especially the reforma physicians of the 1870s, who offered young pregnant women "the salvation that only medicine could provide," Trangay envisioned a priestly kind of obstetrician, one who would offer moral guidance to his patient. In his words, "in the most intimate moments of medical consultation, a physician lends his ears to the suffering of those who confide in him. They [patients] confide their health and corporal well-being to him, and they also put their moral health in his hands, as well. In this way, the surgeon becomes a kind of priest." Yet the doctor was a priest who "did not recur to sophisms," but rather "true occurrences and scientific rationales."[36]

In addition to describing physicians as priestly arbiters of morality, Trangay's manifesto was religiously inflected in that it seemed to respond to each of Pius XI's arguments in turn. It sometimes appeared to have been a direct response inasmuch as Trangay's arguments were structured almost identically to the encyclical. Despite his disdain for Catholicism, the medical student also cited the work of theologians such as St. Thomas Aquinas, though perhaps ironically or ad hominem. The apparent tension between these ideologies—Catholic opposition to eugenics, on the one hand, and medical denunciations of Catholicism, on the other—belie the deep congruence and the continued interpenetration of secular/sacred realms between the viewpoints. Indeed, the young clinician phrased his resistance as a moral issue: in his view, preventing death from starvation should take precedence over saving the unborn from abortion.

These views coincided with concurrent scientific debates about unborn life. When historian and embryologist Joseph Needham published *A History of Embryology* in 1934, he insisted that religious approaches to embryology were questions of the past and that scientists must abandon questions of fetal ensoulment. Nor, it seems, were embryologists in the 1930s substantially concerned with questions about early in-womb development. Surgeons, for their part, were more concerned with a modern liberal conception of "responsible" maternity. This shift became evident in Trangay's discussion, too. His work only briefly approached the question of fetal personhood, and this discussion was primarily concerned with the prioritization of maternal life over fetal survival. Emphasizing the distinction between the "potential life" of sperm, eggs, and recently fertilized embryos, he classified near-term fetuses as "actual life." "The thousands of children who starve to death each year," he wrote, "are actual life."[37] In his mind, only the most amoral authorities would assert that an embryonic life is of more value than an existing one; by the same token, he explained, no husband would wish to see his wife perish during childbirth to save the potential life of an unborn child.

There was no moral reason, the student insisted, to valorize potential fetal life over maternal survival. The obstetrician clarified here that he took issue with many Catholic ideas about reproduction, including the idea that "because the mother is baptized, and the child is not, the death of the woman who is cleansed of the original sin is preferable to condemning a child to limbo and excluding it from God's kingdom." For him, this problem should have been easy to remedy via the performance of either intrauterine baptism or a simple "above the womb" baptism on the stomach. The baptism was symbolic and therefore did not have to be performed in the flesh. "It never fails to shock me," Trangay wrote, "that an obstetrician and a woman's family, even if they are very Catholic, can accept these antiquated beliefs, as if they were in a trance." The child, he insisted, is "unconscious and unknown." He also asserted that "the majority of laicized thinkers agreed that the life of the mother should take precedence." Trangay believed that this would be the most "purely humane" approach and that practitioners must take a more categorical approach than moralists, sociologists, and religious clergy.

Trangay's anticlericalism typified predominant ideologies during Calles's late presidency (1926–28) and the *Maximato* (1928–34), in which authorities believed they could create a state-led alternative that fulfilled people's spiritual needs while rationalizing their behavior and opposing entrenched Church politics. Trangay's anticlerical beliefs reflected the views of some *callista* era hospital administrators that religion had no place in the General Hospital. In 1928, the revised bylaws of the General Hospital outlined this position. In chapter 9 of the bylaws, entitled "Regarding Religious Practices and Rituals, and Regarding Spiritual or Philanthropic Assistance," article 169 stated,

> No form of religious practice will be allowed in the hospital. In certain cases, administrators may grant permission for a patient to be visited by a minister of his or her religion. However, no other patient will be allowed to participate in any act of spiritual worship, nor will they be allowed to receive spiritual assistance. No religious matter will alter the schedules or functions of the Hospital, wing, or ward. The Societies or corporations that wish to provide spiritual services in hospitals are required to have explicit and advance permission from the Director of the hospital at all times.[38]

In 1934, the director of the General Hospital banned religious imagery in patients' rooms as well, an act that was consonant with *callista* school policy. A postcard-sized image of the Virgen de Guadalupe was bound into the archival folder holding this notice because it had been confiscated from a patient in the fifth wing. At the same time, the head administrator sharply notified department heads to keep watch over patients: some had been caught in the front garden "requesting alms."[39]

SOMETIMES WOMEN'S MOTIVES for seeking sterilization shone through the cracks of male-centered writing. In one instance, a married woman asked to be sterilized because her husband had a mental illness. Although this woman wished to practice "responsible maternity," it was her husband who represented the biological threat. Because little political will existed for the sterilization of men who had not committed crimes, Trangay opined that the woman would be better off using birth control under medical supervision. In such situations, obstetricians saw birth control as acceptable because the alternative was often illicit abortions. Medically supervised birth control could allegedly prevent the "tragedy of abortion." "We have seen this problem often in the Hospital de Jesús," Trangay explained, "and fertility control would be the door to salvation for these women."[40] The benefit of using birth control over permanent sterilization would be that if the woman recoupled—with a hereditarily fit man, that is—she would be able to reproduce with him at a later date.

And yet when women came to the hospital asking or begging doctors to help them prevent, interrupt, or manage their pregnancies, doctors obstinately insisted that this authority belonged to them. Apparently it was especially common for free-spirited artists and actresses to resort to medical students for help preventing pregnancies. In one case, Trangay wrote, an artist "sought to annihilate her genetic capability with the pretext that pregnancy might ruin her beauty and cause her to lose her job."[41] Particularly noteworthy here is the medical student's focus on this ambitious woman's genetic potential. This was clearly a biologically essentialist comment about her hereditary and racial worth, and Trangay seemed to wonder if a state could bear responsibility for protecting the beauty of its citizens.

Trangay viewed procreation as much more important than the preservation of one's youth and career, and he wished for the "beautiful" genes of Mexican actresses to enter the pool of Mexican breeding stock.[42] He explained, "The actresses that have become mothers—whether by choice or careless sexual activity—have given healthy children to this country, and those children will always be well-received by the nation." A surgeon would compromise his professional reputation by sterilizing such a woman, so he should recommend abstinence instead, because it was, in his words, "of no collective benefit to sterilize a beautiful artist."[43] The idea behind this statement was forced childbearing and forced maternity in service of the state combined with the assumption that women's professional callings violated the reproductive mandates of her sex.

All this makes it even less surprising that women asked health care providers to help them control their reproductive functions. In the name of gendered sexual mores, Trangay rejected the idea that single women should be able to avoid the consequences of intercourse. Yet what did he make of cases in which married women asked surgeons to assist them in avoiding pregnancy? Even here, sterilization should only be performed only in the interest of scientific medicine and never to capitulate to a woman's desire to control her fertility. Voluntary sterilization seemed just as offensive: "we must never sterilize a woman solely on her whim."[44] The student recognized "a contradiction here, because we accept, as indisputable, the right of all women to be or not to be a mother." "Yes," he continued, "we have accepted this right as indisputable, but now is the opportunity to declare that Medical Science should not be at the unconditional service of this right."[45] Women should cast aside the desire to manage their reproduction in the interest of the state, and only scientific medicine was authoritative enough to prevent certain people from procreating while requiring others to do the same.

Trangay also described feminists who wished to avoid pregnancy "due to a desire to assert feminist autonomy over their sexuality and reproductive capacities." Trangay referred to these women as "the kind of women who wants to put into practice Victor Margueritte's phrase: 'your body is yours,' and so tell the surgeon that she does not wish to be a mother because her true calling is to dedicate herself to a carefree and fun-loving lifestyle.[46] These women end up asking surgeons for some way to temporarily or permanently fulfill their wishes—although we might wish that this scenario was hypothetical, it is all too real."[47] Here, Trangay targeted the *chica moderna*—the 1920s flapper-style "modern girl," who represented the demise of Mexican respectability politics.[48] But his critique was a deeper one because he rejected ideas about women's sexual and reproductive agency, debates of importance during the Progressive Era's liberatory and feminist movements.

Others medical students lashed out against feminist movements as well. Julio Feijóo Peñas, for example, wrote a thesis in 1934 on intersexuality and sexual differentiation in which he noted that "the so-called 'feminist' leagues almost never have a reason for existence, biologically speaking: they are composed of recalcitrant single women, overripe mothers-in-law with the ideas and clothing of a man, and young women who abandon the homes they made into a hellhole." These "feminists" are "just obeying the laws of endocrinology." [49] In a biologically essentialist argument, Feijóo Peñas argued that feminist ideas were irrational mental malfunctions caused by hormonal imbalance.

Although a full analysis of the feminist movements that provoked male medical ire is outside the scope of this chapter, other historians have examined feminist activism in the 1930s. One important organization was Acción Femenina (Feminine Action) a women's activist organization established under President Lázaro Cárdenas and associated with the Partido Nacional Revolucionario (National Revolutionary Party, which would later become the Partido Revolucionario Institucional, the Institutional Revolutionary Party, or the PRI). Another was the Frente Único pro Derechos de la Mujer (United Front for Women's Rights), which built a coalition of eighty-eight organizations with a membership of 50,000. Women achieved hard-won recognition from authorities who—in true populist fashion—appropriated their activism, incorporating it into their platforms whenever possible. Despite some authorities' leftist and populist rhetoric, their appropriation of grassroots movements meant that they could exert more authority over women than before.[50]

While organized left-wing women's activism and volunteerism was relatively novel in the 1920s and 1930s, religious women's activism was not new: by the 1930s Catholic reformers—including those with Acción Católica, or Catholic Action—sought to redeem single women and sex workers, who were perceived as grave threats to national well-being due to their corruption of the public sphere. They founded and ran rehabilitation or "regeneration" houses, where they sought to "retrain" women in domestic, factory-based, and artisanal labors so that they might find employment upon release. In sum, socialists, communists, liberals, and conservatives sometimes engaged in similar types of activism to alleviate the ill-health and suffering of marginalized people, though the ideologies underpinning their advocacy differed considerably. This all contributed to a climate in which medicine and public health were divisive and politicized, especially in relation to gender, race, and religion.[51]

Meanwhile, marginalized people were at the core of the revolution and postrevolutionary state construction, but revolutionary leaders did not always return their loyalty. Despite women's role as soldiers and activists, and despite long-standing and well-coordinated feminist campaigns, many aspects of postrevolutionary law and society continued to constrain women's civic rights. Divorce became legalized, but women were barred from engaging in business or work without their husband's consent. For all the intensity of suffragist movements, citizenship and public office remained male prerogatives. Nevertheless, women undoubtedly influenced politics even when denied the right to vote. In sum, there remained "a de facto patriarchal order," and the politics of pregnancy are best understood as part of the continuation of patriarchy during this rapidly changing landscape.[52]

Trangay and his peers were familiar with social arguments in support of sexual liberation, in part because a group of them had traveled to Copenhagen in 1928 to attend the Second Congress of Sexual Reform. Some in that space supported the platform of sexual liberation, proposing that women's sexual activity should be completely separate from their procreative efforts. Trangay's thesis quoted Jonathan Leunbach, a Danish physician who made a significant but controversial social effort to help women of limited means with sex education, birth control, and abortion. Leunbach was known for developing an iodine and antiseptic paste that, when injected by needle into the uterus, provoked abortion.[53] Trangay quoted the following from Leunbach's more progressive platform: "with the limitation of reproduction, marriage will reach new heights. Fear of pregnancy and disease has ruined society, and now, it is of utmost importance that women decide whether they want to have children, and when they want to do so. Support for voluntary and limited offspring must penetrate even the lowest social classes. The tendency toward promiscuity will decline with acculturation. Birth control is of utmost importance for abolishing prostitution, which facilitates male dominance over women." Although Trangay recognized the validity of these arguments, he did not agree with the logic underpinning them. He promoted a much more conservative eugenic ideology that was particularly insistent on male control over contraception, gestation, and childbirth outcomes.

Trangay's thesis described a range of patients whose reproduction could benefit from control by scientific authorities. One was a married woman who came to him apparently devastated by her struggle with tuberculosis, perhaps somewhat like A. Ríos. The patient had "confessed that her last pregnancy was a disaster," presumably meaning that it ended in abortion or miscarriage. Subsequently, she had "begged the surgeon for a temporary or permanent sterilization." The dictum of responsible maternity made the obstetrician-in-training believe that this mother acted responsibly by requesting sterilization: "any doctor should feel morally obligated to fulfill her request." Unlike Ramírez Elliot, Trangay believed that it was necessary to permanently sterilize many women who suffered from tuberculosis, emphasizing that the disease reduced children's physical size and potential usefulness for the economy.[54] Such an emphasis on "useful" citizens—and especially useful women and children—combined a nineteenth-century emphasis on useful citizens with a kind of ultra-Darwinistic focus on the importance of humans as biological and evolutionary subjects that should advance the race. On this, Trangay quoted his professor, Salazar Viniegra, who insisted, "Women must always be sterilized when their reproduction is presumed to present danger of death to the woman, or danger of extinction to her descendants."[55]

Whereas mid-nineteenth-century reformists sought to make individuals more useful to the nation, this rhetoric was collectivized in postrevolutionary medical literature. In the case of a sick or weakened mother, abstinence should not be recommended because then a male partner could abandon his wife or choose intercourse with another woman. By this logic, a physician should perform sterilization to choose the path of least harm for society. In this way, as in others, his approach emphasized a top-down imposition of moral regimes of reproductive governance.

The social valences of reproductive health care were distinct in Mexico, where contestations primarily concerned the selective incorporation of linguistically and culturally distinct groups into a national polity on the one hand, and battles between Church and state to exert religious and metaphysical influence over women, children, and communities on the other. Tensions abounded between women's desire for reproductive autonomy, scientific efforts to assert control over those choices, and Catholic reactionary responses to fertility control movements. This led some clinicians to promote a form of Catholic-revolutionary eugenics, offering a kind of surgical sterilization that they believed would be acceptable to religious sensibilities. In many ways, this can be read as evidence of intense contestation over women's unwillingness to acquiesce to Catholic patriarchal norms. Some anticlericals viewed eugenic medicine as a means with which to subvert the cultural and political authority of the Catholic Church. All seemed to agree that working-class people exhibited cultural backwardness and promoted efforts to scientifically reform their behavior and their reproductive potential. And yet, while some Mexican eugenicists rejected Catholic attempts to limit women's reproductive agency, they embraced scientific proposals that pursued the same goal. Such issues were pressing for the postrevolutionary state, which aimed to reform and redeem its nation's people.

Contraceptive demands went formally unresolved, despite considerable agitation from radical doctors, women themselves, and feminist activists from various parties, including the communist party. At the same time that Mexico City physicians often asserted that scientific control over reproduction would be an act of rebellion against religion, they sought to reconcile their practices with Catholic perspectives on reproductive control. This was especially the case in the development of temporary sterilization techniques, a practice that this chapter examines as a kind of neo-revolutionary eugenics. Postrevolutionary surgical politics—including anomalous and significant experiments with vaginal bifurcation—were co-produced by competing demands among Church, state, scientific, and popular groups. The women who underwent temporary sterilization were racialized differently, according to their lighter skin; meanwhile, permanent sterilizations continued to be motivated by political, scientific, and cultural ideas that deemed impoverished Mexicans and Indigenous women a threat to the racial and cultural future of the nation.

The meaning of the state was a core theme of obstetricians' debates about gender and reproduction in the 1930s, and the relationship between medical students, the clinical health care system, and the federal government was complex. Doctors simultaneously represented the state by working in state clinics; contested the state by eschewing, disobeying, or resisting policies they disagreed with; and sought to influence the state by making detailed proposals for fertility control policies. Medicine became an even more highly contested sphere of public policy, constructed in moments of contestation and antagonism between federal officials, public health authorities, professors at the medical school, medical students, feminist agitators, and women who sought reproductive services in the health care system. All of these actors took part in the construction of the postrevolutionary project as well as the meanings of cultural revolution: they had personal and social stakes in advocating for particular approaches to reproductive health care, and they used their position to articulate, demand, reinforce, or impose these ideologies within their spheres of dominance. While "the state" is not a static, a priori entity, many of the actors in this history approached it as such: they wrote about the state with great frequency, viewing it as a coordinating mechanism for a widespread effort to reconceptualize the nation and its people. They saw the state as machinery for implementing new social and behavioral codes, and they were determined to exert scientific authority in this milieu.

Postrevolutionary obstetric care shifted in many ways under discourses about maternity, reproduction, and the future of the nation. While eugenics ideologies and programs varied by place, the view that humanity could, and should, be improved—or saved—scientifically was nearly ubiquitous among modern states in the 1930s. States codified, classified, and studied people to bring medicine, immigration, public health, marriage, and reproduction under the remit of rational science. Such racist and hegemonic state discourses sometimes have led historians to characterize doctors as motivated by state prerogatives when they chose to sterilize patients in public hospitals. Although it has long been assumed that Latin American surgeons and eugenicists were less interventionist than their North American and western European counterparts, these chapters have shown that doctors and medical students pushed the boundaries of state eugenics by flouting prohibitions on sterilization and by pursuing it in experimental forms. While the General Hospital was founded with progressive values and as a humanitarian project, clinical medicine was profoundly influenced by the scientific racism and the realities of patriarchy.

Part V

Resistance

CHAPTER NINE

No One Was Decent to Me There

Complaints and Demands for Health Care, 1920s–30s

There were many continuities in nineteenth- and twentieth-century obstetric care: racialized biometrics, paternalistic efforts to control women's access to fertility control, and the persistence of unconsented and sometimes unnecessary surgical procedures. Yet postrevolutionary medical culture brought a significant change: women submitted complaints about their health care experiences in a more systematic manner than ever before.

One of these protestations, penned by the patient herself, was particularly rich in detail. In 1930, an elite woman named Josefina Velásquez Peña sued the former head of the Department of Health, Gabriel Malda.[1] The ordeal began when Velásquez Peña and her husband were experiencing trouble conceiving a child; for that reason, they asked Dr. Malda to come to their home and provide treatment. Velásquez Peña alleged that Malda began to seduce her while insisting that she abstain from intimacy with her husband. Malda even impregnated her, made her sick with a sexually transmitted infection, and then told mutual acquaintances that she had infected him and not vice versa, leading to her successful lawsuit against him for defamation. Although a full analysis of the case is outside the scope of this chapter, Velásquez Peña's testimony is relevant for how it provides rare insight into how she felt about the links between surgery, sexual mores, and cultural, likely class-based, notions of honor.

Velásquez Peña published her account of her relationship with Malda in a small pamphlet. "Dr. Malda," she wrote, "insisted that a surgical operation was indispensable." Eventually she began to question his judgment: "Was the operation necessary? I have asked myself this question many times, and I began to suspect that Dr. Malda used the surgery as a pretext with which he could literally take me into his hands." As Velásquez Peña's relationship with Malda deepened, and as she contemplated his approach to patients, she became increasingly suspicious. In the patient's words, "the surgery put me at his mercy, because I was completely stunned in the physical as well as moral sense. I had the chaste immodesty of a chloroformed woman, a woman who is in the nude, yes, but who has placed herself in the hands of a man who she believes to be a gentleman and a priest of science. She [a chloroformed woman] believes that a surgeon represents true science—a science always chaste, and never destined to become a tool of suffering in the hands of an unscrupulous man."

Velásquez Peña's testimony is provocative for how it imagines the chloroformed woman as a trope, and a gendered and salvational one at that. She believed that although surgical patients were exposed and vulnerable, their honor should have been safeguarded by the surgeon's respectability. An obstetrician must be "priestlike" for women and their families to trust him with personal, corporeal, psychological, and even spiritual forms of betterment and regeneration. By maintaining a kind of professional celibacy, like a priest, a physician could win the respect and loyalty of elite clientele. After all, no head of household would want a lascivious doctor to be his wife's sexual health confidant, especially if that man could provide contraceptives and perform abortions in case of unexpected pregnancy resulting from an affair.

In this example we again see that women's expectations of surgery were cast in religious terms, and they even sometimes expected surgical salvation via therapeutics and personal moral standards. Of course, Josefina Velásquez Peña's initial assumptions about the altruism of male surgeons may have been colored by her status as an elite patient. Because most women in Mexico City's hospitals were impoverished, they were unlikely to have such positive preconceptions as Velásquez Peña, who received private care in her home. Even so, her experience clearly led her to question her preconceptions, and her writing offers meaningful historical insight into the experiential realities resulting from abuses of power.

Other women had similar complaints despite their class differences. Poorer women's writings emphasized that they developed their own notions about the postrevolutionary state's responsibility for their well-being. In this way their discourse corresponded to that of sex workers in Mexico City who declared that poverty and a lack of access to other employment had forced them into selling sex and that they experienced abusive treatment from state authorities. Like those workers, the women in this chapter appealed to authorities' concepts of paternalism and revolutionary morality. Their letters shed light on the complicated perspectives on gender, welfare, and reform that were prominent in postrevolutionary Mexico City.[2]

In her analysis of sex workers, historian Katherine Bliss additionally shows that women understood and acted on "the political currency" of complaints and of reformist rhetoric. In this chapter, too, women's choice to identify themselves as victims of the health care system was not an admission of helplessness. Asserting their agency, patients advocated for change while describing their own life circumstances, defining their own structural vulnerabilities, and pursuing their own participation in postrevolutionary society. Once again, women's bodies and voices were part and parcel of the project to make revolutionary ideals. They spoke in parallel conversations alongside the clinicians who sometimes took into account their agency, but who more often overlooked it in favor of their own understandings. The women featured in this chapter truly understood their own social circumstances whereas doctors were often informed by thin stereotypes of what it meant to be an impoverished person suffering multiple and intersecting oppressions in Mexico.

Beyond highlighting historical women's voices, this chapter sensitizes readers to the experiences of seeking health care in underfunded and overwhelmed systems, even ones ideologically wedded to quality patient care. Though patients demanded and received health care, their treatment continued to be influenced by racialization, class, and gender. One caveat is that I do not take patient complaints at face value or assume that those grievances convey the full nuances of any medical interaction. Still, they are important because they allow for a rare glimpse into patients' perspectives on reproduction. Finally, this chapter explores how medical students and reformers drew on patients' demands and complaints in their own efforts to politicize health care provenance and delivery.

Another prominent theme concerns a deeply rooted cultural conflict over the role of medicine within the newly consolidating state. When revolutionary fervor reached the General Hospital, long-standing obstetric epistemologies came under scrutiny. Resistance from surgical subjects and dissenting surgeons cast a national light on the debates that raged within—about maternity and women's corporeal relationship to the state as well as about fertility control, surgical ethics, scientific experimentation, racial prejudice, and eugenic sterilization. These issues divided students of the medical school and came to be flashpoints in other conflicts, including turnover in the Office of Beneficencia Pública (hereafter, the BP), which oversaw public health in Mexico City.

Surgery, Mortality, and Maternity in the General Hospital: An Overview

From mid-1932 to late 1933, Mexico City's General Hospital entered a period of sustained political conflict. The crisis exploded in 1932 and continued through 1933, when one anonymous informant, "Dr. X," approached local newspapers with allegations of obstetric abuse in the General Hospital.[3] Dr. X claimed that practitioners often performed "unnecessary" and "experimental" hysterectomies in the establishment, and that patients regularly resisted surgeons and escaped the clinic in panic. Dr. X had been expelled during a student revolt in 1932, one year before he shared this scandalous information with the press. This suggests that he or she had their own agenda, both in the revolt and in sharing information with the press.

Protesting what they called "a crisis in clinical ethics," rebellious students in 1932 had staged an armed coup and attempted to oust leading professors of clinical medicine.[4] *La Prensa*'s inflammatory article explained why the students' claims enraged the medical school. They were reportedly told, "In the Hospital General, surgeons are committing premeditated, malicious assassinations, and they are doing so to for their own personal gain."[5] It is important to underscore that *La Prensa* was a sensationalist news source. Furthermore, Dr. X's discontent likely dissuaded him from adding any nuance to his claims, explaining the range of therapeutic and fertility control-based rationales behind some surgeries, or contextualizing maternal mortality rates for different ailments and procedures. Nevertheless, his words must have shocked and preoccupied readers. In addition, and as we saw with the case of the girl from Devil's Alley, some women did die as a result of unconsented surgical procedures.

Potentially unnecessary surgeries incited particular concerns. *La Prensa* quoted Dr. X as saying, "Do not believe for a minute that these operations are performed with altruistic intentions, or that they are recommended by medical science." He continued, "Quite the opposite: the surgeries in question are performed experimentally, and it is clear that a high percentage of them result in death. I insist: surgeons are deliberately murdering women in the maternity ward." The estranged medical student also claimed that patients "try to defend themselves, and flee the hospital screaming." He offered the following description of a scene: "[the women] tell each other about the procedures that await them, and about the probable results of the operations they will endure. When clinicians begin to prepare a woman for an operation, she begins to search desperately for any way to escape. If she is unable to flee, she will defend herself by screaming, and, sometimes, by throwing punches when they strap her to the operating table."[6] While these claims spoke to readers on an emotional level, they are complex and as explained previously, need to be assimilated in light of multiple historical contingencies.

Perhaps women were reluctant or escaped operating theaters because surgery remained dangerous throughout the early twentieth century due to the risk of infection, hemorrhage, puerperal fever, and shock. After all, physicians did not use the first synthetic antibiotics compounds until the 1940s; in the United States, for example, caesarean operations for complicated cases still carried a 34 percent mortality rate in the 1930s. While extremely high, this mortality rate was down from almost 100 percent before the late nineteenth century, and over 50 percent in the late century.[7] Despite these risks, as the previous chapter suggested, women were aware that they could seek contraception at the General Hospital—via hysterectomy, tubal ligation, and vaginal bifurcation—and they sometimes requested these procedures themselves. Other women, racialized and marginalized by class, were not able to exercise the same reproductive agency.

Instead of assessing the veracity of Dr. X's claims that physicians were "deliberately murdering women in the maternity ward," this chapter explores a set of interrelated issues: how women themselves understood, and responded to, issues of coercion in reproductive medicine, and how some doctors debated this issue and its relevance to Mexico's postrevolutionary project.

Several years after Dr. X's complaints, another medical student risked his good standing in the department to offer a similar, if much more measured, critique. Dr. Guillermo Casis Sacre dedicated his thesis to arguing that physicians should exhaust all therapeutic methods before resorting to surgery. Casis Sacre wrote, "The voracious appetite for advancement in surgical techniques transforms our patients: they cease to be subjects of humanitarian attention and medical care. Instead, they become meat for experimentation."[8]

Casis Sacre's stated goal was to "treat some of the many therapeutic problems that present themselves in gynecology." He did not "wish to treat these problems in isolation, but rather, in the context of how they are intimately related to what we confront in medical practice—to social and economic problems." The student also expressed concern for the "future social life of the patients." Even in problems having to do with the inflammation of the fallopian tubes, which was frequently a sign of infection, he said, "I must insist that all therapeutic methods should be tried before surgery. Any unnecessary or precipitous surgery could well be fatal, and this would contribute to what we have already witnessed: an increase in the number of cases that appear incurable."[9]

The General Hospital's registers, which provide statistics regarding admissions, surgeries performed, and mortality rates, can help historians contextualize the claims by Dr. X and Casis Sacre. In the early 1930s, between 13,000 and 14,000 women per year became patients in the Hospital General's obstetrics and gynecology ward. On average, the ward admitted 37 new patients per day, or 1,130 women every month. Of these, and just in the General Hospital, 450 to 750 women underwent surgery on a monthly basis. This means that roughly one-half to two-thirds of patients in the obstetrics and gynecology ward of the General Hospital underwent surgical operations. The average survival rate for these surgeries was quite low, a fact that was repeatedly cited as a source of concern by inspectors from the Secretariat of the BP.[10]

High surgical mortality preoccupied the administrators of other hospitals, too. In the Hospital Juárez, for example, an inspector reported on July 10, 1933, that the clinic had seen a daily average of twenty-three abdominal operations since the beginning of the year. The inspector lamented the total number, which amounted to 4,334 reproductive surgeries performed between January and June. Even he was perturbed by such high operative incidence.[11]

Not all women patients of the General Hospital were pregnant or birthing imminently. In fact, only approximately 19 percent of patients arrived at the hospital because they were in labor. Still, 2,500–3,000 infants were born per year in the General Hospital; in 1936, for example, the hospital saw 2,712 infants born.[12] This translated to enormous patient caseloads, in terms of both pregnant and nonpregnant women. Although most women patients were in the hospital for reasons other than childbirth, the figures still indicate that many of Mexico City's infants began their lives in hospitals, and city births were not attended almost exclusively by midwives. Although midwives predominated everywhere else in Mexico (and much of the world), the nation's capital witnessed a substantial medicalization of childbirth by the 1930s. If the statistics are correct that Mexico City saw the birth of 12,000 to 14,000 children per year between 1922 and 1930, on average almost one-fifth of Mexico City's infants were born in the General Hospital during this decade.[13]

General Hospital records suggest that many women were forcibly interned after having been arrested by the Sanitary Police. For example, in that hospital on September 6, 1914, 194 people resided in the women's ward and 74 women and children were in the maternity wing. Four new women gained admission that day: while one self-admitted voluntarily, the other three came under duress by the Sanitary Police. All took beds in the general medicine ward, not the syphilis ward, meaning it is unclear whether they suffered from sexually transmitted infections.

Of the two women admitted to the maternity wing, one underwent forced admission by the Sanitary Police and the other was the self-admission patient. That day, six women died in the women's ward and four died in the maternity wing. Of those six, two died in surgery, three in the gynecology section, one in general medicine, and four in the maternity wing. These numbers were common. Generally, between four and ten women were admitted each day, with half to two-thirds brought in by the Sanitary Police.[14] As in the nineteenth century, the postrevolutionary state made considerable efforts to find and detain women whom it suspected of selling sex for money without having registered with the Sanitary Inspection and without undergoing regular examinations by the same. The 1932 Sanitary Police regulations had no new provisions; likewise, there was no mention of the criteria for detainment and detention. This suggests that the 1872 criteria for identifying sex workers remained in place.[15]

Over the course of 1931, for example, 195 sanitary agents allegedly made 78,689 home visits to address potential public health concerns throughout the capital city. This is slightly more than one visit per officer per day, presumably for the purpose of identifying ill and destitute people and transporting them to the hospital for treatment and rehabilitation. Even Jorge González, the chief officer of the Sanitary Police, stated that the detentions required "coercive" police action. Sanitary police also collected money by imposing fines on those accused of selling sex. In 1924 the department raised $37,330 from these payments, and in 1925 the much higher sum of $121,583.[16]

In the course of these nearly 80,000 home visits in 1931, the police accused 5,000 women of selling sex for money. However, only 20 percent of those accused were found to have been selling sex (1,000 of 5,000 women), meaning that the majority of women seen in hospitals did not identify as sex workers. Furthermore, many of the women who were detained by the Sanitary Police and interned in Mexico City's hospitals experienced some kind of reproductive surgery. This claim is based on empirical evidence: if one-half to two-thirds of patients in the women's ward were submitted to surgery, and if only one-fifth of them were there to give birth, many of the women must have undergone non-pregnancy-related reproductive surgeries. One wonders if sex workers were being sterilized nonconsensually, having their tubes tied consensually, receiving vaginal bifurcation surgeries, or undergoing ovariotomies or other forms of experimental surgery.

The General Hospital's registers do not show an occupation for most women, who apparently dedicated themselves to household tasks. This suggests that homemakers, potentially including those from the middle or elite classes, increasingly resorted to Mexico City's hospitals for reproductive health care. Others held formal and informal employment outside the home, especially as tortilla makers, cleaners, laundresses, and maids.[17] The majority of patients were impoverished; yet it is also clear that women from all classes received services from Mexico City's public hospitals and clinics.

Having considered how the coercive Sanitary Police influenced the hospital's population, it is fitting to contextualize Dr. X's claims about the high mortality rates within. Because record-keeping on mortality rates did not improve until 1935, the best numbers on that topic are from the years 1935 and 1936. During that time, 20 percent of women patients in the General Hospital died from complications from childbirth and surgery, including uterine rupture (from the application of forceps), puerperal septicemia from postbirth infection, cardiac insufficiency or aneurysm (conditions that generally resulted from anesthesia during surgery), pelviperitonitis, and hemorrhage resulting from childbirth or surgery.

Since only 20 percent of women patients were in the hospital for childbirth, many of the those who died must have experienced other kinds of reproductive surgeries such as abortions, sterilizations, or vaginal bifurcation.[18] For example, thirty-six patients were admitted on July 2, 1936. One, a housewife in labor, was a *pensionista*—she paid a monthly pension to the hospital to guarantee that she would have more satisfactory food and accommodations if hospitalized. The rest were *indigente,* or indigent; lacking resources, indigent patients were dependent on the state for free health care services. Overall, the hospital admitted approximately 928 new patients per month, and of these, 178 patients (19 percent) died. For newborns, the mortality rate was even higher; in 1936, based on the average of 4.6 born per day, of 1,679 total infants 842 died—a 50 percent mortality rate.[19]

Indeed, patients' quality of care varied widely, and especially in accordance with economic status. Eighty to 90 percent of the women in the General Hospital were in the indigent group, not the *pensionista* one. To take an example from just one month, in July 1936, of twenty-nine new patients admitted to the General Hospital, two were insured, and twenty-seven were indigent. Ten of these patients were women admitted for labor or gynecologic concerns, such as metritis and uterine backwardness.[20] Three of the ten women were in labor. Cross-referencing their names (Socorro Escobedo Aguirre, Luz González X, and Catalina Martínez Candilella), with the death records from that month reveals that all three of their infants died within a day of being born. Two of the deaths were attributed to a difficult birth, and the other suffered from hereditary syphilis.[21]

Sometimes women offered much higher sums, 15 to 20 pesos, for specialized operations. Doctors sometimes admitted these patients to the hospital under their own "guarantee of payment" and arranged the charges directly. According to medical students and the newspaper *El Universal,* some women sought hospital care with the precise intention of undergoing a surgical sterilization to control their fertility. Specifically, "influential clinicians had been earning up to 200 pesos per day by performing privately contracted operations in the General Hospital . . . these sometimes caused harm to the patients and reputational damage to the institution."[22] Because the stakes were high, surgeons did not wish to jeopardize their income or their reputation by performing faulty operations. Thus, some obstetricians took advantage of opportunities to practice surgical sterilizations on impoverished patients whose consent was partial or lacking. This allegation was reported by the newspaper *El Universal Gráfico* in August 1932, and it then was echoed by several students, including Dr. X. Because there was a bottom line to be had from wealthy women, the poor ones were at greater risk of abuse.

Sometimes women provided labor to the hospital in exchange for their debt. Those who were uninsured but had some economic means generally exchanged between 20 cents and 1 peso per day for food and services. Wealthy patients paid for higher quality food and medical care, and they resided in reserved rooms. These women generally paid 2 pesos per day. Those who could not pay were at the mercy of the overcrowded hospital system. Hospital inspectors reported terrible overcrowding in obstetrics and gynecology wards, where two women usually occupied each bed simultaneously. When no beds were available, women would lie on wooden pallets; inspectors complained that these were usually covered in bloodstained sheets. Those who did not fit on beds or pallets slept directly on the floor.[23]

It is very difficult for historians to grasp the scope of these massive client loads. Practitioners attended people in fifteen hospitals, three *sanatorios*, six clinics, and twenty shelters, including homeless shelters, insane asylums, elderly care facilities, orphanages, and "reform" homes, all of which housed a mix of voluntary and involuntary occupants. The BP did this with an impressive reserve of 53 million pesos. As of March 1933, 12,206 people lived in their establishments as patients, homeless, and orphans. At least 127,488 people in the city received medical attention, meaning that many, if not most, people were seeking free or reduced-cost treatment instead of paying for private services. Of these, 47,198 individuals sought attention in the *consultorios* (clinics), 97,374 children benefited from the state's budding public education services, and 750 families received 15 pesos of welfare each month.

These numbers underscore the massive undertaking of public health projects in 1930s Mexico City, especially in light of the depression, the repatriation of Mexicans and Mexican Americans from the United States, and postrevolutionary national reconstruction.[24] Given all this, and reflecting the goals of the revolution, Mexico City hospitals pursued more progressive reforms for patient care, including redrafting the regulatory codes to require consent from patients before submitting them to surgery.[25] But although the norms surrounding patient consent changed on paper, in practice they mostly persisted as before—especially because, by and large, the same doctors as before were in charge, so many of the same epistemologies remained.

Women's Complaints and Demands for Medical Care

Women's complaints about surgeons offer insight into the protections that patients demanded and believed they deserved. Perhaps the most affective was a 1929 denunciation by Maria Teodosio, who alleged that hospital authorities had lost her son after she sought refuge with him in the General Hospital.[26] Temporarily unhoused, Teodosio had been loitering near the Castillo de Chapultepec, which was also the residence of the nation's president. Her spatial resistance (loitering) may have even compelled the nation's president to reckon with the plight of his most challenged neighbors. A close friend of hers by the name of Valentina Rios lived and worked in the Castillo de Chapultepec as a domestic servant. When Teodosio began to cry out with labor pains, Rios acted as an impromptu midwife by assisting with the birth of her child and severing his umbilical cord.

Noting that Teodosio was "in a poor state of health," Rios called for the Red Cross and asked them to take Teodosio and her newborn boy to the hospital. However, a problem arose after the nurses removed Teodosio's son from her hospital room: they returned sometime later with a different infant—a girl. Strikingly, the hospital officials attempted to convince Teodosio that she had been mistaken about the sex of her child and that she must accept the new infant as her own. Refusing, Teodosio left the hospital and returned with Rios, who testified that she had witnessed Teodosio give birth to a boy.

A hospital deputy named Fernando García Berne found Rios and Teodosio's testimonies convincing. He wrote to the hospital director, underscoring that "there had been many complaints about this wing of the General Hospital [the women's ward]." Although the deputy requested that this case be investigated thoroughly, with particular attention to the conduct of nurses, the results of that investigation do not appear in the records.

Local papers printed similar reports. In August 1932, *El Popular* reported that while doctors were preparing to administer chloroform to a surgical subject in the Hospital Juárez, the patient "leapt off of the surgical table and took off running in an entirely marathon-like manner." A follow-up article lauded the patient's "spectacular sense of self-preservation," and commented "the patient probably had good reason to be scared."[27] Another journalist lamented that it was "fairly easy to escape from the Hospital Juárez."[28]

One patient who had "received a delicate operation of the abdomen" reportedly became "desperate, leapt out of bed, opened the door to the balcony, and threw herself out of the window before the nurses could react." Her fall resulted in grave injuries to the head, plus "the surgical wound the patient had in her midsection reopened, and this will surely be the cause of her imminent death."[29] Although the circumstances are difficult to discern from the article, the vignette portrays a patient unwilling to continue treatment. Perhaps she had experienced another kind of personal tragedy or had insurmountable depression. No matter the circumstance, her decision to leap from the balcony betrays the embattled hospital environment, in which the levels of physiological, personal, and perhaps collective suffering could become unbearable.

Rather than self-inflicted harm, other women received blows. María Alvarez wrote a letter to the hospital board of directors alleging that when she shifted in pain after a surgeon began to operate, he slapped her across the face and instructed her to keep quiet.[30] Señora Wensceslada Flores, who underwent a curettage and tubal ligation in the General Hospital, complained about similar abuse. She claimed that the nurses were negligent and that they struck two patients for lack of cooperation; in all, she denounced "an absolute lack of professional ethics" in the General Hospital. Flores was also concerned about the material conditions, noting that women who had recently undergone operations had no place to relieve themselves.[31]

Women sometimes raised a collective voice through organized and rebellious actions. Over the course of six years, women staged mass escapes from wards of the General Hospital as well as the Hospital Morelos. They jumped off the roofs, scaled the walls, wrenched security bars from the windows, stole all the medical equipment and linens they could reach, and complained that they were receiving subpar treatment and being subjected to unnecessary surgical interventions.[32] In March 1919, 103 women escaped the Hospital Morelos. Two years earlier, at least seventeen women fled from the same, including four women on March 10, 1917, who jumped from the roof to the top of the neighboring house. The neighbors apparently did not detain them "due to fear." On March 25, eleven more women escaped; on June 20, 1917, another two women escaped through doors that were poorly secured.

On June 27, 1917, the director ordered staff to take funds from the pensionist account to provide the detained women with milk, probably hoping that this would prevent further rebellions and escapes. But it did not work: on October 8, two more women escaped. These women were Soledad García and Celia Hernández. After breaking the handles off of a door, they smashed a window, from which they fled.

In another incident in 1917, thirteen women fled through the windows of the Hospital Morelos, which only had wire that was strong enough to hold them in; what they needed was steel bars. This was the case even though there were fewer women in the Hospital Morelos than there had been during the Porfiriato. Although we do not always know what motivated these women, and although they did not always leave a written record, their embodied resistance was an important symbol of their "weapons of the weak."[33]

On August 5, 1929, a woman wrote a letter to the Señor Licenciado José Almaraz, who was then president of the BP. Unfortunately, the last page of her letter is missing from the folder, so historians do not know her name or title. The woman reportedly journeyed to Mexico City three months prior to writing the letter. She did not mention her home state, but she related that she had chosen to travel to the city because she was "in poor health after undergoing an operation of the uterus."[34] While in the city, the woman exhausted her resources: not only had she had run out of money, but her friends were unable to continue caring for her.

For that reason, she asked volunteers from the Green Cross to take her to the General Hospital, where she was dissatisfied in many ways. She alleged that she was not given food during her first thirty-six hours in the establishment. The patient complained vociferously that her coffee was weak and cold, indicating that perhaps her expectations of public health care were high—likely higher than what could be delivered. She lamented that the eggs prescribed for her diet were unavailable. Presumably the hospital staff fed everyone whatever they could manage. Nevertheless, the patient was angered further when the nurses "woke [her] at six in the morning in an abrupt and rude manner." After she saw the doctor at 10:00 A.M., she was not given any medicine or form of pain control. The patient suffered from diarrhea, and she had to use the one toilet, which was in plain view of the other patients as if they were in a prison cell. Apparently the nurse criticized her for using the toilet so many times, while the other patients laughed at her. Reflecting on these interactions she wrote sadly, "No one was decent to me there."[35]

This patient begged her caretakers to release her the next day because she had received no prescription or medical treatment despite having been interned for seventy-two hours. She wrote, "In all, I have come to the conclusion that even when surgeons fulfill their duties, they do not do so within the necessary timeliness. They also cater unnecessarily to the nurses, who abuse their power completely—in every sense, and by every definition."

When the woman told a doctor why she was leaving the hospital, he reportedly ignored her, and the nurse mocked her. She expressed empathy and pity for the man in the bed next to hers, who had recently undergone an operation. Throughout the night, she wrote, the man called out for something to alleviate his pain. When no nurse attended to him, he began to plead for someone to bring poison instead, saying that he would rather die than continue to suffer. The patient who penned the letter ended her screed on a moving note. She wrote, "It is a shame. Many turn to the hospital as their last option, but there they do not find rest and care—instead, they only encounter scorn and contempt." By means of conclusion, she dramatically added "If I become sick again, and find myself without means, I would prefer to die in the street than to return to that establishment."[36]

Other patients and their families complained about treatments that sometimes seemed dehumanizing or humiliating. In 1929, Juan Viveros Valdez complained to General Juan María Tapía and the BP that his wife's braided hair had been cut off during her stay in the General Hospital, despite her vehement opposition.[37] It is possible that the braid had significance for the patient's Indigenous identity and that its removal was a form of "de-Indianization." This letter was included in a folder of other similar ones, entitled, "Complaints from Clinic Patients Regarding Poor Treatment." That folder also contained a letter addressed "to the head of the Beneficiencia Pública" from a former patient named Ana Hernández. Hernández stated that before seeking medical care she had read objections about the General Hospital in *El Universal Gráfico*, and, she insisted, "unfortunately, they are all true."[38] She reported that nurses had stolen her ring and that the food was deficient; although she had been prescribed fruits and juices for postoperation recovery, she received none.

Sometimes family members complained on behalf of their relatives. In 1928, señora Margarita Saldaña penned an enraged letter regarding her sister's death in the Hospital Juárez.[39] Saldaña reportedly had recommended that her sister give birth in that hospital because one practitioner there had a reputation for being particularly "caring." Her sister was in heavy labor when she was taken as a patient there, and Saldaña reported that "medical negligence" led to her death "even before she underwent a surgical operation."

Saldaña became incensed upon learning that her family would be unable to recover her sister's corpse. She found it shameful that the hospital commissioned the dead to a burial company without acquiring consent from the patients' families. More damning still, she denounced that the hospital director threatened her when she attempted to force the return of her sister's body.

When a journalist from *El Universal Gráfico* investigated the circumstances surrounding her letter of protest, he found that Saldaña's sister had died after ten days in the hospital, during which time she did not receive "any medical treatment." Although the director of the hospital denied that this was the case, *El Universal Gráfico* refused to retract the story.[40]

In the years following, more groups of women investigated the state of the hospital, including Elvia Carrillo Puerto, a socialist politician and feminist activist who founded Mexico's first feminist leagues in 1912.[41] Seventeen women in 1933 wrote a scathing petition about the General Hospital.[42] Complaints included that the food was a crust of bread and moldy cheese in the morning, and cold soup at midday with a thick film of fat on top and no vegetables within. The nurses, they said, forced patients to stand for long periods in the middle of the night under the pretext of changing their sheets, even though they were left without blankets for long periods of time. The women wrote, "In effect, we had heard a great deal about the terror that hospitals inspire among common people, but we attributed it to unfounded prejudices." However, "now that we have palpated the painful circumstances of most patients, we cannot justify such horror." "On the contrary," they wrote, "we deeply regret our powerlessness in the face of this situation."[43]

While it is impossible to know whether nurses and others committed these hostile acts, it is not a historian's task to adjudicate patient complaints or assess their veracity. What is clear is that patients and outsiders had serious concerns about reproductive health care, and that postrevolutionary patients found avenues through which to protest. Perhaps in the legacy of the revolution, there even existed a culture of protest and demands from the disaffected. Such grievances were not only preserved in the national archival record, but they also drew the attention of feminist activists and other revolutionary and postrevolutionary politicians at the time. This postrevolutionary rights-based culture threatened the previous climate of clinical practice.

Perhaps many grievances focused on nurses because they had more interaction with patients. Yet nurses also sometimes voiced trenchant criticisms of their own work environment at the General Hospital. In December 1932, they even sued the hospital for higher wages, shorter shifts, and better working conditions while complaining about sexual harassment and "being treated like slaves at the hands of the doctors." These were claims that General Juan María Tapía, then head of the BP, vehemently denied.[44] The nurses' lawsuit was well-timed, as it immediately followed the news that multi-millionaire

Señora Dolores Sáenz de Lavie had donated 1,400,000 pesos to the General Hospital. Within a month, Tapía responded by organizing subsidized housing for the women workers. He divided them into four classes of employee, with different assignments and pay rates for each group. Finally, he mandated that nurses were only to work eight-hour shifts—instead of the twelve-, fourteen-, or even sixteen-hour shifts that had been common (and unfortunately still are).

Even these decisions were sometimes entwined with the politics of surgical procedures. When Tapía announced that he wished to cultivate a new type of revolutionary nurse—who was to be the opposite of a parochial, backward, or religious one—he declared that they would have the chance to attend surgical operations and develop their medical expertise. In Tapía's words, "Nurses will begin to participate in important clinical instruction, during which doctors will seek to repeat as many surgical operations as possible, for the benefit of the nurses' education."[45] Although complaints about clinical interventions skyrocketed between 1929 and 1933, Tapía still sought to institutionalize the utility of instructional operations. After all, if there were no patients upon which to operate, it would be difficult for Mexican physicians and nurses gain the kind of expertise that would raise the country's scientific profile.

Student Revolt and the Doctor's Strike in the General Hospital, 1932

Patients were not alone in insisting that maternal mortality and patient care were political issues. Medical students invoked these themes often during the tumultuous years of 1932 and 1933, and their writings are key sources for understanding the story of epistemological continuity and revolutionary ruptures in Mexico City's postrevolutionary hospitals and public health and welfare system.

The BP did not undergo major transformations over the course of the immediate revolutionary period (1910–17). The first alteration of Mexico City's hospitals came in 1916, when the BP transferred the maternity wards that had been at the Hospital Morelos and the Hospital Juárez to the General Hospital, which was under the administrative control of the medical school by 1920.[46] This represented a centralization of those services more than a transformation; although women would no longer give birth in the Hospital Morelos and Hospital Juárez at the same rate they had previously, these clinics were still the site of substantial numbers of reproductive surgeries. More importantly, in 1920 the General Hospital was placed under the official direction of the national university's School of Medicine. With the elimination of the long-standing obstetric clinics in Hospital Juárez and Hospital Morelos, the General Hospital became the foremost location for obstetric care in the city. The change may have stemmed from officials' failures to quash repeated rebellions in Hospital Morelos.

A second major change came in 1924 when president General Plutarco Elías Calles restructured the BP and placed it under the direction of the Secretaría de Hacienda. Its services thereafter divided into the following: medical assistance, education and shelter, daytime assistance, and the education of those not seeking shelter. In 1929, the BP was again restructured, this time via the establishment of two new departments that took on greater importance than the others. The first was the Medical Department, and the second was the Department of Social and Educational Action. These were to work together to coordinate and oversee all services and care offered in hospitals, clinics, shelters, and orphanages. In Mexico City, the BP created five new clinics and established new hospitals, shelters, educational centers, public dormitories, and public dining halls.[47] At the same time, however, public health officials lamented that impoverished people often arrived at free hospitals when they had nowhere else to go for food and shelter.[48] Prior to the 1930s, approximately sixty nonpaying patients were admitted per day, but by 1932 the daily number was more than 120.

Even so, the institutional revolution did not send shockwaves through the hospital and welfare system until 1932; before that time, many of the same professors from the 1880s and 1890s continued teaching and practicing largely as before. This entire system was challenged in mid-1932, when the General Hospital and the BP underwent a major internal crisis that was closely related to the politics of surgical operations.[49] This episode is instructive for several reasons, not least of which is that it mirrored in some ways the high revolutionary politics of the early 1930s.

Indeed, Mexico City's hospital system had become thoroughly politicized by this time. Such politicization came to a head in September 1932, when the powerful military general and de facto leader of the nation, *Jefe Máximo* Plutarco Elías Calles, forced Pascual Ortíz Rubio to step down from his position as president of the Republic.[50] Calles had supported Ortíz Rubio's ascent to the presidency but ousted him over ideological disagreements regarding his cabinet appointments. Most notably, Ortíz Rubio had appointed his brother as head of the BP administration in Mexico City. When Calles ousted the Ortíz Rubio brothers from power, therefore, he was able to quash the student rebellion and restore order in the General Hospital.

Historians have long assumed that the conflict between Calles and the Ortíz Rubio brothers was a solely a clash over the appointment of powerful bureaucratic offices.[51] To my knowledge only one historian, Tzvi Medin, has noted the correlation between presidential politics and the medical revolt of 1932. Medin offered a passing comment on the ordeal, noting: "The immediate backdrop was a doctors' strike, which erupted when Estrada Cajigal was ordered by Calles to fire the director of Public Health and Welfare [Beneficencia Pública], Francisco Ortiz Rubio, brother of the President of the Republic."[52]

On July 26, 1932, the BP forced Dr. Escalona to resign from his position as the director of the Hospital General.[53] They sent him a letter saying that they accepted his resignation, but he claimed that he had never submitted one. According to the local press, Calles had ordered Francisco Ortiz Rubio to remove Escalona and appoint Dr. Ignacio González Guzmán in his place.

The press dutifully reported that Calles had Escalona fired because he had begun to challenge doctors in the General Hospital who were performing unethical and experimental operations for profit. In *La Prensa*, Dr. X had made a statement supporting this claim: "All of the physicians and nurses in the hospital are aware of this. When Dr. Escalona was director, he felt compelled to send a strongly worded memorandum instructing surgeons to discontinue these operations, and he even threatened to restrict the access to female patients if they continued to make them into experimental subjects by means of useless operations."[54]

A journalist in *El Universal Gráfico* described a situation of professional conflict over resources and hospital organization. The newspaper reported that there was a "true mafia in the hospital, consisting of three or four professors who are infamous for manipulating the institution while running their own private practices out of the free clinics." The accusation was that these professors accepted payment from wealthy patients while neglecting to tend to the public patients. The report continued, "They have acquired large amounts of privilege and, in exchange for *x* or *y* political favors, the directors agree to spend large sums to purchase top-of-the-line surgical equipment and to construct expensive operating rooms that are inaccessible to the others."[55] Because surgery offered high profit margins, advancements required manipulation of institutional funds and became the site of contention between physicians in the hospital. *El Excelsior* agreed with this characterization. Their correspondent claimed that "some of the old doctors tend to approach the

General Hospital as a site for human experimentation and discount their humanitarian and professional obligations."[56]

Calles believed, conversely, that González Gúzman would be able to reinstate order in the General Hospital by restoring the powers and privileges to the physicians whom Escalona refused to tolerate any longer. Yet Calles's appointee, González Guzmán, only lasted as director of the Hospital General for a few days. By August 4, Dr. Conrado Zuckermann stormed the General Hospital with an armed entourage and seized control of the establishment. Zuckermann had graduated from medical school in 1918 and worked as a gynecologist and surgeon. Zuckermann did not aim to restore the previous status quo, and he immediately "attempted to take a direct intervention in the medical body and the leadership of the BP."[57]

Part of Zuckermann's platform as the new director was to halt student medical experimentations and the performance of operations for profit, which angered the clinicians and their students alike. The student body association took a vote on Zuckermann's leadership: only twenty-eight voted in his favor, whereas 434 opposed him. Twenty-five doctors reportedly resigned the day after Zuckermann's coup d'état, leaving only six of the old faculty members in charge of the hospital wings in the General Hospital.[58] The press, for its part, overwhelmingly supported Zuckermann and seemed to delight in shocking the public with scandalous reports.

It appears that Zuckermann could not handle the political pressure. On August 5, the day after his coup, he temporarily resigned. In his place, the BP appointed Dr. Ernesto Ulrich, who was already head of some wings of the hospital. In other words, Calles meddled in the BP to uphold a high modernist doctors' elite vision, as well as to assert his authority over the Ortíz Rubio clan.

Although Zuckermann temporarily resigned on August 5, the physicians were still in an uproar about the sudden challenge to their power. No government in modern Mexico had challenged the power of the medical authorities, so this affront was probably new and shocking. However, it was in line with *callista* state-building practices: Calles notoriously tried to revolutionize guild-like structures such as churches, schools, and legal guilds.

On August 5, the number of resigned medics went up to thirty-seven, and the press began to speculate that there would be a strike.[59] Francisco Ortiz Rubio, president of the Junta Directiva of the Beneficencia Pública, ordered an immediate investigation of the General Hospital, and the result offered "sufficient data regarding the scandalous machinations of several doctors, who had so many patients that they let their subordinates do what they wished with them."[60] One journalist added, "We speculate that Francisco Ortiz Rubio will pursue legal measures against them to preserve the institution's prestige and commitment to the public." *El Nacional* reported that although the BP had accepted their resignations, they would still remain as professors in the School of Medicine and would continue "carrying out their studies with the support of the student interns in their respective hospitals." Here it was reported that Escalona would return.[61]

The next day brought an unexpected turn. Fifty-three Mexico City doctors joined with dozens of advanced medical students and penned a letter in support of Zuckermann, which they sent to the press. According to *El Excelsior*, the letter celebrated that Zuckermann would "once and for all, eliminate the chaos and privilege of those who have been controlling our hospital, and he will substitute the old system with a regime of equality, justice, and order, which will be of equal benefit to surgeons and patients in public hospitals and the nation at large." The letter continued by responding to the "claim of their opponents," who voiced concern that the "most difficult operations would now have to be performed by inexperienced people." The fifty-three doctors' letter countered that unnecessary operations would be avoided under the future regime.[62]

By August 9, the BP administrators were so angry at the dissenting doctors that they decided to sue a core group for defamation.[63] This was a crucial development, because it shows that Zuckermann's radical regime change enjoyed at least marginal support from the BP, despite General Calles's seeming preoccupation about sudden and drastic challenges to the nation's most esteemed and powerful practitioners. There were other signs of this trend: on August 11, the BP appointed Dr. Anastasio Garza Rios to conduct an investigation in the General Hospital "to protect the patients."[64] The day after the investigations commenced, however, Zuckermann again resigned from his position as director.[65] Dr. Escalona declared that he would not return to his former position as director—in fact, he resigned permanently and announced that he would never again set foot in the General Hospital.[66]

Calles now turned definitively against Zuckermann; by mid-August, he had decided that the doctor's plan to reform the General Hospital was not what he had in mind. Calles ordered the governor of the Federal District, Vicente Estrada Cajigal, to conduct a swift investigation, and the results were disastrous for Zuckermann: Cajigal, under orders from Calles, demanded Zuckermann's resignation and ordered him to name Dr. Luis Méndez as the new director.[67] Delighted, the practitioners who had resigned returned immediately. Not all parties were content with this outcome, however; Calles's intervention provoked the renunciation of Dr. Gastón Melo, who was then head of the Departamento de Salubridad. This followed the resignation of Estrada Cajigal, as the head of the Departamento del Distrito, perhaps because he resented that Calles had forced him to fire Zuckermann.[68] He was instructed to "definitively reorganize the personnel and elaborate on precise instructions for the performance of their duties, and to make, as soon as possible, a regulatory code for the establishment." In the general's written acceptance of Cajigal's resignation, he questioned his "loyalty to the Mexican nation."[69]

The new director of the General Hospital, Dr. Luis Méndez, only lasted one week in the position.[70] In his resignation, Méndez clarified that as the new director he had wished to reinstate some of the doctors who had resigned during the conflict and had succeeded in convincing some to return, but Calles refused to approve their reappointment. Thus, this was a political struggle between Calles and Ortíz Rubio, one waged through hospital appointments and preference to one deeply ideological faction or another.

Because Méndez felt that the president's disapproval extended to him, he resigned in solidarity with the physicians.[71] The faculty who had resigned previously did so again to punctuate their point. This included Dr. Manuel Guevara Oropeza, head of the servicio de propaganda y educación higienica (coordination of hygienic education and public health information), and Salvador Zubirán, head of the servicio de comestibles y bebidas (coordination of food and drink service).[72] At this point, the struggle for preeminence at the BP reached an altogether higher level. Calles managed to push Ortíz Rubio out of his position as president of the BP on August 25; just a few weeks later, in early September, Ortíz Rubio's brother resigned from his position as president of the Republic.[73]

Meanwhile, fifth- and sixth-year students were still performing research in the General Hospital. This is somewhat ironic due to the level of conflict that surrounded their positions. In late 1932 they apparently did this work largely without the supervision of their professors, who were occupied with the chaos of resigning, reaccepting, and then re-resigning from their positions.[74] In the midst of the conflict (in August 1932), the BP decided to open up the instruction clinics for clinicians from other hospitals and clinics, and invited them to come into the General Hospital and begin supervising the students therein.[75]

The dust began to settle by September, first evident when General Juan María Tapía was named the new director of the BP.[76] His appointment broke with tradition and reflected Calles's revolutionizing approach, as Tapía was not a doctor but rather a revolutionary hero. He inspected the General Hospital immediately, declared it to be severely unhygienic, and ordered its total reorganization.[77] The patients, for their part, complained that they were given substandard food, mostly consisting of undercooked beans and cold, unsweetened corn-mush (*atole*). Emphasizing this point, the press highlighted that the BP had a budget surplus of more than 300,000 pesos, so presumably it could have afforded to provide higher quality sustenance. Not everyone was happy with Tapía's appointment: Juan Amezcua—the secretary of the BP—quit.[78] Three days later, his replacement, Dr. Priani, resigned as well.[79]

General Tapía did not waste time addressing the conflict in the General Hospital, and he took similar action on a similar crisis in the Homeopathic Hospital. Tapía fired the director of the latter, Gómez Esparza, and named Dr. Alfredo Araujo in his place. The new director reportedly "followed strict orders from the Department of Medicine in the BP (Departamento Médico de la Beneficencia) to suppress all major surgery—which is alien to the homeopathic healing system—and increase other healing services."[80]

The press appeared quite loyal to Tapía, and generally stopped printing patient and faculty complaints after he took power. Journalists evidently wanted to show that Tapía had pulled the hospital system out of its colonial and Porfirian decadence; once they had conveyed this message, they stopped reporting on the details of the Zuckermann conflict.[81] We only know that in October 1932 Tapía ordered the resigned staff to return to their positions in the General Hospital, and they acceded to his request. The status quo was restored.

Despite the press's propagandistic gloss in 1934, signs of discontent still surfaced. When a large group of medical residents organized and refused to attend a major demonstration in favor of the six-year plan for socialism in Mexico, Tapía fired every one of them from their positions, leaving their medical degrees hanging in the balance.[82] The group of students declared that their resistance was not motivated by their religious opposition to socialist forms of governance; rather, they wanted the freedom to express a diversity of opinions within the BP and felt that being forced to attend a pro-government rally was not in alignment with this priority.[83]

This conflict gained additional significance because it threw into sharp relief the postrevolutionary divisions between the government and the medical school as well as those in the revolutionary elite—divisions that had clearly played a role in the conflict over governance of the General Hospital. In the 1934 incident, the director of the medical school, Fernando Ocaranza, did not let Tapía fire his students. He publicly stated that he would personally grant their degrees—and that if they could not finish their residencies that year, no one would. In fact, he temporarily pulled all residents out of public hospitals in retaliation.[84] In response, Tapía quit after a year of attempting to revolutionize the BP and asked all his subordinates to resign in solidarity with him. In this episode, Fernando Ocaranza (a Porfirian physician and supporter of dissenting students) won the battle over medical education and its relationship to public hospitals.[85]

The federal government dissented, however, inasmuch as president General Lázaro Cárdenas refused to accept Tapía's resignation and demanded that he continue to serve as head of the BP.[86] Cárdenas wanted Tapía to keep fighting to expel the "enemies of the revolution," although it is unclear if he was referring to the professors of medicine as enemies.[87] The resignations, bewildering as they are, nonetheless show how an authoritarian clinical elite who viewed patients as an expendable resource (or one to be co-opted into their rhetoric) made its deal with the revolutionary government and silenced or expelled its internal critics.

At the same time, this era in Mexican history witnessed an unprecedented surge in commentary from the patients themselves about the politics of the General Hospital and the controversies over surgery and reproductive health care within. Any history of surgical politics is incomplete without the voices of patients, but too often historians can only intuit these stories by reading medical sources against the grain. This chapter has highlighted the voices of patients and medical students who lamented that they sometimes found the hospital to be a place of suffering instead of healing. Their insistence on dignified health care and vociferous denunciations of dehumanizing moments foreshadowed the major issues in defining and addressing reproductive injustice today. Reproductive surgery became a deeply divisive topic that represented a range of social issues simultaneously, including the future of the nation and the obligations of the state to provide care for its citizens' bodies. Conflict regarding surgery both reflected, and contributed to, debates about the meaning of the Mexican revolution and concerns about how the new state would revolutionize its citizenry through different kinds of salvation.

CONCLUSION AND EPILOGUE

Patriarchy Is a Judge, and We Are Judged for Being Born

Resistance against Reproductive Injustice in Mexico and Latin America

El Patriarcado es un Juez / Que nos Juzga por Nacer

—Las Tesis, Chile, 2020

In August 2016, a judge in Sonora Mexico refused to allow a thirteen-year-old girl to terminate her pregnancy, which resulted from rape. Although Sonoran state law purportedly allowed for abortion in such cases, a judge decided to classify the assault as only "sexual coercion" and not rape, thereby disallowing the termination.[1] In recent months, news stories such as these have been all too common throughout the Americas. In 2019, a mother in Brazil was excommunicated for seeking an abortion for her nine-year-old daughter, who became pregnant as a result of sexual violence (indeed, any circumstance in which a nine-year-old becomes pregnant involves sexual violence). In response to the Brazilian mother's predicament, Italian Cardinal Giovanni Battista declared that abortion was a sin worse than rape.[2]

A similar tragedy occurred in February 2019 in Tucuman Argentina, where an eleven-year-old girl found herself pregnant after having been raped. Traumatized and scared, the girl and her mother sought an abortion early in the pregnancy, but were stymied by local obstetricians, the mayor, and the governor. As the girl approached twenty-three weeks of gestation, authorities instead resolved to extract the fetus via caesarean operation. This was not an easy decision for obstetrician Cecilia Ousset, who helped to perform the surgery. Dr. Ousset was disturbed by operating on such a young patient. She said, "My legs trembled when I saw her. It was like seeing my younger daughter. The little girl didn't understand completely what was going to happen." One can only imagine how the child herself felt.

Dr. Ousset found other aspects of the case unsettling. She accused Tucumán's governor, Juan Manzur, of exploiting the girl and her fetus for political motives. She claimed that state authorities had "prevented the legal interruption of the pregnancy and forced the little girl to give birth," and that the "11-year-old girl was tortured for a month by the provincial health system."[3] The twenty-three-week fetus died shortly after having been delivered by cesarean section.

The anecdotes above speak to complex and historically rooted problems relating to religion, authority, reproductive autonomy, and violence, themes that are at the heart of this book. Who determines maternal health and fetal life policy, and on the basis of what authority?[4] When do surgeons enforce the law, and when do they subvert it? Whose ideologies should take precedence in reproductive conflicts: those of religious authorities, state officials, families, or individuals? When is an unborn product of conception considered a human, a person, ensouled, or alive, and what role should spiritual and medical authorities play in this debate?

The previous chapters have historicized eras of politicization surrounding both commonplace and emergency obstetric situations. In dialogue with that trend, miscarriages have become increasingly politicized and criminalized in the Americas. Such conflicts reflect the difficulty of differentiating between attempted abortion and miscarriage, and they deepen a trend of surveillance over women's reproduction, with threats of punishment even for circumstances completely out of their control. Last fall in El Salvador, twenty-year-old Imelda Cortez faced twenty years in prison when authorities suspected that she had attempted to provoke a miscarriage. Yet, the young woman had not realized she was pregnant and had not attempted to abort. The complication happened spontaneously, and in fact, the fetus survived.[5] What is jail time for a potential miscarriage—in which the fetus *survived*—other than a message to women that the lives of their fetuses are more valuable or important than their own? In 1991, Susan Bordo phrased this as "Are mothers persons?"[6] Or, as Dorothy Roberts recounted in a recent interview, the seeds of inspiration for her life work took root when she realized, "Oh my God, they can kill her if she's pregnant."[7]

Another example stems from August 2022, in which the state of Texas implemented a trigger law that bans abortion even in cases of ectopic pregnancy or imminent maternal death. Given that an embryo cannot survive an ectopic pregnancy, cruelty seems to be the point of such measures; ample news coverage has highlighted the increased maternal mortality that has resulted from Texan women's inability to access abortion care. Other nations—such as Ecuador and Honduras—have followed the trend of jailing and prosecuting women who suffer miscarriages.[8]

Due to a historical paucity of abortion access, Latin American activists developed a range of legal, activist, and media strategies to highlight the plights of those like the children of Sonora, Brazil, and Tucumán. Now that *Roe v. Wade* has been overturned, activists in the United States have increasingly done the same. Heartbreaking though it is to consider the suffering of abused children, we now see daily reports of young girls who struggle to access abortion. Loretta Ross refers to them as "poster children" for abortion access. Struggles that were previously hidden behind unequal access are now in plain sight, and some women in the United States are turning to Latin American activists for a sense of the path forward.

Since the 1970s, the feminist human rights–based group Grupo de Información en Reproducción Elegida (GIRE) has addressed the intersecting problems of access to fertility control, abortion, obstetric violence, and nonconsented sterilization in Mexico. Their recent report, *The Missing Piece: Reproductive Justice,* shares a wealth of information about these topics. Above all, GIRE argues that a governmental failure to address problems in maternal health care constitutes a web of state violence against women, children, and childbearing people as a whole. They write, "The State has the obligation to promote legislation and public policies designed to transform the health system to ensure the provision of quality obstetric care to eliminate obstetric violence and reduce maternal deaths."[9] GIRE staunchly advocates for abortion access and views a denial of such as forced childbearing. They often accompany survivors of rape and pregnant adolescents to meetings with hospital and state authorities in order to help those women access their constitutionally protected access to the termination of pregnancy.

As mentioned in this book's introduction, GIRE's *Reproductive Justice* report draws on data from Mexico's 2016 national survey on the dynamics of household relationships. The survey received responses from 8.7 million women who experienced pregnancy between 2011 and 2016. Of those 8.7 million, 33.4 percent reported having suffered abuse by their health providers. During the same time period, state bodies received a total of 867 formal complaints of obstetric violence. Rates of violence were highest in public hospitals and lowest in care provided by midwives. States with higher percentages of women reporting obstetric violence include Mexico City (36.5 percent), the State of Mexico (36 percent), Querétaro (34.6 percent), Tlaxcala (34.2 percent), and Morelos (33.7 percent).[10] Women frequently complained about the overmedicalization of childbirth as well as the use of routine procedures without therapeutic justification and without women's consent—two issues repeatedly highlighted in the chapters of this book.

GIRE notes that in Mexico, like in many other countries, clinicians frequently carry out cesarean sections without medical indication. This poses a health risk to childbearing people, especially for those with limited access to comprehensive obstetric care.[11] In 2015, as many as 39.1 percent of births in Mexico were cesarean births. This suggests that there is a high prevalence of unnecessary cesareans in the nation, given that the World Health Organization recommends countries not exceed 10 to 15 cesarean deliveries per 100 live births for optimal maternal and neonatal outcomes. According to the national survey data, 42.8 percent of the women surveyed had experienced a cesarean in their last birth; disturbingly, 10.3 percent did not know the reason for the procedure, and 9.7 percent did not consent to the surgery.[12]

Another form of nonconsented care is the application of contraception without consent. The 2016 national survey indicated that 13.95 percent of women who reported a form of obstetric violence also received a contraceptive method or method of permanent sterilization without prior information, communication, or consent. A large study by Mexico's National University (UNAM) found that of Indigenous women sterilized in Mexico between 2006 and 2012, 27 percent did not consent for the procedure. Still today in Mexico, racism is exacerbated by the economic, cultural, and spatial marginalization of most Indigenous groups, whose languages are not valorized or taught in schools.[13]

Researchers consistently replicate these findings. For example, investigator Gloria López Mora recently estimated that at least 90 percent of mothers in the Mexican state of Veracruz have experienced some form of obstetric violence. In a survey conducted by her team in the Port of Veracruz, seven of ten women interviewed reported having experienced three or more kinds of abuse or mistreatment in the public maternity ward.[14] López Mora defined obstetric violence as physical, verbal, psychological, and institutional abuse that harmed pregnant and postpartum women and their children. Examples included the use of forceps and uterine rasp without pain control and the administration of unnecessary or harmful medicine. Psychological violence comprises dehumanizing treatment, racial discrimination, humiliation, and the all-too-frequent practice of mocking a patient and her children during birth. One's use of voice and freedom of expression appear to be key issues for childbearing people. Indeed, writing about obstetric racism in the United States context, feminists have pointed out that Black women are frequently targeted for their use of tears and their voices to demand attention in a resource-scare environment.[15]

Reproductive health inequities contribute to higher levels of maternal mortality, or the death of a woman from preventable causes during pregnancy, labor/delivery, and the postpartum period. Excessive maternal mortality represents a violation of the rights to life, health, equality and nondiscrimination, "as well as the rights to be free of cruel and inhuman treatment and enjoy the benefits of scientific and technological progress."[16] GIRE tells us that maternal deaths in Mexico disproportionately affect the poorest women, Indigenous women, and women who do not have access to social security because they are employed in informal sectors of the economy.

Indigenous women, in particular, generally live far from health centers, which are usually in poor condition and generally do not have permanent staff or interpreters of local languages.[17] Although Indigenous women only make up 6 percent of the Mexican population, they account for 11.2 percent of all maternal deaths in the country. Girls and adolescents are at particular risk for pregnancy and maternal mortality, and the rates of adolescent pregnancy are higher for Indigenous women. Indeed, up to 50 percent of Indigenous women gave birth as an adolescent. This intersection of youth and racism makes women more vulnerable to death (sadly, perhaps, like for the girl of Devil's Alley in 1884): in 2015, of all maternal deaths, 10.9 percent were those of minors under 19.9 years old.[18] GIRE believes that there is a systematic violation of the reproductive rights of Indigenous and Afro-Mexican women in Mexico, from forced sterilizations, to abuse at health facilities, to a lack of access to culturally sensitive health information and services in their language.

Nongovernmental organizations and activists have issued recommendations to address disparities in health care access. They celebrate state governments' commitment to improving obstetric care services, and they urge the state to continue working for "accessibility, availability, and quality of health care in all regions, particularly rural and remote areas, including improving the infrastructure of the primary health care system," as well as ensuring "that hospitals have enough and adequate medical personnel, infrastructure, and supplies, as well as the necessary medicines for emergencies."[19]

Activists recommend that the Mexican government classify obstetric violence as a form of institutional and gender-based violence and, in particular, that the state take steps to guarantee that medical personnel request a woman's fully informed consent before enacting contraceptive sterilization. GIRE does not support the criminalization of individual health care practitioners for obstetric violence because this would individualize a problem that has its roots in state-based neglect. They also worry that midwives would be criminalized more than medics. Nonetheless, the organization believes that practitioners who perform sterilizations without consent should face penalties and that women who have undergone nonconsensual sterilization receive monetary compensation.

Women throughout Latin American have responded resoundingly to the issues demarcated above. Medical anthropologists like Lina Rosa Berrio Palomo have written a great deal about Indigenous and Afro-Mexicans and the medical and social inequalities they face, from medical neglect to obstetric violence.[20] This scholarly work is deeply informed by street protest, and especially increasing mobilizations by women in Mexico and across Latin America. In the "Purple Spring" protests of 2016 women throughout Latin America denounced obstetric violence and demanded dignity in reproductive health care as well as access to fertility control.[21] Their mobilizations have only increased in recent years.

In the midst of the mass death and economic shock wrought by COVID, activists in Argentina, Chile, and Mexico engaged in months-long street battles to bring attention to gendered violence and reproductive health care. These were epic feminist uprisings that demanded reproductive rights, greater control over local and national institutions, and a halt to the impunity for feminicide and other crimes against women. In Chile, women chanted, "The patriarchy is a judge / and it judges us for being born / And the punishment we face/ is violence that you do not see." Their militant chants rippled throughout the world, and tens of thousands of women joined their intense, angry, perfectly coordinated public performances. The chant went on, "The rapist is you. / He is the police, / the judges, / the state, / the president. / The oppressive state is a violent rapist. / The rapist is you." Chilean feminists' structural analysis of gender violence left the world stunned. They insisted that patriarchal authorities are responsible for—and indeed, take part in—sexual violence against women. Las tesis explained that the chant meant to recall, and critique, the military regime's acts of sexual violence against protestors during Pinochet's military dictatorship of 1973–1990. Women around the world raised their voices in solidarity.

Then, in Argentina, feminists won a protracted and arduous battle to decriminalize abortion. Next the Mexican state of Oaxaca decriminalized abortion in the first trimester. Finally, just days after Texas passed a new "bounty hunter" law that banned abortion after a few days of pregnancy and put a price tag of $10,000 on women's bodies, Mexico's Supreme Court ruled that it is unconstitutional to punish abortion as a crime, a landmark ruling that clears the way for the legalization of abortion across the country. The court took up the issue when eight of eleven justices voted to revoke a law in the state of Coahuila that punished women with up to three years in prison for having an abortion—even in cases of rape. Governors throughout the nation slowly began to release women who were imprisoned for having attempted to end their pregnancies.

Surgery and Salvation has historicized these issues over the *longue durée*, beginning with the relationship between cesarean surgery and religious claims about ensoulment, fetal life, and embryology. In dialogue with the work of inquisitor Francesco Emanuele Cangiamila, a group of priests during the Enlightenment produced a corpus of work regarding "theological embryology." Here it is fitting to emphasize the ironic, and also prescient, words of Joseph Needham, who in the 1930s was both an embryologist and the most prominent modern historian of that discipline. Needham opined that theological embryology had "reach[ed] a climax . . . with Cangiamila's *Embryologia Sacra*." While recognizing that the ideology "liv[es] on embedded in Roman Catholic theology up to our own era," Needham also insisted: "the future holds no place for the discussion of such themes, and what has been called 'theological embryology' is already dead." Needham's concluding remarks on theological embryology were even more direct: "The doctrine," he insisted, "does humanity no credit."[22]

Needham's comments were reflective of a dominant trend in modern science that dismissed the relevance of religious thought and assumed that the epistemological legacies of those traditions would gradually disappear on their own as a result of secularization and modernization. How wrong he was. He could not have predicted the extremely long afterlife of eighteenth-century religious ideas about the importance of saving a fetal soul at all costs, and of weaponizing medical intervention to address metaphysical and social problems while criminalizing women's sexual behavior and punishing them for making health care demands on the state.

As this book has shown, caesarean surgery afforded the Catholic church a unique opportunity to examine the structure and formation of small products of conception. Indeed, Cangiamila and others promoted the idea that women must submit to corporal death in order for products of conception to receive a baptism. Priests were to assume that a woman, dead or alive, was already baptized or was irredeemably lost to paganism, her soul belonging to the devil. This meant that the physical death of her body was of little to no consequence in comparison with the moral death of the infant's soul and its loss of a chance at eternal life. Such ideas signaled an extreme prioritization of the unborn's potential life over its mother's actual life. As the first section of this book demonstrated, the caesarean operation had political value as a way to instill morality in women, curb promiscuity, terrorize Indigenous people, discipline the religious orders, and create a new and individuated subject on the basis of the soul. Surgery made possible the core claims in the Catholic church's modern approach to fetal life.

The second section turned to an examination of hospital administration and the creation of modern medical training after Mexico's independence from Spain. The chapters focus on the medicalization of hysteria and the effort to define normal and pathological phenomena in women's reproductive lives. This all took place within the context of state secularization and the liberalization of Mexican politics. These processes inflected on debates about women's roles as religious hospital administrators as well as rights-based claims on the state.

Scientists and politicians voiced surprising and often contradictory opinions on the cultural dimension of gender relations in postcolonial and reforma-era Mexico. Male politicians invoked stereotypes about the allegedly "hysterical" and "capricious" women who held authority in hospitals. Such language meant to defame the women based on stereotypes about their gender and their alleged hostility to science. Furthermore, a modernized and patriarchal scientific morale was meant to prevent the women from continuing to influence decisions around reproductive medicine. This discourse was gendered in that the religious nurses were accused of denying the country of wives and daughters by means of their participation in health care services.

In 1874, President Sebastián Lerdo de Tejada exemplified the extreme liberal position during the mid-nineteenth century and expelled the religious health care providers. Whereas his predecessor President Benito Juárez had lauded Catholic labor in hospitals, Lerdo de Tejada was willing to risk his political career to demonstrate his intolerance for the sisters. All this was overlain with an interventionist attitude that allowed for the castration, via ovariotomy, of female patients who were deemed insane, hysterical, or immoral, in an era in which authorities valued the utility and productivity of individual and their potential service to the state. Once again, religious and state concerns were strongly linked to conflicts over reproductive surgery.

By the 1870s, medical attention turned to another kind of surgery, in which doctors terminated women's pregnancies when they saw them as unnatural or pathological due to various biological, social, and emotional conditions, including hysteria and out-of-wedlock pregnancy. Historians refer to these procedures as therapeutic abortion, but reforma physicians made them discursively compatible with religion by referring to the procedures as "artificial premature birth." Natural and pathological became contested categorizations that shaped, and were shaped, by social circumstances and contingencies.

Meanwhile, this chapter underscored that there has always been popular demand to terminate pregnancies in Mexico, and that surgeons, midwives, and others have long been willing to fill this demand.

These exclusionary and evolutionary aims were not explicitly racialized during the reforma like they would become during the Porfiriato (1876–1911). Rather, they were couched in behavioral/biological terms about "natural" bodies, "rationally organized bodies," and "weak biology" that led to "moral and emotional suffering." The late nineteenth century, on the other hand, showed the onset of a masculinized notion of scientific progress that prioritized experimental methods over the preservation of both fetal and maternal life. A shift in tone in the late nineteenth-century sources became apparent too. Positivist inquiry and writing was formulaic, obsessed with the quest to find and follow natural laws; thus, Porfirian doctors tended to omit descriptions of women's personal lives and identities. Physicians began to use colder, more objectifying descriptors, a new scientific language that reduced women to their body parts such as "the pelvis" and "the uterus," and referred to fetuses as "the product" as opposed to "the child," as before.

Porfirian medicine witnessed other shifts in cultural, social, biological, and religious issues surrounding reproduction and surgical intervention. Although doctors continued to perform therapeutic abortions, Porfirian physicians no longer wrote about terminating pregnancies due to women's irrational or hysterical mindset. Nor did they discuss fetal baptism as a means with which to prove the individuality of the fetal soul, as in the late colony and early republic. Instead, the battle to stake a cultural claim over reproduction became racialized in ways that it previously had not been.

Racial prejudices continued to affect obstetric surgeries even after Mexico's grassroots and leftist social revolution. Writings on obstetric surgery during this era were dominated by eugenicists, who believed that only sterilization could aid public health officials in achieving the biological regeneration that Mexico needed. They paternalistically emphasized that they alone should control reproduction, and that women should never be free to choose fertility control or abortion for themselves. Like their reforma predecessors, the postrevolutionary eugenicists drew on similar claims for their goal of cultivating "modern" citizens. Promises of surgical perfectability became linchpins because they offered promises of uplifting women, at the same time that they claimed to rationalize and explain ineffable and incomprehensible aspects of human experiences with reproduction and death. Temporary sterilization represented a modernization of patriarchy as well as a reconciliation of scientific and religious claims over women's fertility.

Each era witnessed different kinds of conflict over the idea of "natural" birth. Eighteenth century thinkers believed that God made birth natural, even when priests needed to use surgery to manifest God's will. A priest possessed little medical expertise, but surgical technology made him a more perfect conduit of theology. Then hysteria made women's femininity unnatural and unpredictable, sometimes due to its pathological excess. When doctors performed therapeutic abortions in the 1870s, it was because they believed that pregnancy was made unnatural through maternal suffering, and so needed to end. Likewise, when Trangay sterilized one patient based on racialized criteria, he commented that he did so "in the most natural of manners" in the postrevolutionary period. Racial science had naturalized Mexico's colorist prejudice against Indigenous and Black Mexicans and the lower classes as a whole.

In chapter 8, sterilization "without mutilation" can be read as a claim to "natural" sterilization, in which doctors insisted on the ordinariness of something as extreme as vaginal bifurcation. Although the splitting of the vaginal canal was an invasive and untried procedure, medical student Ramírez Elliot challenged the framework of what could be considered "mutilation" from the surgeon's standpoint. Finally, in chapter 9, practitioners appeared to naturalize obstetric violence and embed it discursively as part of the childbearing experience. Across the centuries, religious and political authorities imbued surgical procedures with distinct meanings, which became particularly contentious in highly politicized environments.

As demonstrated here, reproductive governance and its related surgical interventions have created and responded to legal, popular, and religious tension since at least the eighteenth century, when Spanish colonial authorities began to claim that fetuses were likely ensouled from the moment of conception. Although positions on fetal ensoulment varied throughout the (eighteenth-century religious, nineteenth-century postcolonial, nationalistic, and secular, and twentieth-century revolutionary) eras of Mexican history, there remained the paternalistic insistence that women themselves were not and are not fit to govern the terms of their own fertility.

In each era, authorities pursued reproductive governance in part to acculturate and assimilate individuals and groups selectively into colonial, postcolonial, and revolutionary state projects. These claims were made and remade through discourses around surgery. Like many other places, Mexico now has substantial present-days struggles over reproduction, represented by high maternal mortality rates, a crisis of obstetric violence and unconsented sterilization of Indigenous and Afro-Mexican women, and struggles over abortion, including the imprisonment of more than 4,000 women after they experienced obstetric incidents like miscarriage.

Surgery and Salvation illuminates the history of these struggles, which are dually rooted in religious paternalism and racial prejudice. Examining the historical efforts by religious, state, and medical officials to imbue surgeries with spiritualized, racialized, and politicized meanings provides additional insight into how practices and epistemologies affected—and continue to affect—women's experiences with reproduction, childbirth, and fertility control, while uncovering how women came to be blamed for perpetuating the social conditions that victimized them. In each era of this history, authorities meant for surgery to save the nation from women's rebellious, disorderly, or irrational reproductive choices. Yet, when faced with oppressive coercion over their sexual and reproductive behavior, people consistently responded by asserting their dignity and struggling for justice.

Notes

Introduction

1. Jaffary, *Reproduction and Its Discontents*, 110; On the Girl of Devil's Alley, see Rodríguez, *Memorandum de la operación cesárea*, for the quote referencing her as "the ideal patient for that day's medical lesson," see Rodríguez, page 2.

2. Arrom, *Volunteering for a Cause*; Graham Mooney, *Intrusive Interventions*.

3. Carrillo, "Nacimiento y muerte."

4. Piccato, *City of Suspects*, 226.

5. Carrillo, "La influencia de la bacteriología."

6. Canguilhem, *On the Normal*; Risse, *Mending Bodies*.

7. Weber, *Death Is All around Us*.

8. Morgan and Roberts, "Reproductive Governance," 241.

9. Goodman, McElligott, and Marks, *Useful Bodies*; Comfort, "Prisoner as Model Organism."

10. Lederer, *Subjected to Science*.

11. Many scholars of reproduction have theorized women's constrained choices in reproductive decision-making, including Necochea López, *History of Family Planning*; Lucero, *Race and Reproduction*; Kimball, *Open Secret*; López, *Matters of Choice*.

12. Cházaro, "Pariendo instrumentos médicos"; Briggs, *Reproducing Empire*; Cooper Owens, *Medical Bondage*; Rodriguez, *Female Circumcision*.

13. Ross et al., *Radical Reproductive Justice*; Gurr, *Reproductive Justice*; Combahee River Collective, *Black Feminist Statement*; Theobald, *Reproduction on the Reservation*.

14. Walsh, *Religion of Life*; Sheldon, Ragab, and Keel, *Critical Approaches to Science*.

15. Quattrocchi, *Violencia obstétrica*; one exception is Delay and Sundstrom, "Legacy of Symphysiotomy," 197–218.

16. Sesia, "Naming, framing and shaming through obstetric violence," 222–47.

17. Blundell, "Theory and Practice of Midwifery."

18. O'Brien and Rich, "Obstetric Violence."

19. Grupo de Información en Reproducción Elegida (GIRE), *La pieza faltante*, 109.

20. González-Vélez, "La producción de conocimiento experto."

21. Rodríguez, *Memorándum de la operación cesárea*.

22. Rodríguez, *Memorándum de la operación*, 6. Flores y Troncoso *Historia de la medicina*, vol. 3, 606–609; 745.

23. Gilman, *Difference and Pathology*; Lederer, *Subjected to Science*; Halpern, *Lesser Harms*; Moscucci, *Science of Woman*; Abugideiri, *Gender and the Making of Modern Medicine*; Roberts, *Killing the Black Body*; Schoen, *Choice and Coercion*; Briggs, *Reproducing Empire*.

24. Fuentes, *Dispossessed Lives*.

25. Rodríguez, *Memorandum de la operación cesárea*, 1–5.

26. Gilman, *Difference and Pathology*.

27. Moscucci, *Science of Woman*.

28. Lomnitz, *Death and the Idea of Mexico.*

29. Briggs, *How All Politics.*

30. Davis, "Obstetric Racism."

31. Cooper Owens, *Medical Bondage*; Appelbaum, Macpherson, and Rosemblatt, *Race and Nation.*

32. Roberts, *Fatal Invention.*

33. Martínez, *Genealogical Fictions.*

34. *Gaceta Médica de México* 26, no. 17 (September 1891).

35. Rosemblatt, *Science and Politics of Race.*

36. Andrade, *Acción del Somniféne*, 34–63.

37. Poole, "Image of 'Our Indian,'" 39.

38. Fields and Fields, *Racecraft.*

39. Framptom, *Belly Rippers*, 5; two important exceptions include Cházaro, "Pariendo Instrumentos Médicos"; Roberts, "Scars of Nation." Examples from the rich literature on Mexican women include the following: Socolow, *Women of Colonial Latin America*; Twinam, *Public Lives*; Molyneux and Dore, *Hidden Histories*; Olcott, *Revolutionary Women*; Lavrin, "International Feminisms."

40. Jaffary, *Reproduction and Its Discontents*, 175.

41. Suárez y López Guazo, *Eugenesia y racismo*; Urías Horcasitas, "Eugenesia y aborto."

42. Vaughan, Cano, and Olcott, *Sex in Revolution*; Vaughan, *Cultural Politics*; Rosemblatt, *Gendered Compromises*; Turda and Gillette, *Latin Eugenics*; Walsh, *Religion of Life.*

43. Briggs, "Race of Hysteria"; Schwartz, *Birthing a Slave*; Cooper Owens, *Medical Bondage.*

44. One foundational work on the Atlantic world is Morgan, "Some Could Suckle."

45. Morgan and Roberts, "Reproductive Governance"; Morgan and Roberts, "Rights and Reproduction"; Turner, *Contested Bodies*; Roth, *Miscarriage of Justice*; Fissell, *Vernacular Bodies*; Rivera Garza, "Dangerous Minds."

46. Warren, "Operation for Evangelization"; Few, Tortorici, and Warren, *Baptism through Incision*; Klaeren, "Sacred Embryology"; Few, *For all of Humanity.*

47. Castañeda López and Rodríguez de Romo, *Pioneras de la medicina mexicana*; Carrillo, *Matilde Montoya.*

48. Fissell, "Disappearance of the Patient's Narrative."

49. Hartman, "Venus in Two Acts."

50. Archivo Histórico de la Secretaría de Salubridad y Asistencia (AHSSA), Beneficiencia Pública, Establecimientos Hospitalarios, Hospital General, file 32, exp. 2, 1932: "Investigación practicada por la señora Elvia Carrillo Puerto, acerca de las irregularidades cometidas por un grupo de afanadoras de dicho establecimiento"; On Carrillo Puerto, see Olcott, "Worthy Wives and Mothers" and *Revolutionary Women*, 39–40, 205–6, 208.

51. GIRE, *La pieza faltante*, 84.

Chapter One

1. Blumenfeld-Kosinski, *Not of Woman Born.*

2. Reagan, *When Abortion Was a Crime*; Aristotle, *De Anima*; Christopoulos, *Abortion in Early Modern Italy.*

3. Lehner, *Catholic Enlightenment*, 5.

4. Blumenfeld-Kosinski, *Not of Woman Born*, 1.
5. Blumenfeld-Kosinski, *Not of Woman Born*, 2, 121–22.
6. Blumenfeld-Kosinski, *Not of Woman Born*, 145.
7. Blumenfeld-Kosinski, *Not of Woman Born*, 26.
8. Blumenfeld-Kosinski, *Not of Woman Born*, 25.
9. Blumenfeld-Kosinski, *Not of Woman Born*, 153.
10. Roth and Teixeira, "From Embryotomy to Cesarean."
11. Alcalá y Martínez, *Disertación médico-chirúrgica*.
12. Lanning, *Royal Protomedicato*.
13. Alcalá y Martínez, *Disertación médico-chirúrgica*, 5.
14. Alcalá y Martínez, *Disertación médico-chirúrgica*, 14.
15. Alcalá y Martínez, *Disertación médico-chirúrgica*, 4.
16. Alcalá y Martínez, *Disertación médico-chirúrgica*, 5.
17. Alcalá y Martínez, *Disertación médico-chirúrgica*, 12–13.
18. Alcalá y Martínez, *Disertación médico-chirúrgica*, 8.
19. Cangiamila, *Embriología sagrada*, 144.
20. Dz-Sch. 1184. Cf. also the Constitution "*Apostolicae Sedis*" of Pius IX (Acta Pii IX, V, 55–72; AAS 5 [1869], 305–331; Morgan, "Potentiality Principle"; Silva, "Potentially Human?"
21. Needham, *History of Embryology*, 204.
22. Chapter 2 discusses this in more detail.
23. Cangiamila, *Embriología sagrada*, xxiii–xxviii; Warren, "Operation for Evangelization."
24. Needham, *History of Embryology*, 2.
25. Cangiamila, *Embriología sagrada*, 99.
26. Cangiamila, *Embriología sagrada*, 99.
27. Cangiamila, *Embriología sagrada*, 223.
28. Cangiamila, *Embriología sagrada*, 227 (emphasis in original).
29. Deventer, *Observations importantes*; Needham, *History of Embryology* 205.
30. Owen, *Institutes of Canon Law*; Caffiero, *Forced Baptisms*.
31. Caffiero, *Forced Baptisms*, 205.
32. Cangiamila, *Embriología sagrada*, 56. Park, *Secrets of Women*, 261. Needham, *History of Embryology*, 19.
33. Cangiamila, 225.
34. Aristotle, *De Anima*, book 1, part 1.
35. Aristotle, *De Anima*, book 1, part 2.
36. Aristotle, *De Anima*, book 1, part 2, 75.
37. Needham, *History of Embryology*, 60.
38. Park, *Secrets of Women*, 189–90.
39. Needham, *History of Embryology*, 98; Ladislao Reti, "Two Unpublished Manuscripts."
40. Cangiamila, *Embriología sagrada*, 28.
41. Cangiamila, *Embriología sagrada*, 85.
42. Lehner, *The Catholic Enlightenment*, 85.
43. Cangiamila, *Embriología sagrada*, 27.
44. Cangiamila, *Embriología sagrada*, 106.
45. Cangiamila, *Embriología sagrada*, 140.

46. Vaan, *Etymological Dictionary*; Needham, *History of Embryology*, 105.
47. Rodríguez, *Disertaciones physico-mathematico-medicas*, 56.
48. Rodríguez, *Disertaciones physico-mathematico-medicas*, 69.
49. Medina, *Cartilla nueva útil*. Medina's *Cartilla* was published in Spain in 1750, and reprinted in Mexico in 1806.
50. Medina, *Cartilla nueva útil*, 49.
51. Medina, *Cartilla nueva útil*, 49.
52. Cangiamila, *Embriología sagrada*, 27.
53. González Laguna, *El zelo sacerdotal*, 137.
54. Lehner, *Catholic Enlightenment*; Caffiero, *Forced Baptisms*.
55. González Laguna, *El zelo sacerdotal*, 111.
56. Medina, *Cartilla nueva útil*, 49.
57. Medina, *Cartilla nueva útil*, 49.
58. Bancroft, *California Pastoral*, 87, 89, 23; Sarria, *Descripción de la operación cesárea*, trans. by Cook as "Sarria's Treatise on the Caesarean Section, 1830."
59. Cook, "Sarría's Treatise," Part I, 107.
60. Cook, "Sarría's Treatise," Part III, 250.
61. Cangiamila, *Embriología sagrada*, 76.
62. Needham, *A History of Embryology*, 172.
63. González Laguna, *El zelo sacerdotal*, 117–18; Cangiamila, *Embriología sagrada*, 75.
64. Cangiamila, *Embriología sagrada*, 80.
65. Cangiamila, *Embriología sagrada*, 88.
66. González Laguna, *El zelo sacerdotal*, 101.
67. Cangiamila, *Embriología sagrada*, 101.
68. González Laguna, *El zelo sacerdotal*, 102.
69. González Laguna, *El zelo sacerdotal*, 103.
70. González Laguna, *El zelo sacerdotal*, 104. The meaning of *pullo* in this context is unclear.
71. Lehner, *Catholic Enlightenment*, 109.
72. González Laguna, *El zelo sacerdotal*, 107.
73. González Laguna, *El zelo sacerdotal*, 108.
74. Archivo General de la Nación (AGN), *Reales Cedulas Originales*, GD 100, 1804, vol. 192, exp. 52, foja 4; *Reales Cedulas Originales*, GD 100, 1804, vol. 192, exp. 58, foja 2.
75. Ruiz Castañeda, "La tercera gazeta de la Nueva España," 137–50; Jaffary, *Reproduction and Its Discontents*, 143–45, 150, 152.
76. Castañeda, "La tercera gazeta de la Nueva España," 150; Saladino García, "José Antonio Alzate y Ramírez."
77. Villa, *El presbítero D. José Antonio Alzate Ramírez*.
78. O'Hara, *A Flock Divided*, 98.
79. *Gazeta de México* 10, no. 2 (November 11, 1799), 9.
80. Valdés, editor, *Gazeta de México* 10, no. 24 (September 22, 1800), 191–92.
81. González Laguna, *El zelo sacerdotal*, prologue.
82. Blumenfeld-Kosinski, *Not of Woman Born*, 25.
83. Cangiamila, *Embriología sagrada*, 258–59.
84. Lehner, *Catholic Enlightenment*, 89.

85. Lehner, *Catholic Enlightenment*, 86.
86. Cangiamila, *Embriología sagrada*, 21.
87. González Laguna, *El zelo sacerdotal*, 190–91.
88. Cangiamila, *Embriología sagrada*, 9.
89. Cangiamila, *Embriología sagrada*, 23.
90. Cangiamila, *Embriología sagrada*, 313.
91. Park, *Secrets of Women*, 16, 154.
92. González Laguna, *El zelo sacerdotal*, 112–13.
93. González Laguna, *El zelo sacerdotal*, 114–15.
94. González Laguna, *El zelo sacerdotal*, 114–15.

Chapter Two

1. Cangiamila, *Embriología sagrada*.
2. Keupper Valle, "Cesarean Operation"; Rigau-Pérez, "Surgery at the Service of Theology"; Reid, "Medics of the Soul."
3. Bancroft, *California Pastoral*, 89.
4. Bancroft, *California Pastoral*, 225.
5. Voekel, *Alone before God*.
6. Premo, *Children of the Father King*.
7. Taylor, *Magistrates of the Sacred*; O'Hara, *A Flock Divided*; Mazín Gómez, *Entre dos majestades*.
8. Lehner, *Catholic Enlightenment*, 36.
9. Lehner, *Catholic Enlightenment*, 35, 62.
10. O'Hara, *A Flock Divided*, 110–11.
11. Archivo General de la Nación (AGN), *Bandos*, GD 11, vol. 8, exp. 90, foja 329, March 3, 1772, "Niños nonnatos. Circular para que se les socoxxa [*sic*] por medio de la Operación caesarean quando las madres fallecen."
12. Lehner, *Catholic Enlightenment*, 36.
13. Warren, "Operation for Evangelization," 652.
14. De Demerson, "La cesarea post mortem," 210, 213–16, 218–19.
15. Cangiamila, *Embriología sagrada*, xii; xv–xx.
16. Bobb, *Viceregency of Antonio María Bucareli*, 3.
17. Rodríguez and Ursua, *La caridad del sacerdote*.
18. AGN, *Bandos*, GD 11, vol. 8, exp. 90, foja 329, March 3, 1772, "Niños nonnatos. Circular para que se les socoxxa [*sic*] por medio de la Operación caesarean quando las madres fallecen."
19. Cangiamila, *Embriología sagrada*, 32.
20. AGN, *Reales Cédulas Originales*, GD 100, 1804, vol. 192, exp. 52, foja 4.
21. Bobb, *Viceregency of Antonio María Bucareli*, 38.
22. Bobb, *Viceregency of Antonio María Bucareli*, 40.
23. Peñafort, *El Cardenal Lorenzana*, 52.
24. González Laguna, *El zelo sacerdotal*, 265–66.
25. Venegas, *Manual de párrocos*, 10.
26. AGN, *Inquisición*, Año 1775–1776, GD 61, vol. 1157, exp. 1, fojas 1–80, "El señor Inquisidor Fiscal de este Santo Oficio contra María Guadalupe Sánchez . . ."

27. AGN, *Inquisición*, Año 1707, GD 61, vol. 731, exp. SN, fojas SN 391–401, "Autos sobre un bautismo de muñecos que se celebró en el pueblo de S. Juan Del Rio"; *Inquisición*, Año 1719, GD 61, vol. 777, exp. 63, fojas 472–86, "Autos sobre unos bautismos y casamientos de muñecas efectuados en la ciudad de Zacatecas"; *Inquisición*, Año 1736, GD 61, vol. 753, exp. SN, fojas SN 582, "Certificación de los autos contra manuel de cordova, official de carpintero, y demas complices, por un bautismo de muñecos"; *Inquisición*, Año 1735, GD 61, vol. 872, exp. 27, fojas 395–404, "El Sr. Inquisidor contra Manuel de Cordova, official de carpintero y demás complices en el bautismo de ciertos muñecos"; *Policía y Empedrados*, Año 1799–1800, GD 87, vol. 8, exp. 11, fojas 162–213, "Sobre evitar desórdenes del populacho en los bautismos."

28. Taylor, *Magistrates of the Sacred*, 51–62.

29. AGN, *Inquisición*, Año 1771, GD 61, vol. 1103, exp. 46, fojas 349–52, "Carta del comisario de Guadalajara . . . sobre bautismos de los indios gentiles, en los ranchos, diciéndoles: yo te bautizo en el nombre del Gallo, y de la Gallina, etc. Guadalajara."

30. Huntington Library, HM 4267; Nentvig, *Descripción geógrafica*, 1762.

31. Peñafort, *El Cardenal Lorenzana*, 52.

32. Caffiero, *Forced Baptisms*, 222.

33. April 1, 1823, Santa Cruz Mission, Burial record 01512, Early California Population Database. I did not include the case in table 1.

34. April 8, 1809, SG, 04312, ECPD.

35. February 7, 1837, SBV, Priest Blas Ordaz, ECPD.

36. González Laguna, *El zelo sacerdotal*, 122

37. Kessell, *Friars, Soldiers, and Reformers*, 209.

38. Nentvig, *Rudo Ensayo*.

39. National Park Service, US Department of the Interior, Mission 2000 Database. "Personal Information. Surname: Sagori." http://www.nps.gov/applications/tuma/detail.cfm?Personal_ID=6781.

40. Huntington Library, HM 4267.

41. Nentvig, *Descripción geógrafica*, 1762.

42. Shelton, *For Tranquility and Order*, 43.

43. Weber, *Bárbaros*, 15.

44. Taylor, *Magistrates of the Sacred*, 50.

45. Taylor, *Magistrates of the Sacred*, 50.

46. De Chaparro and Achim, *Death and Dying*.

47. Jackson, "Durán, Fray Narciso (1776–1846)"; Sandos, *Converting California*.

48. Summers, Russell, and Sancho, *Compositor Pione*, 69.

49. *Gazeta de México* 7, no. 2 (Wednesday, January 21, 1795), 11.

50. *Diario de México*, June 6, 1807, 134.

51. "Operación Caesarea," *Diario de Mexico*, February 2, 1810, 168.

52. "Operación Caesarea," *Diario de Mexico*, February 2, 1810, 168.

53. *Gazeta de México* 20, no. 2 (November 11, 1799), 9.

54. *Periódico de la Academia de Medicina en México*, July 15, 1836, 31–32.

55. Reed, *From Soul to Mind*, 81–107.

56. Cook, "Sarría's Treatise," Part III, 250.

57. Jaffary, *Reproduction and Its Discontents*, 86.

58. *El Siglo Diez y Nueve*, June 7, 1844.
59. "Carta Pastoral," *El Siglo Diez y Nueve*, June 11, 1853, 1, 3.
60. "Carta Pastoral," *El Siglo Diez y Nueve*, June 11, 1853, 1, 3.

Chapter Three

1. *Periódico de la Academia de Medicina de Méjico* 5, no. 1 (August 1840): 20–22.
2. Jaffary, *False Mystics*, 156.
3. Archivo Histórico del Arzobispado de México (AHAM), *Religiosas*, Monday, June 10, 1861, "La R. M. Presidenta de Regina dice: que la M. Guadalupe de los cinco señores se halla enferma de ataque nerviosa, y que el facultativo la ha mandado baños Galvánicos; y pide licencia para que entre el que tiene y maneja la máquina."
4. Ríos Molina, *La locura durante la Revolución mexicana*.
5. Moscucci, *Science of Woman*, 1.
6. Ramos, *Breves consideraciones*; Vásquez, *Ligero estudio de algunos*, 24–25.
7. Hernández Sáenz, *Carving a Niche*; Gorbach, "From the uterus," 83–99.
8. Goldstein, "Hysteria Diagnosis."
9. Goldstein, "Hysteria Diagnosis," 236, 239.
10. Ramos, *Bedlam in the New World*.
11. Archivo Histórico de la Secretaría de Salubridad y Asistencia (AHSSA), Consejo Superior de Salubridad, *Guía 4 del Fondo Salubridad Pública*, coord. Javier Morales Meneses, i–ii, 29; AHSSA, SP, P, S, box 2, exp. 44, 1842, "Decreto de Luiz Gonzaga Vieyra, gobernador del Departamento de México, aprobando el Reglamento de Enseñanza y Policía Médicas"; Lanning, *Royal Protomedicato*. "Superior Sanitation Counsel" is how Claudia Agostoni translates *Consejo Superior de Salubridad* in *Monuments of Progress*.
12. AHAM, *Religiosas* [book], 1860, "La M. R. M. Abadesa del Convento de Sta. Ynes, pide licencia para que el facultativo Dn. Jose Ma. Balderas entre a curar las enfermas mientras esta fuera de México el Facultativo que tiene la iguala del Convento" (Tuesday, March 26, 1861); AHAM, *Religiosas* [book], 1861, Wednesday, March 3, 1861: "La R. M. Madera de Sta. Clara pide licencia para que pueda entrar al convento de S. José de Gracia el médico D. Manuel Juárez todas las veces que sea necesario"; and Tuesday, June 10, 1861: "La R. M. Presidenta de Regina dice: que la M. Guadalupe de los cinco snres se halla enferma de ataque nerviosa, y que el facultativo la ha mandado baños Galvánicos; y pide licencia para que entre el que tiene y maneja la máquina."
13. Lehner, *Catholic Enlightenment*, 97; Arrom, "Catholic Philanthropy," 4–5.
14. *El Cosmopolita*, December 10, 1842, 4.
15. Cosio Villegas, *Historia moderna de México*, 406; Cruz Rodríguez, "Los hospitales en la cuidad de México," 9.
16. Fajardo Ortiz, *Breve historia de los hospitales*.
17. Arrom, *Volunteering for a Cause*, 52; "Opinión," *La Unidad Católica*, May 23, 1861; "Las Hermanas de la Caridad," *La Orquesta*, April 27, 1861; "Las Hermanas de la Caridad," *La Orquesta*, June 8, 1865; "Opinión," *Voz de México*, March 12, 1874.
18. AHSSA, SP, IF, box 1, exp. 68, 1852: "Informe sobre la visita realizada al Hospital de San Pablo y las anomalías que se encontraron en la elaboración de las medicinas por las Hermanas de la Caridad"; AHSSA, SP, IF, box 2, exp. 9, 1870, "Lista de la bóticas estableci-

das en el DF"; AHSSA, SP, IF, box 2, exp 11, 1870–1871, "Responsivas de boticas, y cese de responsivas."

19. AHSSA, SP, IF, box 1, exp. 68, 1852: "Informe."

20. *La Unidad Católica*, May 23, 1861, 1.

21. Ceballos Rómulo, *El Hospital Juárez*, 26–32; Del Olmo Araiza, "Medicina en el siglo XIX México," 21–27.

22. Del Olmo Araiza, "Medicina en el siglo XIX México," 22.

23. Reyes Pavón, "Las Hermanas de la Caridad," 35.

24. Archivo Histórico del Distrito Federal, Fondo Ayuntamiento y Gobierno del Distrito: Hospitales en General, año 1861, vol. 2299, exp. 58, "Orden Suprema para que las hermanas de la caridad continuen prestando sus importantes servicios a la humanidad afligida y a la niñez desvalida bajo la inspección del supremo gobierno."

25. No. 5833, February 27, 1863. Dublán and Lozano, *Legislación Mexicana*, 9:595.

26. "Las hermanas de la caridad," *La Orquesta*, April 27, 1861, 2.

27. Marsiske, "Estudiantes universitarios y revolución."

28. Zambrana y Vázquez, *Naturaleza de la infección purulenta*.

29. Salinas y Rivera, *Moral médica*.

30. Salinas y Rivera, *Moral médica*, 15.

31. Salinas y Rivera, *Moral médica*, 15.

32. Salinas y Rivera, *Moral médica*, 16–17.

33. AHSSA, Consejo Superior de Salubridad, *Guía 4 del Fondo Salubridad Pública*, coord. Meneses, 29.

34. AHSSA, SP, SS, box 4, exp. 20, 1871, "Gobierno devuelve una comunicacion por irrespetuosa."

35. AHSSA, SP, SS, box 4, exp. 34, 1872, "Bando . . . que publica el reglamento del Consejo Superior de Salubridad."

36. AHSSA, SP, SS, box 4, exp. 4, foja 2, 1872: "Acuerdo del presidente de la República para que el consejo superior de salubridad se encargue de la administración del ramo de sanidad."

37. Biblioteca Nicolas León, *Catálogo de Tesis*.

38. AHSSA, SP, SP, SS, box 4, exp. 30, 1871, "Borrador de un acta de sesión del consejo superior de salubridad, en la que se trató la situación del Hospital de mujeres dementes y del Monasterio del Guadalupe."

39. AHSSA, SP, SP, SS, box 4, exp. 30, 1871, "Borrador de un acta de sesión . . ."

40. AHSSA, SP, SP, SS, box 4, exp. 30, 1871, "Borrador de un acta de sesión . . ."

41. AHSSA, SP, SP, SS, box 4, exp. 30, 1871, "Borrador de un acta de sesión . . ."

42. AHSSA, SP, SP, SS, box 4, exp. 30, 1871, "Borrador de un acta de sesión . . ."

43. AHSSA, SP, SP, SS, box 4, exp. 30, 1871, "Borrador de un acta de sesión . . ."

44. Salinas y Rivera, *Moral médica*, 15.

45. Ramirez, *La ovariotomia en Mexico*.

46. González Navarro, "Los Positivistas Mexicanos."

47. Warner, *Against the Spirit of System*.

48. Hale, *The Transformation of Liberalism*.

49. Reed, *From Soul to Mind*.

50. Comte, *System of Positive Polity*; Hale, *Transformation of Liberalism*, 23, 141.

51. Barreda, "De la educación moral."

52. Reed, *From Soul to Mind,* 15, 28, 81.
53. Navarro y Cardona, *Del parto prematuro,* 63.
54. Gilman, *Difference and Pathology.*
55. Moscucci, *The Science of Woman,* 4.
56. Reed, *From Soul to Mind,* 144–68.
57. Barreda, *Opúsculos discusiones y discursos,* 111.
58. AHSSA, SP, SP, SP, box 4, exp. 42, 1872, "Acuerdo del presidente de la Republica . . ."
59. Carrillo, "Control sexual"; Agostoni, *Cuidar, sanar, y educar*; Bliss, *Compromised Positions.*
60. AHSSA, SP, SP, box 4, exp. 55, 1873, "Informe . . . concerniente a hygiene publica, en los aspectos científicos y administrativos."
61. AHSSA, SP, SP, box 4, exp. 42, 1872, "El consejo niega haber dado permisos para el tratamiento de prostitutas sifilíticas en sus hogares."
62. AHSSA, SP, IAV, box 2, exp. 17, "Informe de la Inspección de Policia de sanidad . . . sobre el trabajo que realizó la inspección correspondiente a diversos meses de 1873 a 1876."
63. AHSSA, SP, IAV, box 2, exp. 17, "Informe de la Inspección de Policia de sanidad."
64. AHSSA, SP, IAV, box 2, exp. 17, "Informe de la Inspección de Policia de sanidad."
65. AHSSA, SP, IAV, box 2, exp. 17, "Informe de la Inspección de Policia de sanidad."
66. AHSSA, SP, IAV, box 2, exp. 17, "Informe de la Inspección de Policia de sanidad."
67. AHSSA, SP, IAV, box 2, exp. 17, "Informe de la Inspección de Policia de sanidad."
68. AHSSA, SP, IAV, box 2, exp. 16, "Oficio de los médicos del Hospital de San Juan de Dios comunicando que ellos no son responsables de la salida de las enfermas.
69. AHSSA, SP, IAV, box 2, exp.17, "Informe de la Inspección de Policía de sanidad."
70. "Opinión," *Voz de México,* December 5, 1874, 3.
71. "Congreso de la Unión: Sesión del día 3 de Diciembre de 1874," *El Siglo Diez y Nueve,* December 4, 1874, 2.
72. "La Colonia Española y las hermanas de la caridad," *El Monitor Republicano,* December 15, 1974, 1–2.
73. Roldán, "Periódicos Católicos Méxicanos," 85.
74. *El Siglo Diez y Nueve,* December 4, 1874, 2.
75. *Voz de Mexico,* December 10, 1874, 2.
76. "Escandalitos," *La Orquesta,* December 5, 1874, 2–3.
77. "Escandalitos," *La Orquesta,* December 5, 1874, 2–3.
78. "La sesión de anteayer," *Voz de México,* December 5, 1874, 1.
79. *La Luz de Nuevo León,* December 19, 1874, 2–3.
80. "Escandalitos," *La Orquesta,* December 5, 1874, 2–3.
81. *El Foro,* December 22, 1874.
82. *La Orquesta,* December 12, 1874, 5; Cosio Villegas, *Historia moderna de México,* 409.
83. Goldstein, "Hysteria Diagnosis," 231.

Chapter Four

1. Archivo General de la Nación en México (AGN), Indiferente Virreinal, caja 4944-001. Bienes Nacionales. Año 1794, fs. 60; Jaffary, *Reproduction and Its Discontents,* 81.
2. Navarro y Cardona, *Del parto prematuro,* 61–62.
3. Navarro y Cardona, *Del parto prematuro,* 62.

4. Witherspoon, "Reexamining Roe," 29; Smith-Rosenberg and Rosenberg, "Female Animal."

5. Reagan, *When Abortion Was a Crime.*

6. Mijangos y González, *Lawyer of the Church*; Butler, "Liberalism, Anticlericalism," 251–68.

7. Covo, *Las ideas de la reforma*; Stauffer, *Victory on Earth.*

8. Arendt, *Between Past and Future*, 69.

9. Weber, "Science as a Vocation," 139; Eliade, *Sacred and the Profane.*

10. Flores y Troncoso, *Historia de la medicina*, 568.

11. Carrillo, "Nacimiento y muerte."

12. Archivo Histórico de la Secretaría de Salubridad y Asistencia (AHSSA), Beneficencia Pública, Establecimientos Hospitalarios, Hospital de Maternidad e Infancia, leg. 2, exp. 15, 3 fol., 1880; AHSSA, Beneficiencia Pública, Establecimientos Hospitalarios, Hospital de Maternidad e Infancia, leg. 2, exp. 24, 4 fol., 1884.

13. Jaffary, *Reproduction and Its Discontents*, 33, 81.

14. Menocal, *Estudio sobre el aborto*, 19.

15. Menocal, *Estudio sobre el aborto*, 4.

16. Menocal, *Estudio sobre el aborto*, 20.

17. Although 1871 is the date of the first penal code passed in the Federal District and the territory of Baja California, this was not a federal code. Criminal law remained mainly governed by state jurisdictions in Mexico until very recently. After the Federal District passed this code, in the course of the subsequent decade individual states adapted and passed versions of it, generally making small, but sometimes quite significant, modifications. Jaffary, *Reproduction and Its Discontents*, 125; Speckman Guerra, *Del Tigre de Santa Julia.*

18. Murrieta, "Aborto y derechos reproductivos,"182.

19. Jones, *Soul of the Embryo.*

20. Navarro y Cardona, *Del parto prematuro*, 7–8.

21. Navarro y Cardona, *Del parto prematuro*, 15.

22. Navarro y Cardona, *Del parto prematuro*, 42–43.

23. Navarro y Cardona, *Del parto prematuro*, 44–45.

24. Navarro y Cardona, *Del parto prematuro*, 45–46.

25. Navarro y Cardona, *Del parto prematuro*, 47.

26. Navarro y Cardona, *Del parto prematuro*, 48.

27. Navarro y Cardona, *Del parto prematuro*, 48–49.

28. Navarro y Cardona, *Del parto prematuro*, 49.

29. Navarro y Cardona, *Del parto prematuro*, 50.

30. Navarro y Cardona, *Del parto prematuro*, 51.

31. Navarro y Cardona, *Del parto prematuro*, 51.

32. Navarro y Cardona, *Del parto prematuro*, 52–53.

33. Navarro y Cardona, *Del parto prematuro*, 54.

34. Navarro y Cardona, *Del parto prematuro*, 56.

35. Navarro y Cardona, *Del parto prematuro*, 58.

36. Navarro y Cardona, *Del parto prematuro*, 40.

37. Navarro y Cardona, *Del parto prematuro*, 62.

38. Navarro y Cardona, *Del parto prematuro*, 64.

39. Navarro y Cardona, *Del parto prematuro*, 65.
40. Navarro y Cardona, *Del parto prematuro*, 32.
41. Navarro y Cardona, *Del parto prematuro*, 35.
42. Navarro y Cardona, *Del parto prematuro*, 39.
43. Navarro y Cardona, *Del parto prematuro*, 16–17.
44. Navarro y Cardona, *Del parto prematuro*, 19.
45. Navarro y Cardona, *Del parto prematuro*, 80.
46. Navarro y Cardona, *Del parto prematuro*, 21.
47. Navarro y Cardona, *Del parto prematuro*, 15.
48. Navarro y Cardona, *Del parto prematuro*, 25.
49. Navarro y Cardona, *Del parto prematuro*, 26.
50. Navarro y Cardona, *Del parto prematuro*, 28.
51. Navarro y Cardona, *Del parto prematuro*, 14.
52. Navarro y Cardona, *Del parto prematuro*, 28.
53. Navarro y Cardona, *Del parto prematuro*, 28.

Chapter Five

1. Estrada, *La falta de hygiene infantil*, 17.
2. "Predomina en los niños Mexicanos cabeza de forma alargada," *El Imparcial*, April 29, 1911, 8.
3. Hale, *The Transformation of Liberalism*, 3.
4. Padilla Ramos, *Progreso y libertad*.
5. Bliss, *Compromised Positions*; Overmyer-Velázquez, *Visions of the Emerald City*.
6. Buffington, *Criminal and Citizen*, 35; Tenorio-Trillo, *Mexico at the World's Fairs*.
7. Hale, *Transformation of Liberalism*, 3.
8. Hale, *Transformation of Liberalism*, 25–63.
9. Buffington, *Criminal and Citizen*, 156.
10. Markowitz, "Pelvic Politics"; Kapsalis, "Mastering the Female Pelvis."
11. Barahona, "La introducción del darwinismo."
12. Estrada, *La falta de hygiene infantil*, 17.
13. San Juan, *Un caso de anomalía relativa*.
14. Rodríguez, *Breves apuntes*.
15. Rodríguez, *Breves apuntes*, 23.
16. Rodríguez, *Breves apuntes*, 6.
17. Carrillo, "Nacimiento y muerte"; Jaffary, *Reproduction and Its Discontents*, 193.
18. Jaffary, *Reproduction and Its Discontents*, 141–73.
19. Jaffary, *Reproduction and Its Discontents*, 172.
20. Jaffary, *Reproduction and Its Discontents*, 172, citing Gorbach, *El monstruo*, 153.
21. Rodríguez, *Descripción de un monstruo*, 6.
22. Rodríguez, *Descripción de un monstruo*, 25.
23. Rodríguez, *Descripción de un monstruo*, 10, 25–28.
24. Rodríguez, *Descripción de un monstruo*, 26.
25. Rodríguez, *Descripción de un monstruo*, 26.
26. Barnes, "Ernst Haeckel's Biogenetic Law (1866)."

27. Gould, *Ontogeny and Phylogeny*; Gould, *Structure of Evolutionary Theory*; Hopwood, "History of Normal Plates"; Renard, "Problem of the Organic Individual."
28. Weikart, "Progress through Racial Extermination."
29. Gorbach, "Mujeres, Monstruos e Impresiones."
30. Rodríguez, *Descripción de un monstruo*, 25–26. Needham, *History of Embryology*, 204.
31. Rodríguez, *Descripción de un monstruo*, 25.
32. Rodríguez, *Descripción de un monstruo*, 25.
33. Rodríguez, *Descripción de un monstruo*, 28.
34. Esparza, *Breves consideraciones*, 13.
35. Flores, *Ligeros apuntes*.
36. Flores, *Ligeros apuntes*, 10–11.
37. Flores, *Ligeros apuntes*, 10.
38. Flores, *Ligeros apuntes*, 37–38.
39. Flores, *Ligeros apuntes*, 46.
40. Flores y Troncoso, *Historia de la medicina*, 803.
41. Flores, *Ligeros apuntes*, 39.
42. Flores y Troncoso, *Historia de la medicina*, 745.
43. Flores y Troncoso, *Historia de la medicina*, 745.
44. Flores y Troncoso, *Historia de la medicina*, 745.
45. Sánchez Gómez, *Breve estudio sobre la pelvis*, 14.
46. Sánchez Gómez, *Breve estudio sobre la pelvis*, 15.
47. Duque de Estrada, *Contribución al estudio*; Duque de Estrada, *Procedimiento fácil y rápido*.
48. Duque de Estrada, *Contribución al estudio*, 15, 26.
49. Reza, *Acción fisiológica del cuernecillo del centeno*.
50. Stepan, *Hour of Eugenics*.
51. Urías Horcasitas, "El determinismo biológico"; Barahona, "La introducción del darwinismo."
52. McPherson, "Positivism and Religion."
53. Ruiz S., *La herencia en sus aplicaciones*, 6.
54. Ruiz S., *La herencia en sus aplicaciones*, 9.
55. Ruiz S., *La Herencia en sus aplicaciones*, 12.
56. Ruiz S., *La herencia en sus aplicaciones*, 13.
57. Ruiz S., *La herencia en sus aplicaciones*, 10.
58. Ruiz S., *La herencia en sus aplicaciones*, 16.
59. Ruiz S., *La herencia en sus aplicaciones*, 27, 29.
60. Ruiz S., *La herencia en sus aplicaciones*, 20.
61. Ruiz S., *La herencia en sus aplicaciones*, 17–18.
62. Ruiz S., *La herencia en sus aplicaciones*, 18.
63. Orozco, *Comparación de la terapéutica*.
64. Orozco, *Comparación de la terapéutica*, 10.
65. Orozco, *Comparación de la terapéutica*, 29.
66. Orozco, *Comparación de la terapéutica*, 17
67. Orozco, *Comparación de la terapéutica*, 18.
68. Orozco, *Comparación de la terapéutica*, 19.

69. Orozco, *Comparación de la terapéutica*, 30.
70. Orozco, *Comparación de la terapéutica*, 34.
71. Flores, *Educación del médico*.
72. Flores, *Educación del médico*.
73. Flores, *Educación del médico*, 70.
74. Flores, *Educación del médico*, 29.
75. Flores, *Educación del médico*, 65.
76. Flores, *Educación del médico*, 132.
77. Flores, *Educación del médico*, 63.
78. Hankins, *Science and the Enlightenment*, 127–28.
79. Flores, *Educación del médico*, 100.
80. Flores, *Educación del médico*, 28.
81. Flores, *Educación del médico*, 189.
82. Flores, *Educación del médico*, 151.
83. Vyas et al., "Challenging the Use of Race."

Chapter Six

1. Archivo Histórico de la Secretaría de Salubridad y Asistencia (AHSSA), BP, EH, HM, file 2, exp. 18, 1891, "Se queja el director por el crecido numero de enfermas que remite la inspeccion sanitaria."
2. AHSSA, BP, EH, HM, file 2, exp. 31, 1892.
3. Briggs, *Reproducing Empire*.
4. AHSSA, BP, EH, HM, file 2, exp. 31, August 17, 1892.
5. Buffington, *Criminal and Citizen*, 35–36.
6. Cházaro, "Pariendo instrumentos médicos"; Rivera Garza, "Dangerous Minds"; Urías Horcasitas, "El determinismo biológico."
7. Carrillo, "Control sexual para el control social."
8. Gamboa, *Santa*, 106.
9. Gamboa, *Santa*, 106.
10. Montenegro, *Breves apuntes*, 15.
11. Montenegro, *Breves apuntes*, 15.
12. Jaffary, *Reproduction and Its Discontents*, chapter 1.
13. Overmeyer-Velázquez, *Visions of the Emerald City*; Drinot, *Historia de la prostitución*; Bliss, *Compromised Positions*; French and Bliss, *Gender, Sexuality, and Power*; Guy, *Sex and Danger*.
14. Tercero, *Breve consideraciones*; Casillas, *Tratamiento*; Zambrana y Vázquez, "Naturaleza de la infección."
15. AHSSA, BP, EH, HM, file 2, exp. 1, 1882, "Estado que manifiesta el movimiento de enfermos habidos en el expresado, del 1 al 28 del presente mes de febrero 1882"; AHSSA, BP, EH, HM, file 2, exp. 2, 1882, showed similar numbers.
16. AHSSA, BP, EH, HM, file 1, exp. 28, 1881, "Inspección de Sanidad—pide pagar .10c por estancia, por las enfermas que remita como depositadas."
17. AHSSA, BP, EH, HM, file 1, exp. 30, 1881, "Instrumentos—Los pide el señor Dr. San Juan para la sala Ortega que es a su cargo"; AHSSA, BP, EH, HM, file 2, exp. 5, 1882.

18. Horn, *Criminal Body*; Mooney, *Intrusive Interventions.*

19. Montenegro, *Breves apuntes.*

20. Montenegro, *Breves apuntes*, 20.

21. Montenegro, *Breves apuntes*, 16.

22. Montenegro, *Breves apuntes*, 20, 28.

23. Montenegro, *Breves apuntes*, 20.

24. Montenegro, *Breves apuntes*, 27–28.

25. Montenegro, *Breves apuntes*, 31.

26. AHSSA, BP, EH, HM, file 1, exp. 29, 1881; AHSSA, BP, EH, HM, file 1, exp. 30, 1881; AHSSA, BP, EH, HM, file 1, exp. 38, 1881, "Inventorio General."

27. AHSSA, BP, EH, HM, file 2, exp. 18, 1891, "Se queja el director por el crecido numero de enfermas que remite la inspeccion sanitaria."

28. AHSSA, BP, EH, HM, file 2, exp. 18, 1891, "Se queja el director por el crecido numero de enfermas que remite la inspeccion sanitaria."

29. AHSSA, BP, EH, HM, file 2, exp. 18, 1891, "Se queja el director por el crecido numero de enfermas que remite la inspeccion sanitaria."

30. AHSSA, BP, EH, HM, file 2, exp. 20, 1891, "Documentos del fin del mes."

31. AHSSA, BP, EH, HM, file 2, exp. 28, 1891, "Se queja el director por la escasez de algunos artículos de alimentación."

32. AHSSA, BP, EH, HM, file 2, exp. 31, 1892.

33. AHSSA, BP, EH, HM, file 2, exp. 31, 1892.

34. AHSSA, BP, EH, HM, file 2, exp. 31, 1892.

35. AHSSA, BP, EH, HM, file 2, exp. 34, 1893, "Reglamento del Hospital Morelos."

36. AHSSA, BP, EH, HM, file 2, exp. 34, 1893, "Reglamento del Hospital Morelos."

37. AHSSA, BP, EH, HM, file 2, exp. 37, 1893, "Queja del director, por la gente extraña que acude a la fotográfica privada que existe en el hospital"; Overmeyer-Velázquez, *Visions of the Emerald City.*

38. AHSSA, BP, EH, HM, file 2, exp. 36, 1893, "Donativos hechos al establecimiento."

39. AHSSA, BP, EH, HM, file 3, exp. 22, 1897, "Hospital Morelos, Clínica Ginecológica."

40. AHSSA, BP, EH, HM, file 4, exp. 6, 1900, "Movimiento de enfermos habido en dicho establecimiento durante el año de 1900"; AHSSA, BP, EH, HM, file 4, exp. 13, 1901, "Movimiento de enfermos habido en dicho establecimiento durante el año de 1900."

41. AHSSA, BP, EH, HM, file 3, exp. 36, 1899, "Hospital Morelos: Pide el Director que modifique el tipo alimenticio."

42. AHSSA, BP, EH, HM, file 4, exp. 21, 1902, "Consulta sobre aumenta de cien camas"; AHSSA, BP, EH, HM, file 4, exp. 55, 1903, "Documentos del fin de mes."

43. AHSSA, BP, EH, HM, file 4, exp. 25, 1902, "Informe acerca de un artículo publicado por 'El Popular.'"

44. AHSSA, BP, EH, HM, file 4, exp. 20, 1902, "Sobre mejoras del servicios relacionados con la Inspeccion de Sanidad."

45. AHSSA, BP, EH, HM, file 4, exp. 58, 1903, "Pedidos de medicinas."

46. Cházaro, "Pariendo instrumentos médicos," 33; Carrillo, "Nacimiento y muerte de una profesión," 176.

47. Cházaro, "Pariendo instrumentos médicos," 33.

48. Torres Ansorena, *Inconvenientes y peligros.*

49. "Ginecología: La Suspensión Uterina," *Gaceta de la Academia de Medicina* 21, no. 26 (March 31, 1886): 239–45.
50. Fuertes, *Cuatro laparotomías*, 20.
51. Barreiro, *Oportunidad en la aplicación*.
52. Hale, *Transformation of Liberalism*, 24.
53. Barreiro, *Oportunidad en la aplicación*, 10, 14.
54. Barreiro, *Oportunidad en la aplicación*, 8; Carrillo, "Nacimiento y muerte," 183.
55. Carrillo, "Nacimiento y muerte."
56. Barreiro, *Oportunidad en la aplicación*, 15.
57. Barreiro, *Oportunidad en la aplicación*, 22 (emphasis in original).
58. Barreiro, *Oportunidad en la aplicación*, 42.
59. López Hermosa, *Anomalías de las fuerzas*, 4.
60. López Hermosa, *Anomalías de las fuerzas*, 9.
61. López Hermosa, *Anomalías de las fuerzas*, 19.
62. Jaffary, *Reproduction and Its Discontents*, 179.
63. López Hermosa, *Anomalías de las fuerzas*, 15.
64. López Hermosa, *Anomalías de las fuerzas*, 22.
65. López Hermosa, *Anomalías de las fuerzas*, 23.
66. Páez, "Breve estudio."
67. Winter, *Mesmerized*, 166.
68. Páez, "Breve estudio," 24.
69. Páez, "Breve estudio," 24.
70. Páez, "Breve estudio," 21.
71. Páez, "Breve estudio," 13.
72. Páez, "Breve estudio," 14.
73. Páez, "Breve estudio," 14.
74. Páez, "Breve estudio," 14.
75. Páez, "Breve estudio," 14.
76. Rich, "Curse of Civilised Woman," 59–60.
77. Páez, "Breve estudio," 14.
78. "We Bawl So We are Heard."
79. Páez, "Breve estudio," 14.
80. Páez, "Breve estudio," 14.
81. Rich, "Curse of Civilised Woman," 68–71; Briggs, "Race of Hysteria."
82. Páez, "Breve estudio," 9, 15.
83. Páez, "Breve estudio," 29, 25.
84. Páez, "Breve estudio," 30–31.
85. Feliberto, *Breve estudio*.
86. Feliberto, *Breve estudio*, 12–13.
87. Jaffary, *Reproduction and Its Discontents*, 200–201.
88. Márquez, *Algunos datos de estadística obstétrica*.
89. Leal, *Taponamiento vaginal*.
90. Leal, *Taponamiento vaginal*, 13–15.
91. Zárraga, *Brevisimas reflexiones*.
92. Zárraga, *Brevisimas reflexiones*, 9.

93. Zárraga, *Brevisimas reflexiones*, 9–10.
94. Zárraga, *Brevisimas reflexiones*, 13.
95. Zárraga, *Brevisimas reflexiones*, 16.
96. Blundell, "Lectures on the theory and practice of midwifery."
97. Zárraga, *Brevisimas reflexiones*, 30.
98. Zárraga, *Brevisimas reflexiones*, 30.
99. Fuertes, *Cuatro laparotomías.*
100. Fuertes, *Cuatro laparotomias*, 7–8.
101. Fuertes, *Cuatro laparotomias*, 6.
102. Fuertes, *Cuatro laparotomias*, 6.
103. Fuertes, *Cuatro laparotomias*, 7.
104. Ruíz Erdozain, *La responsabilidad médica.*
105. Ruíz Erdozain, *La responsabilidad médica*, 13.
106. Ruíz Erdozain, *La responsabilidad médica*, 13.
107. Ruíz Erdozain, *La responsabilidad médica*, 14.
108. Ruíz Erdozain, *La responsabilidad médica*, 29.
109. Ruíz Erdozain, *La responsabilidad médica*, 41, 50.
110. Ruíz Erdozain, *La responsabilidad médica*, 44.
111. Ruíz Erdozain, *La responsabilidad médica*, 51.
112. "Una calumnia, deshecha," *Revista Católica*, August 24, 1890, 7.
113. Ibañez, *Someras reflexiones.*
114. Ibañez, *Someras reflexiones*, 18.
115. Ibañez, *Someras reflexiones*, 33.
116. Ibañez, *Someras reflexiones*, 11.
117. Ibañez, *Someras reflexiones*, 11.
118. Buffington, *Criminal and Citizen*, 35.
119. Hale, *Transformation of Liberalism*, 30.

Chapter Seven

1. Liceaga and Guayol, "Proyecto de Hospital General," 1.
2. Archivo Histórico de la Secretaría de Salubridad y Asistencia (AHSSA), *Guia 3 de Beneficiencia Pública*, page iii.
3. AHSSA, BP, EH, HJ, file 20, exp. 5, 1933–34, "Reportes de inspección al Hospital y noticias de operaciones quirúrgicas en dicho establecimento"; AHSSA, BP, EH, HJ, file 15, exp. 9, 1928, "Queja por muerte de una parturienta"; "AHSSA, BP, EH, HG, file 28, exp. 6, 1931, "Partes diarios de ingresos de asilados"; AHSSA, BP, EH, HG, file 28, exp. 7, 1931, "Impresos de la sala de maternidad del Hospital General"; AHSSA, BP, EH, HG, file 33, exp. 2, 1933, "Quejas presentadas por asilados del Hospital General"; AHSSA, BP, EH, HG, file 32, exp. 6, 1933, "Partes diarios" (360 pages); AHSSA, BP, EH, HG, file 32, exp. 7, 1933, "Informe de visita practicada en el Hospital General"; AHSSA, BP, EH, HG, file 32, exp. 4, 1933, "Generalidades de quejas presentadas por los enfermos"; AHSSA, BP, EH, HG, file 33, exp. 3, 1933, "Reducción de plazas: se reduce a 1200 el número de enfermos que debe haber en el Hospital General"; AHSSA, BP, EH, HG, file 32, exp. 6, 1933, "Partes diarios del mov-

imiento de enfermos asilados en el Hospital General, correspondiente al presente año"; AHSSA, BP, EH, HG, file 35, exp. 3, 1934, "Que se corrijan las irregularidades: se dispone que sean retirados de las puertas del Hospital General los enfermos que esperan se les admitan"; "Hay graves irregularidades en la Beneficencia," *El Excelsior*, September 21, 1932.

4. Molyneux and Dore, *Hidden Histories of Gender*.

5. Kourí, "Interpreting the Expropriation"; Knight, "Racism, Revolution, and Indigenismo."

6. Rojas Domínguez, "Esterilización humana."

7. Novak et al, "Disproportionate sterilization."

8. Stern, "'The Hour of Eugenics' in Veracruz"; Turda and Gillette, *Latin Eugenics*.

9. Rosemblatt, *Science and Politics of Race*, 4.

10. Turda, *Latin Eugenics in Comparative Perspective*. Suárez, *Eugenesia y Racismo*.

11. Walsh, "Executioner's Shadow."

12. Ramírez, *Esterilización temporal*, 17.

13. Rosemblatt, "Bodies, Environments, and Race."

14. Ramírez, *Esterilización temporal*, 68; AHSSA, SP, SJ, caja 18, leg. 7, 1929–31, "Informe de la investigación realizada al doctor Gutierrez Vásquez, delegado sanitario en Ixtacalco."

15. Carrillo, "Tres problemas Mexicanos de eugenesia," 2.

16. Carrillo, "Tres problemas Mexicanos de eugenesia," 6.

17. Carrillo, "Tres problemas Mexicanos de eugenesia," 6.

18. Carrillo, "Tres problemas Mexicanos de eugenesia," 2.

19. Carrillo, "Tres problemas Mexicanos de eugenesia," 15.

20. Carrillo, "Tres problemas Mexicanos de eugenesia," 14.

21. AHSSA, BP, EH, HJ, file 15, exp. 1, 1926–27, "Relación de tipos de operaciones practicadas, del 8 de Febrero de 1926, al 31 de Enero de 1927." On comparative cesarean rates in the United States, see Wolf, *Cesarean Section*.

22. Ortega Fuentes, "Dieciséis meses de observaciones."

23. Romo Ruíz, "Anotaciones acerca," 57.

24. Sordo Noriega, *Estudios obstétricos*; Flores y Troncoso, *Historia de la medicina*.

25. Duque de Estrada, *Pelviología mexicana*.

26. Souza Vásquez, "Contribución al tratamiento de la fiebre puerperal," 62.

27. Trangay, "La maternidad consciente," 12.

28. AHSSA, BP, EH, HG, file 28, exp. 7, 1931, "Impresos de la sala de maternidad del Hospital General."

29. Mejía Schroeder, *De la esterilidad femenina*, 25.

30. Mejía Schroeder, *De la esterilidad femenina*, 25.

31. Figueroa Ortíz, *La estenosis del diametro bisisquiatico*, 11.

32. García Rodríguez, *Diagnóstico de las estrechez pélvica*.

33. García Rodríguez, *Diagnóstico de las estrechez pélvica*, 19.

34. García Rodríguez, *Diagnóstico de las estrechez pélvica*, 18.

35. García Rodríguez, *Diagnóstico de las estrechez pélvica*, 66.

36. García Rodríguez, *Diagnóstico de las estrechez pélvica*, 35.

37. García Rodríguez, *Diagnóstico de las estrechez pélvica*, 50–51; Torres Septién, "Un nuevo método," 17.

38. Trangay, “La maternidad consciente,” 44.
39. Trangay, “La maternidad consciente,” 9.
40. Trangay, “La maternidad consciente,” 8.
41. Trangay, “La maternidad consciente,” 33.
42. Trangay, “La maternidad consciente,” 76.
43. Trangay, “La maternidad consciente,” 68.
44. Trangay, “La maternidad consciente,” 72.
45. Trangay, “La maternidad consciente,” 16.
46. Trangay, “La maternidad consciente,” 32.
47. Trangay, “La maternidad consciente,” 47.
48. Trangay, “La maternidad consciente,” 24.
49. Trangay, “La maternidad consciente.” Other medical students who reported having sterilized women for eugenic reasons include Torijano y Ritchie, “La ética professional”; Ruíz Culebro, “El problema médico-social”; Rojas Domínguez, “Esterilización humana”; Garza García, *La evolución del hombre*; Navarro Origel, “Orientación en el campo mental”; Figueroa Ortíz, *La estenosis del diámetro bisisquiático*; García Rodríguez, *Diagnóstico de las estreches pélvicas*; Mejía Schroeder, *De la esterilidad femenina*; Pérez, *La propedéutica obstétrica*; Piñeiro Romero, *Escuelas post-operatorias*; Ortega Márquez, *Las técnicas en la histerectomía*; Jolly Hernández, *La retroversión uterina*; Rosales Miranda, “El tratamiento quirúrgico”; Palomino Rojas, “Histerectomía total o subtotal”; Barrón, *Estudió critico*; Caviedes, *Los rayos rubens o infra-rojos*.
50. Trangay, “La maternidad consciente,” 24.
51. Trangay, “La maternidad consciente,” 55–56.
52. Trangay, “La maternidad consciente,” 56.
53. Trangay, “La maternidad consciente,” 24.
54. Vilchis Vilchis, “Consideraciones acerca,” 1933.
55. Trangay, “La maternidad consciente,” 54.
56. Trangay, “La maternidad consciente,” 22.
57. Trangay, “La maternidad consciente,” 53.
58. Trangay, “La maternidad consciente,” 51.
59. Trangay, “La maternidad consciente,” 6.
60. Trangay, “La maternidad consciente,” 28.
61. Trangay, “La maternidad consciente,” 16.
62. Trangay, “La maternidad consciente,” 10.
63. Trangay, “La maternidad consciente,” 41.
64. Blum, *Domestic Economies*, 30.
65. Trangay, “La maternidad consciente,” 6.
66. Trangay, “La maternidad consciente,” 41.
67. Birn, *Marriage of Convenience*, 175.
68. Walsh, “Restoring the Chilean Race”; Rosemblatt, *Science and Politics of Race*; Stern, “The Hour of Eugenics”; Stern, “Responsible Mothers”; Suárez y López Guazo, *Eugenesia y racismo*; Schell, “Eugenics Policy a Practice”; Granados, “¿Quiénes deben procrear?”; Ríos Molina, “Dictating the Suitable Way of Life”; Turda and Gillette, *Latin Eugenics*.
69. Peckham, “Influence of Age and Race”; Harris, “Pregnancy and Labor.”

Chapter Eight

1. Carrillo, "Los modernos minotauro y Teseo."
2. Ramírez Elliot, "Esterilización temporal femenina," 17.
3. Ramírez Elliot, "Esterilización temporal femenina," 40.
4. Ramírez Elliot, "Esterilización temporal femenina," 44.
5. Stepan, *The Hour of Eugenics*, 102–34; Rodriguez, "A Complex Fabric."
6. Rosemblatt, *Gendered Compromises*; Rosemblatt, "What We Can Reclaim"; Walsh, *Religion of Life.*
7. De la Garza Cárdenas, *La mortalidad de las heridas de vientre*; Ramírez, *Traumatología de vientre.*
8. Ramírez Elliot, "Esterilización temporal femenina," frontmatter (no page).
9. Ramírez Elliot, "Esterilización temporal femenina," 23.
10. Ramírez Elliot, "Esterilización temporal femenina," 20.
11. Ramírez Elliot, "Esterilización temporal femenina," 18.
12. Bliss, *Compromised Positions*; French and Bliss, *Gender, Sexuality, and Power*; Mitchell and Schell, *Women's Revolution*; Bliss, "Science of Redemption"; Sonn, "Your Body Is Yours."
13. Islas Hernández, "Aborto no terapéutico," 42.
14. Ramírez Elliot, "Esterilización temporal femenina," 46, 24.
15. Ramírez Elliot, "Esterilización temporal femenina," 16.
16. Souza, *Contribución al tratamiento*, 62.
17. Ramírez Elliot, "Esterilización temporal femenina," 24.
18. Handren, *No Longer Two*; Brind'Amour, "*Casti Connubii* (1930)"; Pius XI, *Carta Encíclica Casti Connubii.*
19. Needham, *History of Embryology*.
20. *Gaceta Oficial del Arzobispado de México, Publicación Mensual* 25, no. 3 (March 1931), no. 4 (April 1931), and no. 5 (May 1931).
21. "Primera carta pastoral del Ilmo. Y Rvmo. Sr. Arzobispado de México, Dr. Don Pascual Díaz," *Gaceta Oficial del Arzobispado de México*, March 1931, 124–25.
22. "Carta Enciclica de S.S.Pio XI Sobre el Matrimonio Cristiano," in the *Gaceta Oficial del Arzobispado de México*, March 1931, "Sobre el matrimonio Cristiana atendidas las actuales circunstancias, necesidades, errors y vicios de la familia y de la sociedad," 131–35.
23. "Primera carta pastoral," 127.
24. "Primera carta pastoral," 127.
25. "Primera carta pastoral," 237.
26. Brind'Amour, "*Casti Connubii* (1930)."
27. "Carta Enciclica de S.S.Pio XI Sobre el Matrimonio Cristiano," 239.
28. "Carta Enciclica de S.S.Pio XI Sobre el Matrimonio Cristiano," 238.
29. "Carta Enciclica de S.S.Pio XI Sobre el Matrimonio Cristiano," 240.
30. "Carta Enciclica de S.S.Pio XI Sobre el Matrimonio Cristiano," 240.
31. "Carta Enciclica de S.S.Pio XI Sobre el Matrimonio Cristiano," 239–40.
32. Ramírez Elliot, "Esterilización temporal femenina," 22–24.
33. Trangay, *La maternidad consciente*, 33.
34. Trangay, *La maternidad consciente*, 4.

35. Trangay, *La maternidad consciente*, 50. Capital "M" on "Morality" in the original, 47.
36. Trangay, *La maternidad consciente*, 15.
37. Trangay, *La maternidad consciente*, 5.
38. Archivo Histórico de la Secretaría de Salubridad y Asistencia (AHSSA), BP, EH, HG, file 27, exp. 3, 1928, "Reglamento interior del establecimiento: Reglamento del Hospital General."
39. AHSSA, BP, EH, HG, file 35, exp. 8, 1934, "Visitas de inspección."
40. Trangay, *La maternidad consciente*, 27.
41. Trangay, *La maternidad consciente*, 19.
42. Trangay, *La maternidad consciente*, 43–44.
43. Trangay, *La maternidad consciente*, 44.
44. Trangay, *La maternidad consciente*, 70–71.
45. Trangay, *La maternidad consciente*, 44.
46. Sonn, "Your Body Is Yours"; Ortiz Rangel, "Feminismo y eugenesia."
47. Trangay, *La maternidad consciente*, 19.
48. Hershfield, *Imagining la Chica Moderna*.
49. Feijóo Peñas, "Intersexualidad y diferenciación sexual," 42.
50. Vaughan, Cano, and Olcott, *Sex in Revolution*, 209–10, 242–69; Olcott, "Worthy Wives and Mothers."
51. Crespo Reyes and Fuentes, "Bodies and Souls"; Sanders, "Women, Sex, and the 1950s."
52. Molyneux and Dore, *Hidden Histories of Gender*, 52.
53. Dutra, "Abortion and Leunbach's Paste."
54. Trangay, *La maternidad consciente*, 19.
55. Trangay, *La maternidad consciente*, 23.

Chapter Nine

1. Archivo Histórico de la Secretaría de Salubridad y Asistencia (AHSSA), Salubridad Publica, Secretaria de Justicia, 22, 12, 1930–31, Folleto impreso titulado "Acusación contra el doctor Gabriel M. Malda, exjefe del Departamento de Salubridad." Unfortunately, the newspaper clipping does not include what publication it comes from. The report was dated February 21, 1931, under the title "El Penoso incidente se ha visto mezclado el Dr. Gabriel Malda."
2. Bliss, *Compromised Positions*, 1–2; Rivera Garza, "She Neither Respected nor Obeyed," 655.
3. "Operaciones criminales en el Hospital General," *La Prensa*, November 6, 1933. AHSSA, BP, EH, HG, file 33, exp. 8.
4. "Operaciones criminales en el Hospital General," *La Prensa*, November 6, 1933. AHSSA, BP, EH, HG, file 33, exp. 8.
5. "Operaciones criminales en el Hospital General," *La Prensa*, November 6, 1933. AHSSA, BP, EH, HG, file 33, exp. 8.
6. "Operaciones criminales en el Hospital General," *La Prensa*, November 6, 1933. AHSSA, BP, EH, HG, file 33, exp. 8.
7. Wolf, *Cesarean Section*, 53.
8. Casis Sacre, "Salpingitis: oportunidad operatoria," 16.
9. Casis Sacre, "Salpingitis: oportunidad operatoria," 16.

10. AHSSA, BP, EH, HJ, file 20, exp. 5, 1933–34, "Reportes de inspección al Hospital y noticias de operaciones quirúrgicas en dicho establecimento"; AHSSA, BP, EH, HJ, file 15, exp. 9, 1928, "Queja por muerte de una parturienta"; *El Excelsior*, September 21, 1932, "Hay graves irregularidades en la Beneficencia"; AHSSA, BP, EH, Hospital General (HG), file 28, exp. 6, 1931, "Partes diarios de ingresos de asilados"; AHSSA, BP, EH, HG, file 28, exp. 7, 1931, "Impresos de la sala de maternidad del Hospital General"; AHSSA, BP, EH, HG, file 33, exp. 2, 1933, "Quejas presentadas por asilados del Hospital General"; AHSSA, BP, EH, HG, file 32, exp. 6, 1933, Partes diarios (360 pages); AHSSA, BP, EH, HG, file 32, exp. 7, 1933, "Informe de visita practicada en el Hospital General"; AHSSA, BP, EH, HG, file 32, exp. 4, 1933, "Generalidades de quejas presentadas por los enfermos"; AHSSA, BP, EH, HG, file 33, exp. 3, 1933, "Reducción de plazas: se reduce a 1200 el número de enfermos que debe haber en el Hospital General"; AHSSA, BP, EH, HG, file 32, exp. 6, 1933, "Partes diarios del movimiento de enfermos asilados en el Hospital General, correspondiente al presente año"; AHSSA, BP, EH, HG, file 35, exp. 3, 1934, "Que se corrijan las irregularidades: se dispone que sean retirados de las puertas del Hospital General los enfermos que esperan se les admitan."

11. AHSSA, BP, EH, HJ, file 15, exp. 1, 1926–27, "Relación de tipos de operaciones practicadas, del 8 de Febrero de 1926, al 31 de Enero de 1927."

12. AHSSA, BP, EH, HG, file 37, exp. 2, 1935, "Enfermedades, estadística de."

13. This analysis is based on birth rates from 1922 through 1930. AHSSA, SP, SJ, 44, 25, 1935, "Expediente relativo a certificados prenupciales. Estadísticas de la natalidad de hijos legítimos e ilegítimos en la República, de 1922 a 1930." They were as follows: 1922: 5,625 legitimate/6,730 illegitimate; 1923: 6,252 /7,643; 1924: 6,763 /7,132; 1925: 6,747 /6,429; 1926: 8,433 /6,438; 1927: 7,597 /5,433.

14. AHSSA, BP; EH; HG; 11; 5, 1914, "Estado de Enfermos"; AHSSA, SP, SJ, 16, 17, 1929, "Expediente relativo a la nota publicada en el periódico *Excelsior* sobre la detención de una mujer dedicada a la prostitución. Contiene informe del inspector de sanidad y recortes del periódico." See also "Una mujer golpeada por un inspector de sanidad: el mal agente, en connivencia con un Chofer, Armó un fuerte escándalo," *El Excelsior*, February 3, 1929; "Acusan de Secuestro a un inspector de sanidad," *El Excelsior de la Tarde*, February 4, 1929.

15. AHSSA, SP, SJ, 30, 12, 1932, "Reglamento de la Policía Sanitaria, Publicado en el Diario Oficial de 31 de Octubre de 1932."

16. From the Jefe de Agentes, Jorge González, on March 11, 1932. Numbers are from 1924 and 1925, respectively: Mujeres inscritas 457 and 1,647; Mujeres prófugas aprehendidas 4,193 and 5,378; Mujeres presentadas por los agentes 1,913 and 4,551.

17. AHSSA, BP, EH, HG, file 37, exp. 2, 1935, "Enfermedades, estadística de."

18. AHSSA, BP, EH, HG, file 39, exp. 1, 1936: "Partes diarios de defunciones de adultos." AHSSA, BP, EH, HJ, file 22, exp. 5, 1935–36: Defunciones en la sala de maternidad, correspondientes al año de 1935. The numbers were as follows: January, 65; February, 45; March, 58; April, 31; May, 101; June, 101; July, 26; August, 23; September, 3; October, 1; November, 192; and December, 196.

19. AHSSA, BP, EH, HG, file 40, exp. 1, 1936, "Partes Diarios de defunciones de niños."

20. AHSSA, BP, EH, HG, file 40, exp. 1, 1936, "Partes Diarios de defunciones de niños."

21. AHSSA, BP, EH, HG, file 40, exp. 1, 1936, "Partes Diarios de defunciones de niños."

22. "Renunciaron en Masa," *El Universal Gráfico*, August 5, 1932.

23. I took samples of 100 patients from each set of mortality rate charts in the following folders in AHSSA: BP, EH, HG, file 37, exp. 3, 1935, "Mortalidad del Hospital General correspondiente al mes de enero del presente año"; BP, EH, HG, file 37, exp. 5, 1935, "Informes de estadística de defunciones registradas en el hospital"; BP, EH, HG, file 37, exp. 7, 1935, "Relativo a las anamolías en admisiones que existen en el Departamento de illionn del Hospital General"; BP, EH, HG, file 39, exp. 1, 1936, "Partes diarios de defunciones de adultos"; BP, EH, HG, file 39, exp. 3, 1936, "Partes diarios de los ingresos de asilados por primera vez"; BP, EH, HG, file 39, exp. 3, 1936; "Partes diarios de los ingresos de asilados por primera vez"; BP, EH, HG, file 40, exp. 1, 1936, "Partes Diarios de defunciones de niños"; BP, EH, HG, file 40, exp. 2, 1936, "Partes diarios de las defunciones, correspondientes al año de 1936"; BP, EH, HJ, file 22, exp. 3, 1934, "Queja sobre maltrato de enfermos"; BP, EH, HJ, file 22, exp. 5, 1935–1936, "Defunciones en la sala de maternidad, correspondientes al año de 1935."

24. These statistics about the services offered by the Beneficencia Pública are available in "El Estado y la Caridad," *El Mundo*, August 7, 1933.

25. AHSSA, BP, EH, HG, file 27, exp. 3, 1928, "Reglamento interior del establecimiento: Reglamento del Hospital General."

26. AHSSA, BP, EH, HG, file 27, exp. 14, 1929, "Reclamación presentada por la señora Maria Teodosio, que estuvo internada en el Pabellón número 30, referente a que le fue cambiado el niño que dió a luz, por una niña."

27. AHSSA, BP, EH, HJ, file 22, exp. 3, 1934, "Queja sobre maltrato de enfermos."

28. "Es bastante facil para los reos escaparse del Hospital Juárez," *El Excelsior*, August 17, 1932; "Ninguna Seguridad en el Hospital Juárez," *El Excelsior*, August 19, 1932.

29. "Se arroja desde un balcón de Hospital Juárez," *El Gráfico*, October 15, 1932.

30. AHSSA, BP, EH, C3, file 21, exp. 1, 1935, "Queja presentada contra el personal del consultorio." María Álvarez filed this complaint with the director of the Beneficencia Pública.

31. AHSSA, BP, EH, HG, file 32, exp. 7, 1933, "Informe de visita practicada en el Hospital General"; complaints about nurses: AHSSA, BP, EH, HG, file 27, exp. 11, 1929, "Acusaciones en contra de las enfermeras del Hospital y artículos publicados en la prensa que se relacionan con el Establecimiento."

32. AHSSA, BP, EH, HM, file 18, exp. 12, 1916–18, "Asuntos diversos de asilados correspondientes al año fiscal de 1916 a 1917"; AHSSA, BP, EH, HM, file 14, exp. 19, 1919, "Articulos publicados en la prensa indicando que a las asiladas de dicho establecimiento no se les illionnt alimentos"; AHSSA, BP, EH, HM, file 14, exp. 20, 1919, "Reja de fierro que se instala para evitar la evasion de las enfermas"; AHSSA, BP, EH, HM, file 18, exp. 13, 1916, "Solicita se gestione que las enfermas que se dan de alta como curadas, no sufran nuevo examen en las oficicinas de la inspeccion de sanidad"; AHSSA, BP, EH, HM, file 18, exp. 18, 1920, "Se solicita de la inspeccion general de policia dos gendarmes para evitar la fuga de las enfermas detenidas"; AHSSA, BP, EH, HM, file 18, exp. 19, August 24, 1920, "Informa haberse fugado trece enfermas de las detenidas, llevándose once camisones."

33. Nugent and Joseph, *Everyday Forms of State Formation*.

34. BP, EH, HG, file 27, exp. 11, 1929, "Acusaciones en contra de las enfermeras del Hospital y artículos publicados en la prensa que se relacionan con el Establecimiento."

35. BP, EH, HG, file 27, exp. 11, 1929, "Acusaciones en contra de las enfermeras del Hospital y artículos publicados en la prensa que se relacionan con el Establecimiento."

36. BP, EH, HG, file 27, exp. 11, 1929, "Acusaciones en contra de las enfermeras del Hospital y artículos publicados en la prensa que se relacionan con el Establecimiento."

37. "Graves quejas de enfermas del Hospital General," *La Prensa,* February 21, 1933; AHSSA, BP, EH, C5, file 1, 1929, exp. 8, "Queja de los pacientes del Consultorio por malos tratos."

38. BP, EH, HG, file 27, exp. 11, 1929, "Acusaciones en contra de las enfermeras del Hospital y artículos publicados en la prensa que se relacionan con el Establecimiento."

39. AHSSA, BP, EH, HJ, file 15, exp. 9, 1928, "Queja por muerte de una parturienta."

40. "Queja sobre el Hospital Juárez," *El Universal Gráfico,* September 19, 1928.

41. AHSSA, BP, EH, HG, file 32, exp. 2, 1932, "Investigación practicada por la señora Elvia Carrillo Puerto, acerca de las irregularidades cometidas por un grupo de afanadoras de dicho establecimiento"; Olcott, *Revolutionary Women,* 111, 165–205.

42. AHSSA, BP, EH, HG, file 32, exp. 4, 1933, "Generalidades de quejas presentadas por los enfermos." The women were Consuelo Melendez, Teódula Dominguez de Rosas, Justina Forres de R., Esperanza Peña, Paula Zavala, Francisca Espindola, Juliana Suarez de C., Mariana Valdes, Abigail Soldado, Amanda Báeza, Evangelina Ruiz, Esperanza Perez, Severina Carrillo, Felipa Camacho, Carmen Jiménez, Carolina Jovan de Mendoza, and María López.

43. AHSSA, BP, EH, HG, file 32, exp. 4, 1933, "Generalidades de quejas presentadas por los enfermos"; AHSSA, BP, EH, HG, file 33, exp. 2, 1933, "Quejas presentadas por asilados del Hospital General."

44. "Más de un million de pesos para socorrer a los indigentes," *El Excelsior,* December 3, 1932.

45. "Las enfermeras tendrán sus casas y mejorarán en las pesadas tareas," *El Nacional,* March 2, 1933; "Casas par alas enfermeras de los hospitals," *El Universal Gráfico,* March 2, 1933.

46. AHSSA, BP, EH, HG, file 16, exp. 4, 1916, "Relativo al traslado de los departamentos de maternidad de los hospitales Juárez y Morelos al Hospital General"; AHSSA, BP, EH, HG, file 23, exp. 11, 1920, "Acuerdo por el cual el Hospital General pasa a depender de la Escuela de Medicina."

47. AHSSA, BP, EH, HM, file 11, exp. 3, 1917, "Participa haberse fugado varias asiladas por las ventanas por lo que solicita se le pongan rejas para mayor seguridad." The director general agreed the new bars were necessary and authorized them immediately. In 1919, the same occurred: AHSSA, BP, EH, HM, file 14, exp. 15, 1919, "Participa haberse fugado 35 enfermas, las cuales se llevaron varias prendas de ropa."

48. "Hay congestion de enfermos en los hospitales," *El Excélsior,* April 5, 1933.

49. "No fue aceptada la renuncia del personal medico," *El Excelsior,* October 7, 1932; "Los médicos del Hospital General que renunciaron, tornan al puesto," *El Gráfico,* October 7, 1932; "No se acepta la renuncia," *El Universal Gráfico,* October 7, 1932.

50. Arciniega, *Querella por la cultura "revolucionaria"*; Soto Laveaga, "Bringing the Revolution to Medical Schools."

51. Meyer, "La etapa formativa"; Córdova, *La revolución en crisis*; Semo, "El Cardenismo Revisado"; Medina Peña, *Hacia el nuevo estado.*

52. Medin, *El minimato presidencial,* 114.

53. *El Excelsior,* July 26, 1932.

54. "Operaciones criminals en el Hospital general," *La Prensa,* November 6, 1933. AHSSA, BP, EH, HG, file 33, exp. 8.

55. *El Universal Gráfico*, July 28, 1932.

56. "Se Serena la Contienda en el Hospital: No Saldrá Ningún Médico de Prestigio, pero la Institución no Servirá más para Provecho Meramente Personal de Otros Facultativos," *El Excelsior*, August 14, 1932.

57. "Reina Anarquia en la AHSSA, BP," *La Época*, August 21, 1932.

58. "Renunciaron en Masa," *El Universal Gráfico*, August 5, 1932. There were thirty-one wings in the General Hospital.

59. "Renunciaron en Masa," *El Universal Gráfico*, August 5, 1932.

60. "Renunciaron en Masa," *El Universal Gráfico*, August 5, 1932.

61. "Renunciaron en Masa," *El Universal Gráfico*, August 5, 1932; "Se aceptó la renuncia del personal medico del Hospital General," *El Nacional*, August 6, 1932.

62. "Fué aceptada la Renuncia a los Facultativos del Hospital General," *El Excelsior*, August 6, 1932.

63. "Los medicos que hacen cargos a la Beneficencia Pública, fueron consignados ayer al procurador: el asunto pasará a una corte penal o a la Controlaría," *El Excelsior*, August 9, 1932.

64. "Se Estudiará el Caso del Hospital General: El Dr. Anastasio Garza Ríos fue comisionado para hacer un detenido studio," *El Nacional*, August 11, 1932; "En El Hospital Se Instalará el Dr. Garza Ríos para Dar su Dictamen: La Beneficencia Pública ha determinado que él sea quien tome la opinion del personal y de los enfermos del plantel," *El Gráfico*, August 11, 1932.

65. "Fue Solucionado el Conflicto del Hospital General con la Renuncia del Dr. Zuckermann," *El Excelsior*, August 13, 1932.

66. "Fue Solucionado el Conflicto del Hospital General con la Renuncia del Dr. Zuckermann," *El Excelsior*, August 13, 1932; "Funcionarios, no Incondicionales," *El Univeral Gráfico*, August 9, 1932, opinion piece by lic. Eduardo Pallares.

67. "Reina anarquia en la AHSSA, BP," *La Época*, August 21, 1932.

68. "Fue Solucionado el Conflicto del Hospital General con la Renuncia del Dr. Zuckermann," *El Excelsior*, August 13, 1932.

69. "Se Aceptó la renuncia del Sr. E. Cajigal," *El Excelsior*, August 20, 1932.

70. "Mas funcionarios renuncian a sus cargos: ha dimitido el Jefe del Depto. De Salubridad. Resignaron también sus puestos el director y médicos del hospital general," *El Excelsior*, August 20, 1932.

71. "Se aceptó su renuncia al doctor Melo; Dimitió el Dr. Méndez," *El Nacional*, August 1932.

72. "Renuncio el Jefe del Depto. De Salubridad: Los médicos que habían separado del Hospital General y volvieron, dimiten nuevamente," *El Universal Gráfico*, August 20, 1932; "La renuncia del Dr. Melo fue aceptada," *El Universal Gráfico*, August 21, 1932; "Renuncias a Granel Hay en Diversas Dependencias," *El Gráfico*, August 23, 1932.

73. "Renunció a la Presidencia de la Beneficencia Don F. Ortiz Rubio," *El Popular*, August 26, 1932; "Dimitio el Presidente de la Beneficencia Pública: por las dificultades surgidas en el Hospital General," *La Prensa*, August 26, 1932.

74. "Esta pendiente la renuncia de los 28 médicos," *El Excelsior*, August 22, 1932.

75. "Contestación al Dr. Méndez," *El Nacional*, August 23, 1932.

76. "El nuevo director de la Beneficencia," *El Universal Gráfico*, August 9, 1932.

77. "Total reorganizacion del Hospital General," *El Nacional*, August 14, 1932; "Visita del Gral. Tapia al Hospital General: Encontró que casi todos los pabellones están en pésimo estado," *El Excelsior*, September 15, 1932.

78. "Hay graves irregularidades en la Beneficencia," *El Excelsior*, September 21, 1932; "Se descubrieron irregularidades en el Manicomio," *El Excelsior*, September 21, 1932; "El Manicomio, Eden de Placer y de Lujuria: Funcionaba allí un garito y se comitia todo género de irregularidades y de actos inmorales que ya se han reprimido," *La Prensa*, September 21, 1932; "Orgías de empleados y enfermas guapas del manicomio general," *El Excelsior*, September 22, 1932; "Se castigará todo acto de dishonor en el Manicomio," *El Gráfico*, September 23, 1932.

79. "Por qué renunció el Dr. Priani," *El Universal Gráfico*, September 26, 1932.

80. "Gran Actividad en el Hospital Homeopático: cerca del 50 por ciento de consultas gratuitas han aumentado en un mes," *El Nacional*, January 31, 1933; "Nuevo director del Hospital Homeopático," *El Nacional*, October 8, 1932; "Mas de 10,000 personas reciben atenciones médicas gratuitas," *La Prensa*, February 1, 1933.

81. "Los médicos del Hospital General que renunciaron, tornan al puesto," *El Gráfico*, October 7, 1932.

82. "Ceses en los hospitales: Los estudiantes que hacían en ellos sus ractices no fueron a la manifestacion," *El Universal Gráfico*, November 6, 1934.

83. "Los ceses de practicantes," *El Universal Gráfico*, November 7, 1934.

84. "La exclusion de los hospitales a practicantes," *El Excelsior*, November 9, 1934; "Un conflicto en la Beneficiencia," *El Excelsior*, November 14, 1934.

85. "Renuncia el Gral. Tapia: Circular a los Jefes," *El Nacional*, November 17, 1934; "Dimisiones en el personal de la Beneficencia," *La Prensa*, November 17, 1934; "Renunciará el General Tapia: ha girado una circular para que los empleados de la AHSSA, BP presenten también la dimisión de los cargos que desempeñan," *El Universal Gráfico*, November 17, 1934.

86. "Quedará el General Tapia como presidente de las directivas de las juntas de Beneficencia: el presidente de la república no aceptó la renuncia que presentó aquel funcionario en vista de su Buena Labor," *El Excelsior*, December 8, 1934; "Seguirá el Gral. Tapia," *El Universal Gráfico*, December 10, 1934.

87. "La obra del Comité de Salud Pública," *El Nacional*, December 11, 1934.

Conclusion and Epilogue

1. Nina Lakhani, "Mexican Rape Victim, 13, Denied Access to Abortion," *The Guardian*, August 1, 2016.

2. "'Violar a una niña es menos grave que un aborto,' afirma Cardenal," *El Excelsior*, May 8, 2019.

3. Daniel Politi, *New York Times*, "An 11-Year-Old in Argentina Was Raped: A Hospital Denied Her an Abortion," March 1, 2019; "Girl, 11, Gives Birth to Child of Rapist after Argentina Says No to Abortion," *The Guardian*, March 1, 2019.

4. Roberts, *God's Laboratory*; Morgan and Roberts, "Reproductive Governance"; Tuñón, *Enjaular los cuerpos*; Morgan, *Icons of Life*.

5. Nina Lakhani, "Woman who bore rapist's baby faces 20 years in El Salvador jail," *The Guardian*, November 12, 2018.

6. Bordo, "Are Mothers Persons?"

7. Carmon, "Dorothy Roberts Tried to Warn Us," *Intelligencer Report,* September 6, 2022.

8. Zoë Carpenter, "Ecuador's Crackdown on Abortion Is Putting Women in Jail," *The Nation,* May 7, 2019.

9. Grupo de Información en Reproducción Elegida (GIRE), *La pieza faltante,* 95.

10. GIRE, *La pieza faltante,* 86.

11. GIRE, *La pieza faltante,* 87.

12. GIRE, *La pieza faltante,* 87.

13. Fernández and Castro, *Estudio nacional sobre las fuentes,* 37.

14. Andrea Ramírez, "9 de cada 10 mujeres sufren violencia obstétrica en Veracruz," *El Dictamen,* December 18, 2017.

15. Maurice, "We Bawl So We Are Heard."

16. GIRE, *La pieza faltante,* 115.

17. GIRE, *La pieza faltante,* 117.

18. GIRE, *La pieza faltante,* 117.

19. GIRE, *La pieza faltante,* 94.

20. Palomo, "Cuerpos intervenidos, violencias naturalizadas."

21. Williams, Jerez, Klein, Correa, Belizán, Cormick, "Obstetric violence."

22. Needham, *History of Embryology,* 204.

Bibliography

Archives

Archivo de La Escuela Antigua de Medicina
Archivo Histórico del Arzobispado de México (AHAM)
Archivo Histórico del Distrito Federal (AHDF)
Archivo General de la Nación (AGN)
Archivo Histórico de la Cuidad de México
Archivo Histórico de la Secretaría de Salubridad y Asistencia (AHSSA)
Benson Latin American Collection, University of Texas at Austin
La Biblioteca Dr. Nicolás León, UNAM
La Hemeroteca Nacional de México, UNAM
The Huntington Library and Collections, San Marino, California
The Newberry Library, Chicago, Illinois

Periodicals

Diario de Mexico
La Gazeta de México
Periódico de la Academia de Medicina en México
El Siglo Diez y Nueve
Periódico de la Academia de Medicina de Méjico
El Cosmopolita
Legislación Mexicana
La Orquesta
Voz de México
El Monitor Republicano
La Luz de Nuevo León
El Foro
El Imparcial
Gaceta de la Academia de Medicina
Revista Católica
Gaceta Oficial del Arzobispado de México
La Prensa
El Excelsior
Excelsior de la tarde
El Universal
El Mundo
El Gráfico
El Universal Gráfico
El Nacional
La Época
El Popular
The Guardian
The Nation
The New York Times
The Intelligencer Report
El Dictamen
The Nation

Printed Primary Sources

Alcalá y Martínez, Jaime. *Disertación médico-chirúrgica, sobre una operación cesárea ejecutada en muger, y feto vivos esta Ciudad de Valencia*. Valencia: Por la Viuda de Geronimo Conejos, 1753.

Andrade, Jesús. *Acción del somniféne en los dolores del parto*. Mexico City, 1927.

Bancroft, Hubert Howe. *California Pastoral: 1769–1848*. Cambridge, MA: Harvard University, 1888.

Barreda, Gabino. "De la educación moral" (1863). In *Opúsculos, discusiones y discursos coleccionados y publicados por la Asociación metodófila Gabino Barreda*, 117. Mexico City: Imprenta del Comercio de Dublán y Chavéz, 1877.

———. *Opúsculos discusiones y discursos*. Mexico City: Imprenta de Dublán y Chávez, 1877.

Barreiro, Manuel. *Oportunidad en la aplicación de forceps*. Mexico City: Tipografía de B. Nichols, 1885.

Barrón, Juán. *Estudió critico de algunas de las indicaciones de la histerectomía fúndica*. Mexico City, 1935.

Cangiamila, Francesco Emmanuelle. *Embriología sagrada*. Madrid: Imprenta de Pantaleón Aznar, 1774.

Carrillo, Rafael. "Tres problemas Mexicanos de eugenesia: etnografia y etnologia, herencia e inmigración." *Revista Mexicana de Puericultura: Organo de la Sociedad Mexicana de Puericultura* 3, no. 25 (November 1932): 1–14.

Casillas, Tomás. *Tratamiento de las manifestaciones secundarias de la sifilis por inyecciones subcutáneas de preparaciones mercuriales*. Mexico City: Imprenta de Jens y Zapiain, 1876.

Casis Sacre, Guillermo. "Salpingitis: oportunidad operatoria y factor social del tratamiento." Licenciatura thesis, Universidad Nacional Autónoma de México, Facultad de Medicina, 1936.

Caviedes, Luis. *Los rayos rubens o infra-rojos como tratamiento de las anexitis rebeldes*. Mexico City: Imprenta Universal, 1932.

Comte, Auguste. *System of Positive Polity, or, Treatise on Sociology: Instituting the Religion of Humanity*. Translated by John Henry Bridges, Frederic Harrison, Edward Spencer Beesly, Richard Congreve, and Henry Dix Hutton. London: Longmans, Green and Co., 1875.

Cook, Sherburne. "Sarría's Treatise on the Cesarean Operation, 1830: Part I." *California and Western Medicine* 47, no. 2 (1937): 107–11.

———. "Sarría's Treatise on the Cesarean Operation, 1830: Part II." *California and Western Medicine* 47, no. 3 (1937): 187–89.

———. "Sarría's Treatise on the Cesarean Operation, 1830: Part III." *California and Western Medicine* 47, no. 4 (1937): 248–50.

Deventer, Henrik van. *Observations importantes sur le manuel des accouchements*. Translated by Jacques-Jean Bruier d'Ablaincourt. Paris, 1734.

Dublán, Manuel, and José Maria Lozano, eds. *Legislación mexicana, ó, Colección completa de las disposiciones legislativas expedidas desde la independencia de la República*. Vol. 9. Mexico City: Imprenta del Comercio de Dublán y Chavéz, 1878.

Duque de Estrada, Juan. *Contribución al estudio de las deformaciónes pélvicas en México por el Dr. Duque de Estrada*. Mexico City: Tipografía y Litografía "La Europea," de J. Aguilar Vera y Compañia, 1901.

———. *Pelviología mexicana: Descripción de una pelvis infundibuliforme de tipo infantil*. Mexico City: n.p., 1917.

———. *Procedimiento fácil y rápido para la medición del diametro bis-isquiatico, gran importancia clínica de este diámetro, y estudios hechos en la antigua casa de la maternidad de México en los años de 1898–1902, por el Dr. Juan Duque de Estrada*. 2nd ed. Mexico City: Imprenta del Museo Nacional, 1911.

Esparza, Carlos M. *Breves consideraciones sobre la herencia normal y patológica*. Mexico City: Imprenta de Horcasitas, Hermanos, 1881.

Estrada, Ramon. *La falta de hygiene infantil en México, y sus relaciones con la degeneración de la raza*. Mexico City: Escuela correc, 1888.

Feijóo Peñas, Julio. "Intersexualidad y diferenciación sexual." Licenciatura thesis, Universidad Nacional Autónoma de México, Facultad de Medicina, 1934.

Feliberto, Benito Soriano. *Breve estudio sobre el empleo del cloroformo en los partos naturales*. Mexico City: Tipografía Literaria de Filomento Mata, 1884.

Figueroa Ortíz, José. *La estenosis del diámetro bisisquiático en México*. Mexico City: n.p., 1934.

Flores, Florencio. *Ligeros apuntes de pelvimetría comparada*. Cuernavaca: Imprenta del Gobierno del Estado, 1881.

Flores, Manuel. *Educación del medico: Tésis inaugural*. Mexico City: Imprenta de Ignacio Escalante, 1880.

Flores y Troncoso, Francisco de Asís. *Historia de la medicina en México*, Tomo III. Mexico City: Oficina de Tipografía de la Secretaría de Fomento, 1888.

Fuertes, Ricardo. *Cuatro laparotomías por Ricardo Fuertes*. Mexico City: Imprenta de Guillermo Veraza, Calle de la Canda, número 6 1/4, 1886.

García Rodríguez, Rufino. *Diagnóstico de las estreches pélvicas y operación cesárea clásica*. Mexico City, 1936.

Garza García, José Mario. *La evolución del hombre*. San Luis Potosí: [Universidad Autónoma de San Luis Potosí, Facultad de Medicina], 1936.

González Laguna, Francisco. *El zelo sacerdotal para con los niños no-nacidos*. Lima: Imprenta de los Niños Expósitos, 1781.

Harris, John. "Pregnancy and Labor in Young Primiparae." *Johns Hopkins Hospital Bulletin* 33 (1922): 12–21.

Ibáñez, Joaquín. *Someras reflexiones sobre el aborto obstetrical, el parto prematuro y la gastrohisterotomía*. Puebla: Imprenta de Ibañez y Lamarque, 1882.

Islas Hernández, Alfredo. "Aborto no terapéutico, su aspecto social y legal." Licenciatura thesis, Universidad Nacional Autónoma de México, 1933.

Jolly Hernández, Gustavo. *La retroversión uterina y la ligamentopexia de Arce*. Mexico City: 1936.

Leal, Manuel. *Taponamiento vaginal en obstetricia*. Mexico City: Oficina Tipografía De la Secretaría de Fomento, 1887.

León, Nicolás. *La obstetricia en México: Notas bibliográficas, etnicas, históricas, documentarias y críticas, de los orígenes históricos hasta el año 1910*. Mexico City: Viuda de Diaz de Leon, 1910.

Liceaga, Eduardo, and Roberto Gayol. "Proyecto de Hospital General de la Ciudad de México." In *Memorias del 2 Congreso Médico Pan-americano verificado en la Ciudad de México, D.F., Noviembre 16, 17, 18, 19 de 1896*. Mexico City: Hoeck y Compañía, 1896.

López Hermosa, Alberto. *Anomalías de las fuerzas expulsivas y su tratamiento: Estudio que para el concurso de profesor adjunto a la clase de Clinica de Obstetricia presenta al jurado de calificacion*. Mexico City: Imprenta y Litografía de F. Diaz de Leon Sucesores, S.A., 1895.

Márquez, Miguel. *Algunos datos de estadística obstetrica: Tesis inaugural*. Mexico City: Imprenta de Horcasitas Hermanos, 1881.

Medina, Antonio. *Cartilla nueva útil y necesaria para instruirse a las matronas que vulgarmente se llaman comadres en el oficio de Partear*. Mexico City: Doña María Fernanda Jauregui, 1806.

Mejía Schroeder, Alfonso. *De la esterilidad femenina: Su etiología*. Mexico City: Imprenta Mundial, 1935.

Menocal, Francisco de S. *Estudio sobre el aborto en México: Tesis para el concurso á la plaza de adjunto á la cátedra de clínica de obstetricia de la Escuela de Medicina de Mexico*. Mexico City: Imprenta de José M. Lara, 1869.

Montenegro, Francisco. *Breves apuntes sobre la pornografía en la capital*. Mexico City: 1880.

Navarro Origel, José. "Orientación en el campo mental, normal y patológico." Licenciatura thesis, Universidad Nacional Autónoma de México, Facultad de Medicina, 1936.

Navarro y Cardona, Eduardo. *Del parto prematuro en México y de las maneras con que se le ha provocado: Tésis inaugural que presenta al jurado de calificacion*. Mexico City: Imprenta de Diaz de Leon y White, 1873.

Nentvig, Juan. *Descripción geógrafica natural y curiosa de la provincia de Sonora*. Sonora: n.p., 1762.

Orozco, Carlos. *Comparación de la terapeútica y la hygiene, bajo el punto de vista social: Estudio de filosofia médica*. Mexico City: Imprenta de E. Orozco y Comp., 1880.

Ortega Fuentes, Francisco. "Dieciséis meses de observaciones en un servicio de ginecologia." Licenciatura thesis, Universidad Nacional Autónoma de México, Facultad de Medicina, 1917.

Ortega Márquez, Tomás. "Las técnicas en la histerectomía vaginal y su estudio comparativo." Licenciatura thesis, Universidad Nacional Autónoma de México, Facultad de Medicina, 1936.

Owen, Robert. *Institutes of Canon Law*. London: J. T. Hayes, 1884.

Páez, Gonzalo. "Breve estudio acerca de la acción del cloroformo sobre la mujer en trabajo de parto y de sus indicaciones." Licenciatura thesis, Universidad Nacional Autónoma de México, Facultad de Medicina, 1886.

Palomino Rojas, Jesús. "Histerectomía total o subtotal." Licenciatura thesis, Universidad Nacional Autónoma de México, Facultad de Medicina, 1935.

Peckham, C. H. "The Influence of Age and Race on the Duration of Labor." *American Journal of Obstetrics and Gynecology* 24, no. 5 (1932): 744–50.

Pérez, Alfonso. *La propedéutica obstétrica*. Mexico City, 1936.

Piñeiro Romero, Benito. *Escuelas post-operatorias en las intervenciones del vientre*. Mexico City, 1936.

Pius XI (pope). *Carta Encíclica Casti Connubii del Papa Pío XI Sobre el Matrimonio Cristiano*. Vatican City: Dicastero per la Comunicazione, Libreria Editrice Vaticana, 1930. https://www.vatican.va/content/pius-xi/es/encyclicals/documents/hf_p-xi_enc_19301231_casti-connubii.html.

Ramirez, Román. *La ovariotomia en Mexico: Tésis para el exámen profesional de medicina, cirujia y partos*. Mexico City: Imprenta Poliglota, 1874.

Ramírez Elliot, Genaro. "Esterilización temporal femenina sin mutilación." Licenciatura thesis, Universidad Nacional Autónoma de México, Facultad de Medicina, 1932.

Ramos, Manuel. *Breves consideraciones sobre la eclamsia puerperal: Principalmente bajo el punto de vista de su patogenia y tratamiento*. Mexico City: Ti. Literaria de F. Mata, 1880.

Reza, Agustín. *Acción fisiológica del cuernecillo de centeno y el zihuatlpatl durante y después del parto*. Mexico City: Tipografía "El Socialista," 1887.

Rodríguez, Antonio Joseph. *Disertaciones physico-mathematico-medicas sobre el gran problema de la respiracion, y modo de introducir los medicamentos por las venas: Con una pieza de historia philosofica*. Madrid: En la Oficina de Manuel Martin, 1760.

Rodríguez, José Manuel, and Antonio Bucareli Ursua. *La caridad del sacerdote: Para con los niños encerrados en el vientre de sus madres difuntas, y documentos de la utilidad, y necesidad de su práctica*. Mexico: La Oficina del Br. D. Joseph Fernandez Jauregui, 1772.

Rodríguez, Juan María. *Breves apuntes sobre la obstetricia en México: Tésis sostenida por Juan María Rodriguez como candidato para la plaza de adjunto a la Catedra de Clínica de Obstetricia de la Escuela de Medicina*. Mexico City: Imprenta de José M. Lara, 1869.

———. *Teratologia: Descripción de un monstruo humano cuádruple, nacido en Durango el año de 1868: Memoria escrita por encargo de la dirección de la Escuela de Medicina, y leida ante la Sociedad Médica de México, el dia 27 de enero de 1870*. Mexico City: Imprenta de José Mariano Fernandez de Lara, 1870.

———. *Memorándum de la operación cesárea y amputación útero-ovárica, ejecutada por la primera vez en México*. Mexico City: Imprenta de Ignacio Escalante Bajos de San Agustín, Número 1, 1884.

Rojas Domínguez, Jacinto. "Esterilización humana." Licenciatura thesis, Universidad Nacional Autónoma de México, Facultad de Medicina, 1934.

Romo Ruíz, Manuel. "Anotaciones acerca del tratamiento quirurgico de las retroversiones uterinas." Licenciatura thesis, Universidad Nacional Autónoma de México, Facultad de Medicina, 1929.

Rosales Miranda, Fernando. "El tratamiento quirúrgico de la retroversión uterina." Licenciatura thesis, Universidad Nacional Autónoma de México, Facultad de Medicina, 1935.

Ruíz Culebro, Ciro. "El problema médico-social del aborto." Licenciatura thesis, Universidad Nacional Autónoma de México, Facultad de Medicina, 1936.

Ruíz Erdozain, Alfonzo. *La responsabilidad médica ante del código penal del Distrito Federal y territorio de la Baja California*. Mexico City: Imprenta de Francisco Díaz de León Calle de Lerdo número 3, 1887.

Ruiz S., Gustavo. *La herencia en sus aplicaciones medico-legales*. Mexico City: Imprenta del Comercio de Dublán y Chavéz, 1877.

Salinas y Rivera, Alberto. *Moral médica*. Tesis para el examen profesional de medicina, cirujía y obstetricia, Escuela Nacional de Medicina, México. Mexico City: Imprenta de la V. é hijos de Murguia, Portal del Águila de Oro, 1871.

Sánchez Gómez, José de Jesús. *Breve estudio sobre la pelvis*. Mexico City: Officina Tipografía de la Secreteria de Fomento, 1891.

San Juan, Nicolás. *Un caso de anomalía relativa a la ausencia de órganos únicos*. Mexico City: 1880.

Souza Vásquez, Guillermo. "Contribución al tratamiento de la fiebre puerperal: La histerectomía vaginal." Licenciatura thesis, Universidad Nacional Autónoma de México, Facultad de Medicina, 1932.

Tercero, Rosendo. *Breve consideraciones acerca de la inyección uterina*. Mexico City: Imprenta de Eduardo Dublan, 1899.

Torijano y Ritchie, Jorge. "La ética profesional en la maternidad consciente." Licenciatura thesis, Universidad Nacional Autónoma de México, Facultad de Medicina, 1936.

Torres Ansorena, José. *Inconvenientes y peligros que presenta la anteversión y anteflexión uterinas para el embarazo, parto y puerperio: Trabajo presentado para el exámen general de medicina, cirugía y obstetricia*. Mexico City: Imprenta de Francisco Diaz de Leon, 1884.

Torres Septién, Juan Antonio. "Un nuevo método de pelvigrafía." Licenciatura thesis, Universidad Nacional Autónoma de México, Facultad de Medicina, 1934.

Trangay, Gustavo Adolfo. "La maternidad consciente y la clínica." Licenciatura thesis, Universidad Nacional Autónoma de México, Facultad de Medicina, 1931.

Vásquez, Isaac. *Ligero estudio de algunos de los accidentes de la gran histeria*. Mexico City: Imprenta del Comercio, de Dublan y Compañia, 1882.

Venegas, Miguel. *Manual de párrocos, para administrar los santos sacramentos, y executar las demás sagradas funciones de su ministerio*. Mexico City: La Oficina de los Herederos del Lic. D. Joseph de Jauregui, 1803.

Vilchis Vilchis, José. "Consideraciones acerca de la esterilización definitiva." Licenciatura thesis, Universidad Nacional Autónoma de México, Facultad de Medicina, 1933.

Villa, Galindo. *El presbítero D. José Antonio Alzate Ramírez: Apuntes biográficos y bibliográficos*. Mexico City: Imprenta del Gobierno, 1890.

Zambrana y Vázquez, Santiago. "Naturaleza de la infección purulenta." *El Observador Medical* 2 (1872–74): 304–12.

Zárraga, Fernando. *Brevisimas reflexiones sobre las causas de las desgracias de la cirugía*. Mexico City: Imprenta de G. Horcasitas, 1884.

Secondary Sources

Abugideiri, Hibba. *Gender and the Making of Modern Medicine in Colonial Egypt*. Farnham, United Kingdom: Ashgate, 2010.

Agostoni, Cláudia. *Cuidar, sanar y educar: Enfermedad y sociedad en México: Siglos XIX y XX*. Mexico City: UNAM, 2008.

———. *Monuments of Progress: Modernization and Public Health in Mexico City, 1876–1910*. Calgary, Alberta: University of Calgary Press, 2003.

Appelbaum, Nancy, Anne Macpherson, and Karin Alejandra Rosemblatt, eds. *Race and Nation in Modern Latin America*. Chapel Hill: The University of North Carolina Press, 2003.

Arciniega, V. D. *Querella por la cultura "revolucionaria" (1925)*. Mexico City: Fondo de Cultura Economica, 1985.

Arendt, Hannah. *Between Past and Future*. Cleveland: Meridian, 1963.

Aristotle. *De Anima*. Translated by J. A. Smith. Cambridge, MA: Classics Department, Massachusetts Institute of Technology, 2009. http://classics.mit.edu//Aristotle/soul.html.

Arrom, Silvia. "Catholic Philanthropy and Civil Society: The Lay Volunteers of Saint Vincent de Paul in Nineteenth- Century Mexico." *Vincentian Heritage Journal* 27, no. 1 (2007): article 1.

———. *Volunteering for a Cause: Gender, Faith, and Charity in Mexico from the Reform to the Revolution*. Albuquerque: University of New Mexico Press, 2016.

Barahona, Ana. "La introducción del darwinismo en México." *Teorema: Revista Internacional de Filosofía* 28, no. 2 (2009): 201–14.

Barnes, M. Elizabeth. "Ernst Haeckel's Biogenetic Law (1866)." In *Embryo Project Encyclopedia*. Tempe: School of Life Sciences, Arizona State University, May 3, 2014. http://embryo.asu.edu/handle/10776/7825.

Berrio Palomo, Lina Rosa. "Cuerpos intervenidos, violencias naturalizadas: Reflexiones sobre la violencia obstétrica e institucional experimentada por mujeres indígenas en Guerrero." *Antropologías feministas en México: Epistemologías, éticas, prácticas y miradas diversas*, edited by Berrio Palomo et al., 431–61. Mexico City: UNAM, Universidad Autónoma Metropolitana; Universidad Nacional Autónoma de México; Bonilla Artigas Editores, 2020.

Birn, Anne-Emanuelle. *Marriage of Convenience: Rockefeller International Health and Revolutionary Mexico*. Rochester, NY: University of Rochester Press, 2006.

Bliss, Katherine. *Compromised Positions: Prostitution, Public Health and Gender Politics in Revolutionary Mexico City*. University Park: Pennsylvania State University Press, 2001.

———. "The Science of Redemption: Syphilis, Sexual Promiscuity, and Reformism in Revolutionary Mexico City." *Hispanic American Historical Review* 79, no. 1 (1999): 1–40.

Blum, Ann. *Domestic Economies: Family, Work, and Welfare in Mexico City, 1884–1943*. Lincoln: University of Nebraska Press, 2009.

Blumenfeld-Kosinski, Renate. *Not of Woman Born: Representations of Caesarean Birth in Medieval and Renaissance Culture*. Ithaca, NY: Cornell University Press, 1990.

Blundell, James. "Lectures on the Theory and Practice of Midwifery." *Lancet* 8, no. 1 (1827): 673–81.

Bobb, Bernard. *The Viceregency of Antonio María Bucareli in New Spain, 1771–1779*. Austin: University of Texas Press, 1962.

Bordo, Susan. "Are Mothers Persons? Reproductive Rights and the Politics of Subjectivity." In *Unbearable Weight: Feminism, Western Culture, and the Body*, 71–97. Berkeley: University of California Press, 1993.

Briggs, Laura. *How All Politics Became Reproductive Politics: From Welfare Reform to Foreclosure to Trump*. Berkeley: University of California Press, 2018.

———. "The Race of Hysteria: 'Overcivilization' and the 'Savage' Woman in Late Nineteenth-Century Obstetrics and Gynecology." *American Quarterly* 52 (2000): 246–73.

———. *Reproducing Empire: Race, Sex, Science, and U.S. Imperialism in Puerto Rico*. Berkeley: University of California Press, 2002.

Brind'Amour, Katherine. "*Casti Connubii* (1930), by Pope Pius XI." In *Embryo Project Encyclopedia*. Tempe: School of Life Sciences, Arizona State University, January 20, 2009. http://embryo.asu.edu/handle/10776/1749.

Buffington, Robert. *Criminal and Citizen in Modern Mexico*. Lincoln: University of Nebraska Press, 2000.

Butler, Matthew. "Liberalism, Anticlericalism, and Anti-religious Currents in the Nineteenth-Century." In *Cambridge History of Religions in Latin America*, edited by Virginia Garrard-Burnett and Paul Freston, 251–68. Cambridge: Cambridge University Press, 2016.

Caffiero, Marina. *Forced Baptisms: Histories of Jews, Christians, and Converts in Papal Rome*. Translated by Lydia Cochrane. Berkeley: University of California Press, 2012.

Canguilhem, Georges. *On the Normal and the Pathological*. Translated by Carolyn R. Fawcett. Dordrecht, the Netherlands: D. Reidel/Springer, 2012. Originally published in 1978.

Carrillo, Ana María. "Control sexual para el control social: La primera campaña contra la sífilis en México." *Espaço Plural* 11, no. 22 (2010): 65–77.

———. "La influencia de la bacteriología francesa en la mexicana en el periodo de su institucionalización." *Quipu. Revista Latinoamericana de Historia de las Ciencias y la Tecnología* 14, no. 2 (2012): 193–219.

———. "Los modernos minotauro y Teseo: La lucha contra la tuberculosis en México." *Estudios: Centro d Estudios Avanzados* 1 (2012): 85–101.

———. *Matilde Montoya: Primera médica mexicana*. Mexico City: DEMAC, 2002.

———. "Nacimiento y muerte de una profesion: Las parteras tituladas en México." *Dynamis* 19 (1999): 167–90.

Castañeda López, Gabriela, and Ana Cecilia Rodríguez de Romo. *Pioneras de la medicina mexicana en la UNAM: Del porfiriato al nuevo régimen, 1887–1936*. Madrid: Ediciones Díaz de Santos, 2011.

Ceballos Rómulo, Velazco. *El Hospital Juárez*. Mexico City: Talleres gráficos de la Nación, 1934.

Cházaro, Laura. "Pariendo instrumentos médicos: Los forceps y pelvímetros entre los obstetras del siglo XIX en México." *Dynamis* 24 (2004): 27–51.

Christopoulos, John. *Abortion in Early Modern Italy*. Cambridge, MA: Harvard University Press, 2021.

Combahee River Collective. "The Combahee River Collective Statement." 1977. US Library of Congress Web Archive, 2015. https://www.loc.gov/item/lcwaN0028151.

Comfort, Nathaniel. "The Prisoner as Model Organism: Malaria Research at Stateville Penitentiary." *Studies in History and Philosophy of Biological and Biomedical Sciences* 40, no. 3 (2009): 190–203.

Cooper Owens, Dierdre. *Medical Bondage: Race, Gender, and the Origins of American Gynecology*. Atlanta: University of Georgia Press, 2017.

Córdova, Arnaldo. *La revolución en crisis: La aventura del maximato*. Mexico City: Cal y Arena, 1995.

Cosio Villegas, Daniel et al., *Historia moderna de México: La República restaurada. La vida política*. Mexico City: Editorial Hermes, 1955.

Covo, Jacqueline. *Las ideas de la reforma en México (1855–1861)*. Mexico City: Universidad Nacional Autónoma de México, Coordinación de Humanidades, 1983.

Crespo Reyes, Sofía, and Pamela J. Fuentes. "Bodies and Souls: A Fight between the Revolutionary State and Catholic Women over the Sexuality of Prostitutes in the 1920s." *Mexican Studies/Estudios Mexicanos* 36, no. 1–2 (2020): 243–69.

Cruz Rodríguez, Soledad. "Los hospitales en la cuidad de México: De la caridad cristiana a la seguridad social." *Sociología: Revista del Departamento de Sociología de la Universidad Autónoma Metropolitana Azcapotzalco* 2, no. 4 (1987): 1064.

Davis, Dána-Ain. "Obstetric Racism: The Racial Politics of Pregnancy, Labor, and Birthing." *Medical Anthropology* 38, no. 7 (2019): 560–73.

De Chaparro, Martina Will, and Miruna Achim, eds. *Death and Dying in Colonial Spanish America*. Tucson: University of Arizona Press, 2011.

De Demerson, Paula. "La cesarea post mortem en la España de la ilustracion." *Asclepio; archivo iberoamericano de historia de la medicina y antropologia medica* 28 (1976): 185–233.

Delay, Cara, and Beth Sundstrom. "The Legacy of Symphysiotomy in Ireland: A Reproductive Justice Approach to Obstetric Violence." In *Reproduction, Health, and Medicine*, edited by Elizabeth M. Armstrong, Susan Markens, and Miranda R. Waggoner, 197–218. Bingley, Ireland: Emerald Publishing, 2019.

Del Olmo Araiza, Consuelo. "Medicina en el siglo XIX México: El Hospital Juárez, 1847–1898." BA thesis, Universidad Nacional Autónoma de México, 1999.

Drinot, Paulo. *Historia de la prostitución en el Perú (1850–1956)*. Lima: CreaLibros Ediciones, 2022.

Dutra, Frank. "Abortion and Leunbach's Paste." *JAMA* 111, no. 6 (1938): 535.

Eliade, Mircea. *The Sacred and the Profane*. New York: Harper Torchbooks, 1961.

Fajardo Ortiz, Guillermo. *Breve historia de los hospitales de la cuidad de México*. Mexico City: Asociación Mexicana de Hospitales, 1980.

Fernández, Florinda Riquer, and Roberto Castro. *Estudio nacional sobre las fuentes, orígenes y factores que producen y reproducen la violencia contra las mujeres*. Mexico City: Secretaría de Gobernación, Comisión Nacional para Prevenir y Erradicar la Violencia contra las Mujeres, 2012.

Few, Martha. *For All of Humanity: Mesoamerican and Colonial Medicine in Enlightenment Guatemala*. Tucson: University of Arizona Press, 2015.

Few, Martha, Zeb Tortorici, and Adam Warren. *Baptism through Incision: The Postmortem Cesarean Operation in the Spanish Empire*. University Park: Pennsylvania State University Press, 2021.

Fields, Barbara, and Karen Fields. *Racecraft: The Soul of Inequality in American Life*. New York: Verso, 2022.

Fissell, Mary. "The Disappearance of the Patient's Narrative and the Invention of Hospital Medicine." In *British Medicine in an Age of Reform*, edited by Roger French and Andrew Wear, 92–109. London: Routledge, 1991.

———. *Vernacular Bodies: The Politics of Reproduction in Early Modern England*. Oxford: Oxford University Press, 2004.

Frampton, Sally. *Belly Rippers, Surgical Innovation and the Ovariotomy Controversy*. London: Palgrave Macmillan, 2018.

French, William, and Katherine Elaine Bliss, eds. *Gender, Sexuality, and Power in Latin America since Independence*. Lanham, MD: Rowman & Littlefield, 2006.

Fuentes, Marisa. *Dispossessed Lives: Enslaved Women, Violence, and the Archive*. Philadelphia: University of Pennsylvania Press, 2016.

Gamboa, Federico. *Santa*. Translated by John Chasteen. Chapel Hill: The University of North Carolina Press, 2010. Originally published in 1903.

Gilman, Sander. *Difference and Pathology: Stereotypes of Sexuality, Race, and Madness*. Ithaca, NY: Cornell University Press, 1985.

Goldstein, Jan. "The Hysteria Diagnosis and the Politics of Anticlericalism in Late Nineteenth-Century France." *Journal of Modern History* 54, no. 2 (1982): 209–39.

González Navarro, Moisés. "Los Positivistas Mexicanos en Francia." *Historia Mexicana* 9, no. 1 (1959): 119–29.

González-Vélez, Ana Cristina. "La producción de conocimiento experto: Un eje central en la implementación del aborto legal en Colombia." Supplement, *Cadernos de Saúde Pública* 36, no. S1 (2020).

Goodman, Jordan, Anthony McElligott, and Lara Marks, eds. *Useful Bodies: Humans in the Service of Medical Science in the Twentieth Century*. Baltimore: Johns Hopkins University Press, 2003.

Gorbach, Frida. "From the Uterus to the Brain: Images of Hysteria in Nineteenth-Century Mexico." *Feminist Review* 79, no. 1 (2005): 83–99.

———. *El monstruo, objeto imposible: Un estudio sobre teratología Mexicana, siglo xix*. Mexico City: Itaca, 2008.

———. "Mujeres, Monstruos e Impresiones en la medicina mexicana del siglo XIX." *Relaciones: Estudios de Historia y Sociedad* 21, no. 81 (2000): 40–55.

Gould, Stephen. *Ontogeny and Phylogeny*. Cambridge, MA: Harvard University Press, 1977.

———. *The Structure of Evolutionary Theory*. Cambridge, MA: Harvard University Press, 2002.

Granados, Marta Saade. "¿Quiénes deben procrear? Los médicos eugenistas bajo el signo social (México, 1931–1940)." *Cuicuilco* 11, no. 31 (2004): 1–36.

Grupo de Información en Reproducción Elegida. *La pieza faltante: Justicia reproductiva*. Mexico City: GIRE, 2018.

Gurr, Barbara. *Reproductive Justice: The Politics of Health Care for Native American Women*. New Brunswick, NJ: Rutgers University Press, 2014.

Guy, Donna. *Sex and Danger in Buenos Aires: Prostitution, Family, and Nation in Argentina*. Lincoln: University of Nebraska Press, 1991.

Hale, Charles. *The Transformation of Liberalism in Late Nineteenth-Century Mexico*. Princeton, NJ: Princeton University Press, 2014.

Halpern, Sydney. *Lesser Harms: The Morality of Risk in Medical Research*. Chicago: University of Chicago Press, 2006.

Handren, Walter. *No Longer Two: A Commentary on the Encyclical "Casti Connubii" of Pius XI*. Westminster, MD: Newman Press, 1955.

Hankins, Thomas. *Science and the Enlightenment*. Cambridge: Cambridge University Press, 1995.

Hartman, Saidiya. "Venus in Two Acts." *Small Axe: A Caribbean Journal of Criticism* 12, no. 2 (2008): 1–14.

Hernández Sáenz, Luz María. *Carving a Niche: The Medical Profession in Mexico, 1800–1870*. Montreal: McGill-Queen's Press, 2018.

Hershfield, Joanne. *Imagining la Chica Moderna: Women, Nation, and Visual Culture in Mexico, 1917–1936*. Durham, NC: Duke University Press, 2008.

Hopwood, Nick. "A History of Normal Plates, Tables, and Stages in Vertebrate Embryology." *International Journal of Developmental Biology* 51 (2007): 1–26.

Horn, David. *The Criminal Body: Lombroso and the Anatomy of Deviance*. London: Routledge, 2015.

Jackson, Robert H. "Durán, Fray Narciso (1776–1846)." In *Encyclopedia of Latin American History and Culture*, vol. 2, edited by Jay Kinsbruner and Erick D. Langer, 2:871. Detroit: Charles Scribner's Sons, 2008.

Jaffary, Nora. *False Mystics: Deviant Orthodoxy in Colonial Mexico*. Lincoln: University of Nebraska Press, 2004.

———. *Reproduction and Its Discontents in Mexico, 1750–1905*. Chapel Hill: The University of North Carolina Press, 2016.

Jones, David Albert. *The Soul of the Embryo: An Enquiry into the Status of the Human Embryo in the Christian Tradition*. New York: Continuum International, 2004.

Kapsalis, Terri. "Mastering the Female Pelvis: Race and the Tools of Reproduction." In *Skin Deep, Spirit Strong: The Black Female Body in American Culture*, edited by Kimberly Wallace-Sanders, 263–300. Ann Arbor: University of Michigan Press, 2002.

Kessell, John. *Friars, Soldiers, and Reformers: Hispanic Arizona and the Sonora Mission*. Tucson: University of Arizona Press, 1976.

Keupper Valle, Rosemary. "The Cesarean Operation in Alta California during the Franciscan Mission Period (1769–1833)." *Bulletin of the History of Medicine* 48, no. 2 (1974): 265–75.

Kimball, Natalie. *An Open Secret: The History of Unwanted Pregnancy and Abortion in Modern Bolivia*. New Brunswick, NJ: Rutgers University Press, 2020.

Klaeren, George. "Sacred Embryology: Intrauterine Baptisms and the Negotiation of Theology and Health Sciences across the Eighteenth-Century Spanish Empire." In *Health and Healing in the Early Modern Iberian World: A Gendered Perspective*, edited by Sarah E. Owens and Margaret E. Boyle, 219–40. Toronto: University of Toronto Press, 2021.

Knight, Alan. "Racism, Revolution, and Indigenismo: Mexico, 1910–1940," in *The Idea of Race in Latin America, 1870–1940*, edited by Richard Graham, 71–113. Austin: University of Texas Press, 1990.

Kourí, Emilio H. "Interpreting the Expropriation of Indian Pueblo Lands in Porfirian Mexico: The Unexamined Legacies of Andrés Molina Enríquez." *Hispanic American Historical Review* 82, no. 1 (2002): 69–117.

Lanning, John Tate. *The Royal Protomedicato: The Regulation of the Medical Professions in the Spanish Empire*. Durham, NC: Duke University Press, 1985.

Lavrin, Asunción. "International Feminisms: Latin American Alternatives." *Gender and History* 10, no. 3 (1998): 519–34.

Lederer, Susan. *Subjected to Science: Human Experimentation in America before the Second World War*. Baltimore: Johns Hopkins University Press, 1997.

Lehner, Ulrich. *The Catholic Enlightenment: The Forgotten History of a Global Movement*. Oxford: Oxford University Press, 2016.

Lomnitz, Claudio. *Death and the Idea of Mexico*. New York: Zone Books, 2005.

López, Iris Ofelia. *Matters of Choice: Puerto Rican Women's Struggle for Reproductive Freedom*. New Brunswick, NJ: Rutgers University Press, 2008.

Lucero, Bonnie. *Race and Reproduction in Cuba*. Atlanta: University of Georgia Press, 2022.

Markowitz, Sally. "Pelvic Politics: Sexual Dimorphism and Racial Difference." *Signs: Journal of Women in Culture and Society* 26, no. 2 (2001): 389–414.

Marsiske, Renate. "Estudiantes universitarios y revolución mexicana: de la élite cultural a la élite política y económica." In *Grupo marginados de la educación (siglos XIX y XX)*, edited by María de Lourdes Alvarado and Rosalina Ríos Zúñiga, 191–219. Mexico City: Instituto de Investigaciones sobre la Universidad y la Educación (IISUE), 2011.

Martínez, María Elena. *Genealogical Fictions: Limpieza de Sangre, Religion, and Gender in Colonial Mexico*. Stanford, CA: Stanford University Press, 2008.

Maurice, Rochelle. "We Bawl So We Are Heard: The Stories We Must Tell About Obstetric Racism." *Sexual and Reproductive Health Matters*, forthcoming.

Mazín Gómez, Oscar. *Entre dos majestades: El obispo y la Iglesia del Gran Michoacán ante las reformas borbónicas, 1758–1772*. Zamora de Hidalgo: El Colegio de Michoacán, 1987.

McPherson, Thomas. "Positivism and Religion." *Philosophy and Phenomenological Research* 14, no. 3 (1954): 319–31.

Medin, Tzvi. *El minimato presidencial: Historia política del maximato (1928–1935)*. Mexico City: Ediciones Era, 1982.

Medina Peña, Luis. *Hacia el nuevo estado: México, 1920–2000*. Mexico City: Fondo de Cultura Económica, 2014.

Meyer, Lorenzo. "La etapa formativa del estado Mexicano contemporáneo (1928–1940)." *Foro Internacional* 17, no. 4/68 (1977): 453–76.

Mijangos y González, Pablo. *The Lawyer of the Church: Bishop Clemente de Jesús Munguía and the Clerical Response to the Mexican Liberal Reforma*. Lincoln: University of Nebraska Press, 2015.

Mitchell, Stephanie, and Patience A. Schell, eds. *The Women's Revolution in Mexico, 1910–1953*. Lanham, MD: Rowman & Littlefield, 2006.

Molyneux, Maxine, and Elizabeth Dore, eds. *Hidden Histories of Gender and the State in Latin America*. Durham, NC: Duke University Press, 2000.

Mooney, Graham. *Intrusive Interventions: Public Health, Domestic Space, and Infectious Disease Surveillance in England, 1840–1914*. Rochester, NY: Boydell & Brewer, 2015.

Morgan, Jennifer. "'Some Could Suckle over Their Shoulder': Male Travelers, Female Bodies, and the Gendering of Racial Ideology, 1500–1770." *William and Mary Quarterly* 54, no. 1 (1997): 167–92.

Morgan, Lynn M. *Icons of Life: A Cultural History of Human Embryos*. Berkeley: University of California Press, 2009.

———. "The Potentiality Principle from Aristotle to Abortion." In "Potentiality and Humanness: Revisiting the Anthropological Object in Contemporary Biomedicine," edited by Karen-Sue Taussig, Klaus Hoeyer, and Stefan Helmreich. Supplement, *Current Anthropology* 54, no. S7 (2013): S15–S25.

Morgan, Lynn M., and Elizabeth F. S. Roberts. "Reproductive Governance in Latin America." *Anthropology and Medicine* 19, no. 2 (2012): 241–54.

———. "Rights and Reproduction in Latin America." *Anthropology News* 50, no. 3 (2009): 12–16.

Moscucci, Ornella. *The Science of Women: Gynaecology and Gender in England, 1800–1929*. Cambridge: Cambridge University Press, 1990.

Murrieta, Alicia Márques. "Aborto y derechos reproductivos, leyes y debates públicos." In *Los grandes problemas de México. VII. Relaciones de género*, edited by Ana María Tepichin, Karine Tinat, and Luzelena Gutiérrez, 179–200. Mexico City: El Colegio de México, 2010.

Necochea López, Raúl. *A History of Family Planning in Twentieth-Century Peru*. Chapel Hill: University of North Carolina Press, 2014.

Needham, Joseph. *A History of Embryology*. 2nd ed. New York: Abelard-Schuman, 1959. First edition published in 1934.

Nentvig, Juan. *Rudo Ensayo: A Description of Sonora and Arizona in 1764*. Translated and annotated by Alberto Francisco Pradeau and Robert R. Rasmussen. Tucson: University of Arizona Press, 1980. https://web.archive.org/web/20170525014932/https://library.arizona.edu/exhibits/swetc/rudo/index.html.

Novak, Nicole L., Natalie Lira, Kate E. O'Connor, Siobán D. Harlow, Sharon LR Kardia, and Alexandra Minna Stern. "Disproportionate Sterilization of Latinos under California's Eugenic Sterilization Program, 1920–1945." *American Journal of Public Health* 108, no. 5 (2018): 611–13.

Nugent, Daniel, and Gilbert Joseph. *Everyday Forms of State Formation: Revolution and the Negotiation of Rule in Modern Mexico*. Durham, NC: Duke University Press, 1994.

O'Brien, Elizabeth, and Miriam Rich. "Obstetric Violence in Historical Perspective." *Lancet* 399, no. 10342 (2022): 2183–85.

O'Hara, Matthew. *A Flock Divided: Race, Religion, and Politics in Mexico, 1749–1857*. Durham, NC: Duke University Press, 2009.

Olcott, Jocelyn. *Revolutionary Women in Postrevolutionary Mexico*. Durham, NC: Duke University Press, 2006.

———. "'Worthy Wives and Mothers': State-Sponsored Women's Organizing in Postrevolutionary Mexico." *Journal of Women's History* 13, no. 4 (2002): 106–31.

Ortiz Rangel, Andrea. "Feminismo y eugenesia en México: Articulaciones posrevolucionarias en Yucatán, Veracruz y Tabasco, 1915–1935." MA thesis, El Colegio de México, 2016.

Overmeyer-Velázquez, Mark. *Visions of the Emerald City: Modernity, Tradition, and the Formation of Porfirian Oaxaca, Mexico*. Durham, NC: Duke University Press, 2006.

Padilla Ramos, Raquel. *Progreso y libertad: Los yaquis en la víspera de la repatriación*. Hermosillo: Programa Editorial de Sonora, 2006.

Park, Katherine. *Secrets of Women: Gender, Generation, and the Origins of Human Dissection*. New York: Zone Books, 2006.

Peñafort, Luisa Zahino, ed. *El Cardenal Lorenzana y el IV Concilio Provincial Mexicano*. Ciudad Real, Spain: La Universidad de Castilla-La Mancha, 1999.

Piccato, Pablo. *City of Suspects: Crime in Mexico City, 1900–1931*. Durham, NC: Duke University Press, 2001.

Poole, Deborah. "An Image of 'Our Indian': Type Photographs and Racial Sentiments in Oaxaca, 1920–1940." *Hispanic American Historical Review* 84, no. 1 (2004): 37–82.

Premo, Bianca. *Children of the Father King: Youth, Authority, and Legal Minority in Colonial Lima*. Chapel Hill: University of North Carolina Press, 2006.

Quattrocchi, Magnone. *Violencia obstétrica en América Latina: Conceptualización, experiencias, medición y estrategias*. Buenos Aires: EDUN La Cooperativa, 2020.

Ramos, Christina. *Bedlam in the New World: A Mexican Madhouse in the Age of Enlightenment*. Chapel Hill: The University of North Carolina Press, 2022.

Reagan, Leslie. *When Abortion Was a Crime: Women, Medicine, and Law in the United States, 1867–1973*. Berkeley: University of California Press, 1997.

Reed, Edward. *From Soul to Mind: The Emergence of Psychology from Erasmus Darwin to William James*. New Haven, CT: Yale University Press, 1997.

Reid, Anne Marie. "Medics of the Soul and the Body: Sickness and Death in Alta California, 1769–1850." PhD diss., University of Southern California, 2013.

Renard, Ruth. "The Problem of the Organic Individual: Ernst Haeckel and the Development of the Biogenetic Law." *Journal of the History of Biology* 14 (1981): 249–75.

Reti, Ladislao. "The Two Unpublished Manuscripts of Leonardo da Vinci in the Biblioteca Nacional of Madrid-II." *Burlington Magazine* 110, no. 779 (1968): 81–91.

Reyes Pavón, Leonor Eugenia. "Las Hermanas de la Caridad: Su labor asistencial y educativa en Yucatán, 1865–1875." BA thesis, Universidad Autónoma de Yucatán, 2013.

Rich, Miriam. "The Curse of Civilised Woman: Race, Gender and the Pain of Childbirth in Nineteenth-Century American Medicine." *Gender and History* vol. 28, no. 1 (2016): 57–76.

Rigau-Pérez, José G. "Surgery at the Service of Theology: Postmortem Cesarean Sections in Puerto Rico and the Royal Cédula of 1804." *Hispanic American Historical Review* 75, no. 3 (1995): 377–404.

Ríos Molina, Andrés. "'Dictating the Suitable Way of Life': Mental Hygiene for Children and Workers in Socialist Mexico, 1934–1940." *Journal of the History of the Behavioral Sciences* 49, no. 2 (2013): 142–66.

———. *La locura durante la Revolución mexicana: Los primeros años del Manicomio General La Castañeda, 1910–1920*. Mexico City: El Colegio de México, 2007.

Risse, Guenter. *Mending Bodies, Saving Souls: A History of Hospitals*. Oxford: Oxford University Press, 1999.

Rivera Garza, Cristina. "Dangerous Minds: Changing Psychiatric Views of the Mentally Ill in Porfirian Mexico, 1876–1911." *Journal of the History of Medicine and Allied Sciences* 56, no. 1 (2001): 36–67.

———. "'She Neither Respected nor Obeyed Anyone': Inmates and Psychiatrists Debate Gender and Class at the General Insane Asylum La Castañeda, Mexico, 1910–1930." *Hispanic American Historical Review* 81, no. 3–4 (2001): 653–88.

Roberts, Dorothy. *Fatal Invention: How Science, Politics, and Big Business Re-create Race in the Twenty-First Century*. New York: New Press, 2011.

———. *Killing the Black Body: Race, Reproduction, and the Meaning of Liberty*. New York: Vintage Books, 1999.

Roberts, Elizabeth. *God's Laboratory: Assisted Reproduction in the Andes*. Berkeley: University of California Press, 2012.

———. "Scars of Nation: Surgical Penetration and the Ecuadorian State." *Journal of Latin American and Caribbean Anthropology* 17, no. 2 (2012): 215–37.

Rodriguez, Julia. "A Complex Fabric: Intersecting Histories of Race, Gender, and Science in Latin America." *Hispanic American Historical Review* 91, no. 3 (2011): 409–29.

Rodriguez, Sarah. *Female Circumcision and Clitoridectomy in the United States: A History of a Medical Treatment*. Rochester, NY: Boydell & Brewer, 2014.

Roldán, Adriana Pacheco. "Periódicos católicos mexicanos del siglo XIX: Conformación de la madre de familia durante la República Restaurada para trabajar por el otro México." *Tinkuy: Boletín de Investigación y Debate* 21 (2014): 75–90.

Rosemblatt, Karin Alejandra. "Bodies, Environments, and Race: Roots and Branches of Eugenic Nationalism in the Long Twentieth Century." In *Handbook of the Historiography of Latin American Studies on the Life Sciences and Medicine*, edited by Ana Barahona, 1–20. Cham, Switzerland: Springer Nature, 2022. https://doi.org/10.1007/978-3-030-48616-7_31-1.

———. *Gendered Compromises: Political Cultures and the State in Chile, 1920–1950*. Chapel Hill: The University of North Carolina Press, 2003.

———. *The Science and Politics of Race in Mexico and the United States, 1910–1950*. Chapel Hill: The University of North Carolina Press, 2018.

———. "'What We Can Reclaim of the Old Values of the Past'": Sexual Morality and Politics in Twentieth-Century Chile." *Comparative Studies in Society and History* 43, no. 1 (2001): 149–80.

Ross, Loretta, Erika Derkas, Whitney Peoples, Lynn Roberts, and Pamela Bridgewater, eds. *Radical Reproductive Justice: Foundation, Theory, Practice, Critique*. New York: CUNY Press, 2017.

Roth, Cassia. *A Miscarriage of Justice: Women's Reproductive Lives and the Law in Early Twentieth-Century Brazil*. Stanford, CA: Stanford University Press, 2020.

———, and Luiz Antônio Teixeira. "From Embryotomy to Cesarean: Changes in Obstetric Operatory Techniques in Nineteenth-and Twentieth-Century Urban Brazil." *Bulletin of the History of Medicine* 95, no. 1 (2021): 24–52.

Ruiz Castañeda, María del Carmen. "La tercera gazeta de la Nueva España: *Gazeta de México* (1784–1809)." *Boletín del Instituto de Investigaciones Bibliográficas* (1971): 137–50.

Saladino García, Alberto. "José Antonio Alzate Ramírez: Máxima figura de la cultura novohispana del siglo XVIII." *La Colmena* 21 (1999): 83–90.

Sanders, Nichole. "Women, Sex, and the 1950s Acción Católica's Campaña Nacional de Moralización del Ambiente." *Mexican Studies/Estudios Mexicanos* 36, no. 1–2 (2020): 270–97.s

Sandos, James. *Converting California: Indians and Franciscans in the Missions*. New Haven, CT: Yale University Press, 2004.

Schell, Patience. "Eugenics Policy a Practice in Cuba, Puerto Rico, and Mexico." In *The Oxford Handbook of Global Eugenics*, edited by Allison Bashford and Philippa Levine, 477–92. New York: Oxford University Press, 2010.

Schoen, Johanna. *Choice and Coercion: Birth Control, Sterilization, and Abortion in Public Health and Welfare*. Chapel Hill: The University of North Carolina Press, 2005.

Schwartz, Jenkins. *Birthing a Slave: Motherhood and Medicine in the Antebellum South*. Cambridge, MA: Harvard University Press, 2010.

Semo, Ilán. "El cardenismo revisado: La tercera vía y otras utopías inciertas." *Revista Mexicana de Sociología* 55, no. 2 (1993): 197–223.

Sheldon, Myrna Perez, Ahmed Ragab, and Terence Keel, eds. *Critical Approaches to Science and Religion*. New York: Columbia University Press, 2023.

Shelton, Laura M. *For Tranquility and Order: Family and Community on Mexico's Northern Frontier, 1800–1850*. Tucson: University of Arizona Press, 2010.

Silva, José Filipe. "Potentially Human? Aquinas on Aristotle on Human Generation." *British Journal for the History of Philosophy* 23, no. 1 (2015): 3–21.

Smith-Rosenberg, Carroll, and Charles Rosenberg. "The Female Animal: Medical and Biological Views of Woman and Her Role in Nineteenth-Century America." *Journal of American History* 60, no. 2 (1973): 332–56.

Socolow, Susan. *The Women of Colonial Latin America*. Cambridge: Cambridge University Press, 2015.

Sonn, Richard. "'Your Body Is Yours': Anarchism, Birth Control, and Eugenics in Interwar France." *Journal of the History of Sexuality* 14, no. 4 (2005): 415–32.

Sordo Noriega, Antonio. *Estudios obstétricos del profesor Doctor D. Juan Duque de Estrada, publicados de 1897 a 1919*. Mexico City: Imprente Mercevia, 1955.

Soto Laveaga, Gabriela. "Bringing the Revolution to Medical Schools: Social Service and a Rural Health Emphasis in 1930s Mexico." *Mexican Studies/Estudios Mexicanos* 29, no. 2 (2013): 397–427.

Speckman Guerra, Elisa. *Del Tigre de Santa Julia, la princesa italiana y otras historias: Sistema judicial, criminalidad y justicia en la ciudad de México (siglos XIX y XX)*. Mexico City: INACIPE, 2014.

Stauffer, Brian. *Victory on Earth or in Heaven: Mexico's Religionero Rebellion*. Albuquerque: University of New Mexico Press, 2019.

Stepan, Nancy. *The Hour of Eugenics: Race, Gender, and Nation in Latin America*. Ithaca, NY: Cornell University Press, 1991.

Stern, Alexandra Minna. "'The Hour of Eugenics' in Veracruz, Mexico: Radical Politics, Public Health, and Latin America's Only Sterilization Law." *Hispanic American Historical Review* 91, no. 3 (2011): 431–43.

———. "Responsible Mothers and Normal Children: Eugenics, Nationalism, and Welfare in Post-revolutionary Mexico, 1920–1940." *Journal of Historical Sociology* 12, no. 4 (1999): 369–97.

Suárez y López Guazo, Laura Luz. *Eugenesia y racismo en México*. Mexico City: Universidad Nacional Autónoma de México, 2005.

Summers, William J., Craig H. Russell, and Antoni Gili. *J. B. Sancho: Compositor pioner de Califòrnia*. Palma, Spain: Universitat de les Illes Balears, 2007.

Taylor, William. *Magistrates of the Sacred: Priests and Parishioners in Eighteenth-Century Mexico*. Stanford, CA: Stanford University Press, 1996.

Tenorio Trillo, Mauricio. *Mexico at the World's Fairs: Crafting a Modern Nation*. Berkeley: University of California Press, 1996.

Theobald, Brianna. *Reproduction on the Reservation: Pregnancy, Childbirth, and Colonialism in the Long Twentieth Century*. Chapel Hill: The University of North Carolina Press, 2019.

Tuñón, Julia, ed. *Enjaular los cuerpos: Normativas decimonónicas y feminidad en México*. Mexico City: El Colegio de México, 2008.

Turda, Marius, and Aaron Gillette. *Latin Eugenics in Comparative Perspective*. Bloomsbury, 2016.

Turner, Sasha. *Contested Bodies: Pregnancy, Childrearing, and Slavery in Jamaica*. Philadelphia: University of Pennsylvania Press, 2017.

Twinam, Ann. *Public Lives, Private Secrets: Gender, Honor, Sexuality, and Illegitimacy in Spanish America*. Stanford, CA: Stanford University Press, 1999.

Urías Horcasitas, Beatriz. "El determinismo biológico en México: Del darwinismo social a la sociología criminal." *Revista Mexicana de Sociología* 58, no. 4 (1996): 99–126.

———. "Eugenesia y aborto en México (1920–1940)." *Debate Feminista* 27 (2003): 305–23.

Vaan, Michiel de. *Etymological Dictionary of Latin and the Other Italic Languages*. Leiden, the Netherlands: Brill, 2008.

Vaughan, Mary Kay. *Cultural Politics in Revolution: Teachers, Peasants, and Schools in Mexico, 1930–1940*. Tucson: University of Arizona Press, 1997.

Vaughan, Mary Kay, Gabriela Cano, and Jocelyn Olcott, eds. *Sex in Revolution: Gender, Politics, and Power in Modern Mexico*. Durham, NC: Duke University Press, 2007.

Voekel, Pamela. *Alone before God: The Religious Origins of Modernity in Mexico*. Durham, NC: Duke University Press, 2002.

Vyas, Darshali A., David S. Jones, Audra R. Meadows, Khady Diouf, Nawal M. Nour, and Julianna Schantz-Dunn. "Challenging the Use of Race in the Vaginal Birth after Cesarean Section Calculator." *Women's Health Issues* 29, no. 3 (2019): 201–4.

Walsh, Sarah. "The Executioner's Shadow: Coerced Sterilization and the Creation of 'Latin' Eugenics in Chile." *History of Science* 60, no. 1 (2022): 18–40.

———. *The Religion of Life: Eugenics, Race, and Catholicism in Chile*. Pittsburgh: University of Pittsburgh Press, 2022.

———. "Restoring the Chilean Race: Catholicism and Latin Eugenics in Chile." *Catholic Historical Review* 105, no. 1 (2019): 116–38.

Warner, John Harley. *Against the Spirit of System: The French Impulse in Nineteenth-Century American Medicine*. Baltimore: Johns Hopkins University Press, 2003.

Warren, Adam. "An Operation for Evangelization: Friar Francisco González Laguna, the Cesarean Section, and Fetal Baptism in Late Colonial Peru." *Bulletin of the History of Medicine* 83, no. 4 (2009): 647–75.

Weber, David. *Bárbaros: Spaniards and Their Savages in the Age of Enlightenment*. New Haven, CT: Yale University Press, 2005.

Weber, Jonathan. *Death Is All around Us: Corpses, Chaos, and Public Health in Porfirian Mexico City*. Lincoln: University of Nebraska Press, 2019.

Weber, Max. "Science as a Vocation." In *From Max Weber: Essays in Sociology*, edited and translated by Hans Heinrich Gerth and Charles Wright Mills, 129–56. New York: Oxford University Press, 1946.

Weikart, Richard. "Progress through Racial Extermination: Social Darwinism, Eugenics, and Pacifism in Germany, 1860–1918." *German Studies Review*, 26, no. 2 (2003), 273–94.

Williams, C. R., C. Jerez, K. Klein, M. Correa, J. M. Belizán, and G. Cormick. "Obstetric Violence: A Latin American Legal Response to Mistreatment during Childbirth." *BJOG* 125, no. 10 (2018): 1208–11.

Winter, Alison. *Mesmerized: Powers of Mind in Victorian Britain*. Chicago: University of Chicago Press, 1998.

Witherspoon, James S. "Reexamining Roe: Nineteenth-Century Abortion Statutes and the Fourteenth Amendment." *St. Mary's Law Journal* 17, no. 1 (1985): 29–71.

Wolf, Jacqueline. *Cesarean Section: An American History of Risk, Technology, and Consequence*. Baltimore: Johns Hopkins University Press, 2018.

Index

Please note that: (i) page numbers in *italics* denote tables; (ii) countries are placed according to their status as nations at the time of publication, rather than under "Spanish Empire," "New Spain" or similar; (iii) persons generally appear under suitable headings where the index directs the reader to thoughts about all or part of that group, such as "patients" and so on. Where there is no such heading, individual people again appear in their own right; and (iv) no titles are given to medical practitioners, who may have held several during their lifetimes. An exception has been made for medical practitioners referred to in primary sources as "Dr.", without given names.

Printed in the USA
CPSIA information can be obtained
at www.ICGtesting.com
LVHW041254071223
765824LV00001B/55

9 781469 675879